CARDIOLOGY

CARDIOLOGY
The Evolution of
the Science and the Art

Edited by

Richard J. Bing, MD
Huntington Medical Research Institutes
Pasadena, California

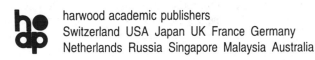

harwood academic publishers
Switzerland USA Japan UK France Germany
Netherlands Russia Singapore Malaysia Australia

Harwood Academic Publishers

Post Office Box 90
Reading, Berkshire RG1 8JL
United Kingdom

Glinkastrasse 13–15
O–1086 Berlin
Germany

58, rue Lhomond
75005 Paris
France

Emmaplein 5
1075 AW Amsterdam
Netherlands

5301 Tacony Street, Drawer 330
Philadelphia, Pennsylvania 19137
United States of America

3–14–9, Okubo
Shinjuku-ku, Tokyo 169
Japan

Private Bag 8
Camberwell, Victoria 3124
Australia

Library of Congress Cataloging-in-Publication Data

Bing, Richard J., 1909–
    Cardiology : the evolution of the science and the art / Richard J. Bing.
        p.   cm.
    includes index.
    ISBN 3–7186–0549–X (hardcover)
    1. Cardiology—History.   I. Title.
    [DNLM: 1. Cardiology—history.   2. Physicians—biography.   WG
11.1 B613c]
    RC666.5.B56   1992
    616.1'2'009—dc20
    DNLM / DLC
    for Library of Congress   92–1542
                                                                           CIP

To the memory of Mary Whipple Bing

CONTENTS

CONTENTS

ILLUSTRATIONS

Figures

PREFACE

In the conception of a scientific or artistic creation, emotional involvement is the generating force. Both artists and scientists are driven by the desire to meet an emotional challenge, the former responding with an urge to reveal an image of his inner self, the latter by a desire to explore the unknown. The scientist may possess some artistic characteristics when a romantic element in his personality propels him to explore nature; the artist may also be motivated by scientific impulses if the search for structure and form are predominant. In either case the genetic makeup and the environmental challenges determine the course. It is the opinion of some scientists that emotion and scientific facts should be separate; at least the emotional element should be out of sight. But unavoidably, newly introduced scientific facts frequently evoke emotions through newly developed intellectual concepts.

In any case, it is the personality of the artist or scientist that determines the ultimate character of his work. Therefore, for a historian, the personality of the artist or scientist must be an essential element of study. The historian can do this by recording the impact of a person on his time and future and by tracing his fleeting shadow during his lifetime. Without the human element, history becomes a colorless recitation of facts. This is even more true when dealing with medical science, which has as its final goal the application of science to human beings. The goals of the physician are primarily humanistic.

Therefore, in writing a history of cardiology we have stressed the source of ideas which have guided cardiology to the present, and we have dwelled on the mind and emotions, on the lives of the scientists and physicians, their successes and failures, their struggles and disappointments. We have at the same time attempted to achieve a balance between the scientist and his work, even though some chapters recount more facts, while others dwell more on personalities.

As Ralph Waldo Emerson wrote in his essay on experience: "As I am so I see; use whatever language we will, we can never say anything but what we are." This applies to the artist and to the scientist, and yes, to all human beings.

Appreciation is expressed to Medtronics, Minneapolis, Minnesota, Dr. Henry Lee of San Marino, California, and particularly to the

PREFACE

Commonwealth Fund, New York, New York, for their support in the preparation of this book. Special appreciation to the Huntington Medical Research Institutes and its executive director, Mr. William Opel, for his patience; Halaine Maccabee Rose and Elizabeth Wood for their editorial assistance; and particular gratitude to my secretary, Linda DeChaine, who carried the main burden of preparing this book for publication.

R.J. Bing, MD

CONTRIBUTORS

Dr. Walter Abelmann, Professor Emeritus of Medicine, Harvard Medical School, Boston, Massachusetts; Senior Physician, Beth Israel Hospital, Boston, Massachusetts

Dr. I. Babotai, Herzzentrum Hirslanden Zurich, Switzerland

Dr. Donald Baim, Director of Invasive Cardiology, Beth Israel Hospital, Boston, Massachusetts; Associate Professor of Medicine, Harvard Medical School, Boston, Massachusetts

Dr. John Baldwin, Professor and Chief Cardiothoracic Surgery, Yale University, New Haven, Connecticut

Dr. Tirone David, Professor of Surgery, University of Toronto, Canada; Head, Division of Cardiovascular Surgery, The Toronto Hospital, Canada

Dr. Richard DeWall, Professor Emeritus of Surgery, Wright State University School of Medicine, Dayton, Ohio

Dr. Pamela Douglas, Associate Professor of Medicine, Harvard Medical School, Boston, Massachusetts; Director of Noninvasive Cardiology, Beth Israel Hospital, Boston, Massachusetts

Dr. Raymond Heimbecker, Professor Emeritus of Surgery, University of Western Ontario, London, Canada

Dr. Herman Hellerstein, Professor Emeritus of Medicine, Case Western Reserve University School of Medicine, Cleveland, Ohio; Attending Physician, University Hospitals of Cleveland, Ohio

Dr. Arnold M. Katz, Professor of Medicine and Head of Cardiology Division, University of Connecticut, Farmington

Dr. Alexander Nadas, Emeritus Chief of Cardiology, Senior Associate in Cardiology, The Children's Hospital, Boston, Massachusetts;

Professor Emeritus of Pediatrics, Harvard Medical School, Boston, Massachusetts

Dr. Oglesby Paul, Professor Emeritus of Medicine, Harvard Medical School, Boston, Massachusetts; Senior Physician Emeritus, Brigham and Women's Hospital, Boston, Massachusetts

Dr. Juan Sanchez, Resident in Cardiothoracic Surgery, Yale University, New Haven, Connecticut

Dr. Heinrich Schelbert, Professor of Radiological Sciences, Division of Nuclear Medicine and Biophysics, University of California, Los Angeles

Dr. Ake Senning, Professor Emeritus of Surgery, University of Zurich, Switzerland

Appreciation of others who have been of immeasurable help:

Dr. Konrad Bloch, Higgins Professor Emeritus of Biochemistry, Department of Chemistry, Harvard University, Boston, Massachusetts, Nobelist

Dr. Howard Burchell, Professor Emeritus of Medicine, University of Minnesota, Minneapolis

Dr. P.A.N. Chandraratna, Martin Luther King Hospital, Los Angeles, California

Dr. James Dalen, Vice Provost for Medical Affairs, Dean, College of Medicine, University of Arizona, Tucson

Dr. Peter Edwards, Associate Professor, Departments of Biological Chemistry and Medicine, University of California, Los Angeles

Dr. Jack Matloff, Chairman, Department of Thoracic and Cardiovascular Surgery at Cedars-Sinai Medical Center in Los Angeles, California

Dr. Eli Milgalter, Assistant Professor, Division of Cardiothoracic Surgery, University of California, Los Angeles

Dr. Neil Moran, Professor of Pharmacology, Emory University School of Medicine, Atlanta, Georgia

Dr. Carter Printup, Huntington Memorial Hospital, Pasadena, California

Dr. John Simpson, Stanford, California

Chapter 1

Cardiac Catheterization

D. BAIM AND R.J. BING

Cardiac catheterization over the last 50 years is staggering. Well over 1 million such procedures are performed in the United States each year. Precise anatomic and physiologic cardiac diagnoses are made in less than one hour in a lightly sedated patient who is frequently able to return home six hours after the procedure. Drawing on the techniques developed by Dotter and Gruentzig, another 300,000 patients undergo catheter correction on the underlying problem using only percutaneous femoral artery puncture with local anesthesia, rather than open surgical thoracotomy.

Claude Bernard was the first to catheterize the heart in animals, motivated by purely basic physiological considerations (1,2). The argument had not been settled at that time, whether cellular metabolism takes place in the lung as proposed by Antoine-Laurent Lavoisier, or in the tissue as suggested by Gustav Magnus. Bernard's studies are described in two volumes, the first "Chaleur Animale," and the second "Physiologie Operatoire," published in 1876 (1,2). In his straightforward manner, Bernard conceived an experiment to answer this question. If the temperature in the right and the left ventricle are equal, heat production could not have primarily taken place in the lung. Since Bernard found the temperature of the blood in the left ventricle to be slightly elevated, he concluded that Lavoisier was in error: the body heat is due to cellular metabolism taking place in all tissues. Bernard had considered and discarded the idea of making an open window for direct inspection of the heart or to exteriorize the heart, but preferred insertion of a catheter because it was relatively non-invasive. He used a catheter made of lead to give it the

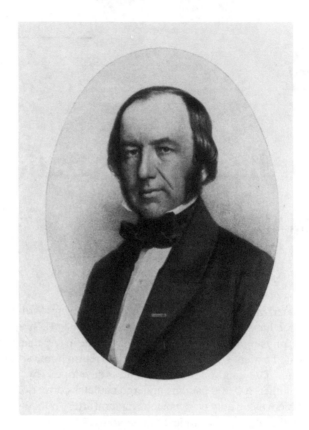

Figure 1.   Claude Bernard (*Courtesy of the New York Academy of Medicine*)

right curvature, a forerunner of the pre-formed catheter of today. Bernard's thinking and writing are characterized by clarity and by directness of approach (3). He was a master at finding ingenious solutions which went straight to the "heart" of the problem and he disliked scientific speculations. As he wrote, "The best philosophical system for the working scientist is not to have any at all!" Bernard was a master of the new science, experimental physiology, and had an unbending devotion to his work despite immense personal difficulties (3; Figure 1).

In 1861, A. Chaveau and Etienne Jules Marey published their work on the measurement of intracardiac pressure (4,5; Figure 2). Their paper is on the graphic determination of the relationship between the apex beat and the movement of the atrium and ventricles, respectively. By means of pressure

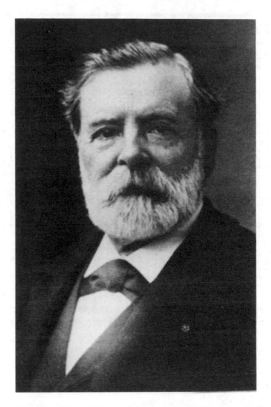

Figure 2. Etienne Jules Marey (*Courtesy of the New York Academy of Medicine*)

tracings they found that "la systole du ventricule et la pulsation cardiaque (choc du coeur) commencent et finissent toute deux simultanement," that is, ventricular systole and apical beat commence and terminate completely simultaneously (Figure 3). Chaveau and Marey also achieved the first recorded simultaneous measurement of pressure in the left ventricle and in the central aorta (4,5). They defined the influence of left ventricular systole upon the contour of the central aortic pressure curve. Moreover, they were the first to refer to the isometric phase of the left ventricular contraction. Marey set forth the technical procedure in detail: the recording instrument, and the graphic tracings (Figure 3,4,). Anticipating the concerns of later physicians as to the application of catheterization of the heart, Marey wrote in a footnote of his book on the effect of catheterization of the heart of horses, "One can be reassured of the innocuity of this method by examining the horse, which is

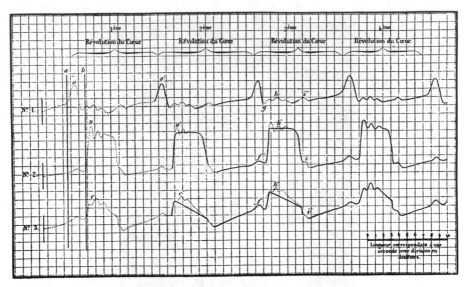

Figure 3. Intracavitary tracings of atrial (1), ventricular pressures (2) and apical impulse (3). Time is indicated in the abscissa. (*Courtesy of H.A. Snellen, Kooyker Scientific Publications, Rotterdam, The Netherlands*)

scarcely disturbed, walks and eats as usual. In only a few instances is the pulse rate slightly increased, especially at the time of introduction of the catheter within the heart cavities (6)."

Bernard paid tribute to Marey for his development of instruments to graphically record events of the circulation and of biological phenomena. He wrote, "It is true that efforts had been made in the same direction by Herman von Helmholtz, Carl Friedrich Ludwig, etc., before Marey but they were not amenable to general application and they were doomed to remain personal

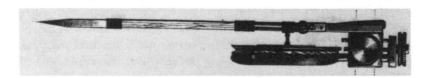

Figure 4. Recording device used by Marey (Marey's Capsule). (*Courtesy of H.A. Snellen, Kooyker Scientific Publications, Rotterdam, The Netherlands*)

procedures (7)." He also discussed Marey's work on the relationship of the apical beat to the cardiac cycle. To quote Bernard, "Two opinions existed: An old one which stems from William Harvey and was accepted with a few modifications by an eminent member of your commission, according to which the heart beat results from the contraction of the ventricles; and the other, which is more recent and at first seems simpler and more satisfactory and attributes the phenomenon to the propulsion from the apex of the heart through the surge of blood from the auricular systole. The graphic method provided the answer. An examination of the resultant graphs completely eliminated uncertainty. The relationship between the beat of the heart and the contraction of the ventricle was demonstrated by the synchronous upward movement of the two levers and by the simultaneous elevation in the two curves they recorded (7)."

Bernard's statement, in which he mentions Marey's third book entitled "La Machine Animale," is significant. This work deals with Marey's investigation of locomotion of animals on land and in the air, "a subject which only became experimentally approachable with the advent of the ingenious instrument to record events that the eyes of the observer cannot follow." Bernard concludes his recommendation to the academy by writing, "In conclusion it is evident that Marey has accomplished a considerable task with which his name will always be identified (7)."

Marey's investigations on the movements of animals clearly show that he was primarily concerned with the application of physical techniques to physiology. Some have credited Marey with the invention of cinematography, primarily because he advised the brothers Lumiere, the acknowledged inventors of cinematography, in the utilization of his methods. However, long before Marey took out a patent on this invention in 1893 and before he communicated his findings to the Academy of Sciences, other patents for similar discoveries were awarded, one in 1888 from England even mentions perforation of films (5).

One of the questions which occupied scientists at that time concerned the movement of horses. What happens when a horse gallops? How many feet are on the ground at any one time? Marey's instrumentation made it possible to state that a galloping horse placed first one then three then two and again one foot on the ground. It is likely that the governor of California, Leland Stanford, who was an enthusiastic horseman saw some of Marey's illustrations (6). He therefore requested Edward Muybridge, an Englishman, who was a land surveyor in California, to repeat Marey's photographic studies. Muybridge accomplished this by placing, in series, 24 photographic apparatus which were activated by a galloping horse moving in front of these cameras. Thus, a photographic series originated which demonstrated the movements of the horse in all details. In 1881, Muybridge came to Paris and delivered a lecture in Marey's laboratory. Marey had closely followed the development of Muybridge's methodology but he considered it inadequate for his own experimentation. For instance, Marey was aware that Muybridge's methods were inadequate for the study of the flight of birds. In order to accomplish this goal, Marey constructed, in 1882, his "photographic gun (6)." The technique for this invention goes back to Pierre Jules Janssen, an astronomer, working in Paris, who in 1874 was able to take 17 rapid pictures of the passage of Venus by the sun. Both investigators, the astronomer, and physiologist never fought for the patent rights: Janssen was interested in astronomy, Marey in physiological exploration, and for both the rapid firing photographic gun was a means to accomplish their goals. Marey was particularly interested in establishing the fundamental conditions for human flight by photographing birds in flight. Finally, he was able to take 24 pictures per second of the flight of birds and increased the speed of exposure to 1/1400 of a second.

To summarize, Marey's scientific work originated from an application of engineering skill to physiological goals. It was this combination which made him a unique figure in the history of medicine.

More than 50 years later, Werner Forssmann introduced the era of the clinical application of intracardiac catheterization (Figure 5). Forssmann was born in 1904 in Berlin and died in 1979 after two myocardial infarctions. Forssmann's life, personality, and character, are unusual even in the field of science where unusual personalities abound. The inspiration for Forssmann's discovery was the work of Marey. In his book, "Experiments on Myself" Forssmann wrote, "It is strange how an early impression can remain firmly implanted! As a student, I saw the reprint of an old etching in a textbook of physiology. It originated in a paper of Marey's which showed a touching, naive presentation of a man standing before a horse and holding a tube which had been introduced through a jugular vein into the heart of the animal. In the ventricle, the lumen of the tube was closed by a rubber balloon, which transmitted the changes in pressure to a Marey "tambour" and thence to a pen which described the pressure curves. This picture has excited me to such a degree that it pursued me by day and night. Even today I see it exactly as it was even when I close my eyes. The words of these classical French physiologists have convinced me that their experimental studies could be performed in man without any danger (8)."

Thus, in the early summer of 1929, Forssmann's plans came to fruition. He presented them to his superior, Professor Schneider, but as he said, his good old chief turned him down because, "For this sort of work I cannot permit you to work on any one of my patients. Of course, I think your idea is excel-

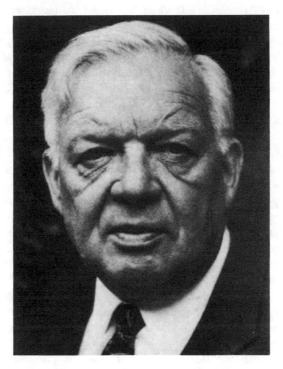

Figure 5. Werner Forssmann (*Courtesy of the New York Academy of Medicine*)

lent and that it will contribute much to future work. And possibly the whole thing is completely without danger just as you think in your youthful enthusiasm." He suggested more animal experimentation, but Forssmann said that that was not necessary. "Well then, I will prove that this experiment is without danger and will do it on myself." But that too was vetoed by Schneider (8).

Despite these warnings, Forssmann went ahead and persuaded a nurse, Gerda Ditz, to help him. She offered to undergo heart catheterization herself, but Forssmann who was determined to do it on himself, tricked her, tying her to the operating table to prevent her from interfering. Then, after local anesthesia of his left antecubital fossa, he inserted a ureteral catheter about 30 cm deep into his vein. He then untied the nurse and asked her to call the nurse in charge of x-rays. Forssmann had to walk down to the basement with the catheter in his heart where nurse Eva took several x-ray pictures showing the catheter in his right ventricle. His chief, Schneider, an understanding and obviously patient physician, told him, "Forssmann, you have done something really great and I want to congratulate you but I believe that your place is not here in this little hospital; you should work in a larger institution," and recommended him through friends to Professor Ferdinand Sauerbruch, the Director, or Dictator, of the surgical clinic at the University of Berlin. It's main hospital, the Charite, accepted him as a surgical assistant. Schneider advised him not to talk about his work until it had been published. The paper appeared in the Klinische Wochenschrift in November, 1929 in an article called "Die Sondierung des rechten Herzens (9)." It shows a picture of the catheter in the right atrium. But instead of getting praise from Sauerbruch, he got fired. As he wrote, "Late in the evening I was asked to see the Geheimrat. He was well prepared and on his desk lay the Klinische Wochenschrift as well as a newspaper and a letter from Unger who apparently had complained that Forssmann had plagiarized his work. He sternly looked at Forssmann for a while in silence and then he yelled: "This is a shameful thing you did and in addition to that you have stolen the priority from one of my most esteemed senior surgeons and why did you not mention that this scientific study was carried out in my department?" Forssmann answered with a short and, as he thought, well rehearsed lecture on the future of cardiac catheterization. Sauerbruch answered with disdain, "That work has no place in surgery. These are purely questions for the internist and physiologist." Forssmann meekly suggested that this work might make it possible for him to "habilitate," that is, to enter the academic career. Sauerbruch answered, "With such circus tricks you never can obtain a position in a decent German clinic. Do you want to be an internist or a surgeon?" Forssmann answered softly, "But I do not know that, Herr Geheimrat, I just am nine months out of medical school and I just do not know what I am good for." That was the last straw. Sauerbruch yelled at him, "For a real surgeon there is only one thing, to operate, to operate, to operate. Get out and leave the clinic immediately." Forssmann writes that rather than submitting to depression, he left the interview elated. Obviously he was relieved and felt justified that he had done the right thing regardless of the prejudice of his "betters (8)."

Soon afterwards, Forssmann conceived an even more daring idea: the injection of contrast material into the heart in order to "improve cardiac diagnosis." First he used the rabbit but soon found that this species was unsuitable and therefore he proceeded to perform his experiments on dogs. The problem was that none of the hospitals to which Forssmann had access, had quarters to house dogs for experimental purposes. It was then that his mother came into the breach and took care of the animals in her own apartment (8). Forssmann injected morphine into the dog as basal narcosis, placed the dog into a sack and drove it to the hospital. Ether narcosis deepened the anesthesia and under aseptic conditions the catheter could be introduced through the external jugular vein into the right ventricle. Contrast material was then injected while x-ray pictures were taken. The animal was then returned to his mother's care where it was kept in the bathtub, a convenient location since the animals were often incontinent. The animal was then replaced by another dog and the experiments were repeated. Forssmann mentioned that the greatest difficulty was his mother's and grandmother's attachment to the animals. After having taken care of them for a while, they were loath to part with them and according to Forssmann many tears were shed.

The next step was to attempt the injection of contrast material into the human heart. Again, Forssmann accomplished this by self experimentation. He admits that he had some anxious moments because this was different from simply putting a catheter in his heart; the injection of contrast material meant that a foreign substance was circulating in his blood with unknown consequences. He attempted to see whether he was sensitive to the iodine by "filling a small test tube with the contrast material and pressing the opening for hours against his buccal mucosa." Since there was no reaction he concluded that the inside of the heart was equally tolerant. Thus, after having placed the catheter in his heart he injected the contrast material while pictures were taken. Unfortunately, the technique was not sufficient to obtain clear pictures of the passage of contrast material, but Forssmann found the technique safe since he experienced only slight symptoms such as a brief dizziness and transient diminution of vision. Prior to publication, it was arranged that Forssmann would present his findings before the illustrious Surgical Congress of 1931, but his speaking time was cut from eight to four minutes. During his lecture there was little attention and his presentation was accompanied by murmurs of ridicule and snickers of derision. The discouraged Forssmann was consoled by his uncle, a country doctor, with these words, "Don't get angry. Those idiots don't understand what you have in mind. One day you will get the Nobel Prize." His uncle had spoken the truth.

Despite the local adverse reaction, four weeks after the publication of Forssmann's paper in 1931 (10), O. Klein, in Prague, published a preliminary paper and six months later a definite report on the determination of cardiac output according to Fick's principle (11). This article first describes the indirect methods of determining cardiac output, then refers to the work of Forssmann which made it possible to determine the cardiac output by direct means. Klein performed 18 catheterizations in man, determining the oxygen and carbon dioxide content of arterial and mixed venous blood and calculated a cardiac output of 4.5 liters/min. He described the procedure as simple and without incident (11).

Despite a few references to Forssmann's work in the literature, his work was forgotten after the war, and his whereabouts were unknown. Forssmann owes his resurrection after the war to his English colleagues, but primarily to Sir John MacMichael, who invited him to England once his whereabouts were known. Forssmann never became chairman of a department of surgery, a goal which he would have appreciated; he did become Honorary Professor in several German universities; he made friends with several German medical men, particularly Grosse-Brockhoff, Chairman of the Department of Medicine in Duesseldorf in 1965. I (RJB) met Forssmann and his wife for the first time at a party given by Grosse-Brockhoff, in 1968. Both were charming people; Forssmann himself impressed me by his wit and sense of humor.

Forssmann's last years were characterized by research into medical problems not connected with cardiology or science, but with euthanasia, truth at the bedside, cardiac transplantation, etc. (12). He became an opponent of the death penalty; he did consider himself, as he wrote me, a "medical fossil." In the last letter I received from him in 1978 from Wies-Wambach, nine months before his death, he apologized for not being able to attend a meeting in which I was to talk about cardiac catheterization. He wrote that he had nothing to say about modern cardiology except platitudes, and that he was not willing to talk about the history of cardiology because he realized, "how deep I am already in the shadow of the past." He also wrote that it "nauseates" him when his self-experimentation is described as an act of heroism, "This it was not!! I had thought very carefully about whether the method of catheterization would lead to a clinical routine procedure." He had, he wrote, "to rule out the risk to patients, otherwise, it would have become a circus stunt, as I was accused by Sauerbruch and Nissen in their conceit (12)."

H. Schadewaldt, Professor of History of Medicine at the University of Duesseldorf, wrote in his eulogy of Forssmann, "Men of spirit and zest who love science are most certainly not in need of rules and regulations. The force which pushes them onward lies within themselves, urging them to go forward; they themselves are a law within themselves (13)."

Forssmann shared the Nobel Prize with two American scientists, Andre Cournand and Dickinson Richards. Cournand was born in France and Richards was a New Englander (Figure 6). Their cooperation began in 1932. As Cournand wrote, "In 1932, Dickinson Richards, then at Columbia Presbyterian Medical Center and I, Chief Resident of the Chest Service of Bellevue Hospital in New York, agreed on a systemic and comprehensive examination of cardiopulmonary function in normal and diseased man. The lungs, heart, and circulation form a single system for the exchange of respiratory gases between the atmosphere and the tissues of the organism (14)." In 1940, they first attempted to catheterize a patient's heart, but failed because

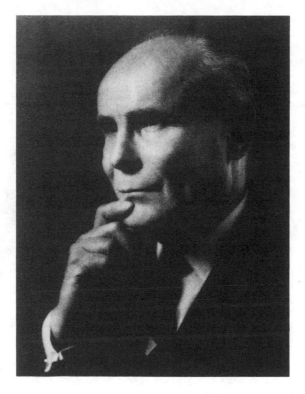

Figure 6. Andre Cournand (*Courtesy of The New York Academy of Medicine*)

the catheter was obstructed at the level of the axilla. Not long afterwards a new opportunity presented itself (14). Homer W. Smith, the renal physiologist, novelist, and Professor of Physiology at the New York University College of Medicine, was planning to measure cardiac output in hypertensive patients. In a first report published in 1941, Cournand and H.A. Ranges reported the results of the initial catheterization (15). The report emphasized the necessity for a steady state, for simultaneous and prolonged blood and air sampling, the value of the checking provided by comparing results based on application of the Fick principle to O_2 data, the reproducibility of the results and finally proof that cardiac catheterization was innocuous. New catheters were designed and a new manometer (not electronic!) for measurement of pressure was built. Cournand and Richards and their co-workers studied many clinical conditions in man including hypertension, circulatory shock,

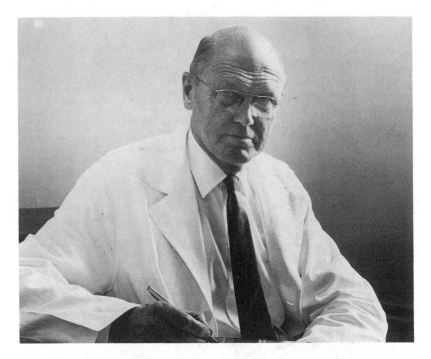

Figure 7. Dickinson Richards (*Courtesy of The New York Academy of Medicine*)

and chronic lung disease. Richards and Cournand made an ideal team. Richards, a great clinician, was a quiet and reserved individual with a keen intellect and compassion for his fellow man (Figure 7). Cournand was a meticulous worker, with a passion for accuracy.

Cournand clearly outlined his motivation for catheterization of the heart at that time (16). His interest stemmed from an investigation of the study of ventilation pertaining to perfusion. He was stimulated by "Something important, which could only be revealed in disease: the relationship between alveolar ventilation and perfusion." The lead was given to Cournand and Richards very early in their study on the basis of the application of the Fick principle. This work led them from the study of cardiac output and pulmonary blood flow to a study of the unequal distribution of blood flow.

At Richard's death in 1973, Cournand wrote a moving eulogy (17). He described Richards' background, his New England family, his student days at Yale, his passion for patients, and his dedication to improve the lot of patients at Bellevue Hospital by consistently recommending the building of a new hospital. His editorship with A.P. Fishman of a book, *Circulation of the Blood, Men and Ideas* (18), and a small volume "Medical Priesthoods and Other Essays" (19) are examples of his knowledge of the history of medicine and his passion for truth. His philosophy is best expressed in a letter he wrote to Cournand: "Man's potentiality, or in these days his survival, will depend on his consciousness, more specifically his conscience, more specifically still, the ability of the leaders and their followers to change character, into more merciful beings (19)."

Why was cardiac catheterization developed at the Columbia division of Bellevue? There were two reasons. The main one was that Dickinson Richards was head of the Columbia division of the Medical Service at Bellevue Hospital, and Bellevue was a progressive inner-city hospital, with medical services run by Columbia, New York and Cornell Universities. Richards was the ideal man to promote progressive research. A tolerant and cultured New Englander, he promoted as well as participated in new research. In addition, New York University's Medical Service, which interacted with Richards' department, was one of the most progressive and imaginative centers in the country. With Tillet as departmental chairman, and with Homer Smith, Chairman of the Department of Physiology, whose name is synonymous with renal physiology, and with Drs. Goldring and Chasis who applied Smith's method to the bedside, this was the right environment to accept and execute ideas.

Despite its early purposes as a scientific instrument, the catheter became more and more a diagnostic tool, particularly for selective coronary arteriography and for continuous hemodynamic monitoring (the Swan-Ganz catheter).

The idea for the Swan-Ganz catheter originated with the appreciation of the need to conduct cardiac catheterization in sick patients without fluoroscopy and without moving the critically ill patient (Figure 8). The idea was developed by H.J. Swan, watching the spinnaker on a sailboat; the first suggestion in 1967 was to place a sail or a parachute at the end of a soft catheter and have that device drag the catheter into the pulmonary artery (20). This, Swan writes, was the outcome of a series of coincidences, namely that he had been Director of the Cath Lab at the Mayo Clinic and that Ron Bradley from London had been a student of his in 1950. Bradley had developed the concept of a very fine soft tubing which sometimes "regrettably and frequently" would spontaneously float into the pulmonary artery; however, the idea of a sail or parachute was technically difficult. The other chance phenomenon, which resulted in the introduction of a balloon catheter, was through his connection with a laboratory which built heart valves. He was able to persuade them to attach a balloon to the catheter (20,21). William Ganz evaluated it in

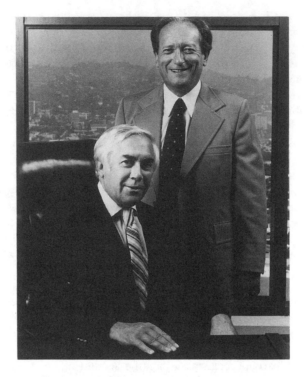

Figure 8. William Ganz (*standing*) and Jeremy Swan.

animal experiments and confirmed the validity of the pulmonary capillary wedge pressure (21,22). Ganz's outstanding contribution was the incorporation of the measurement of cardiac output by thermodilution, a matter which had occupied him for many years and which further increased the clinical impact of the catheter. As Swan wrote "Hence, we have effective hemodynamic monitoring today (1980), applied (correctly or incorrectly, rightly or wrongly, efficaciously or harmfully) to approximately two to three million patients per annum."

The study of cardiac metabolism by catheterization was started in 1946, when I (RJB) found that the catheter slipped several times inadvertently into a region of the heart which under the x-ray looked like a portion of the right ventricle but actually was the coronary sinus; when the blood was withdrawn it was much blacker than that obtained from the right ventricle. Others had already observed that the coronary sinus could be catheterized. In 1941, as told by J.H. Comroe, in attempting to catheterize the right ventricle, Cournand obtained a sample of blood with lower oxygen content than right atrial blood (23). Because the fluoroscopic picture showed that the catheter tip was misplaced and was possibly in the coronary sinus (by mere chance), Cournand was concerned with possible damage to the lining of the coronary sinus, and hastily withdrew the catheter (23). Gene Stead had trouble with three patients because the sample of the blood from the right heart had a very low oxygen content; they concluded that the catheter must have slipped into the coronary sinus, and discarded the data (23). Sosman, a radiologist in Boston, listed among his "failures and errors" unexpected location of the catheter tip and published in one of his figures an x-ray film showing a catheter tip in the coronary venous sinus (23). In 1947, my (RJB) group at Johns Hopkins Hospital, originally organized to study congenital heart disease wrote, "When the catheter is in the coronary sinus, it is seen curved upwards to the base of the heart. In the first cases, intubation of these vessels was fortuitous (24)." In the remaining four cases, catheterization of the sinus was carried out deliberately. All our energy was now devoted to the new rewarding field of coronary blood flow and cardiac metabolism in man. Fortunately S. Kety and E.F. Schmidt had devised a method for determining coronary blood flow using nitrous oxide (N_2O); one was therefore in a position to measure not only the myocardial extraction of food stuffs by the heart, but also their usage. One of many findings was that the heart in the fasting state preferentially extracted free fatty acids but could also use amino acids and ketones; in human heart failure no changes in utilization of substrates could be detected (25,26,27).

In congenital heart disease it was Cournand's group, particularly with A. Himmelstein and the group of Lewis Dexter at Harvard, and the Johns Hopkins Hospital team of R.J. Bing which defined procedures for the diagnosis of congenital heart disease by intracardiac catheterization (28,29,30). Formulae derived from the oxygen content of blood made it possible to calculate regional blood flow such as the effective pulmonary blood flow, the direction and size of the intracardiac shunt, and vascular resistances in the pulmonary and systemic circulation (30). This use of the catheter in congenital heart disease owes its main impetus to the advent of cardiac surgery in the 1940's, primarily the work of Blalock at Hopkins, Robert E. Gross at Harvard and Clarence Craaford in Stockholm. The fact that children with congenital heart disease could now be helped by surgery made the catheter an essential tool in clinical diagnosis. The abundance of patients who underwent surgery by Blalock provided a wealth of material to study the circulation in these children. The use of the catheter also made possible the recognition and importance of pulmonary hypertension (31) and initiated studies on the adaptation to hypoxia of cyanotic children (32). Every week brought new surprises and new revelations in a field which heretofore had been considered of theoretical importance only (*see also Chapter on Congenital Heart Disease*).

Of great importance was the discovery of Dexter at Harvard that by wedging the catheter into a pulmonary artery it is possible to record the height of left atrial pressure (29). Without this pioneering study, the work of Ganz and Swan would not have been possible.

CORONARY ARTERIOGRAPHY

Forssmann had shown that it was safe to inject contrast (radio-opaque) material into the human heart (10). But it was a long way from this discovery to satisfactory visualization of the coronary arteries in man. It was the Swedish school which in the late 40's pioneered this field, with Stig Radner, B. Broden, J. Karnell and G. Jonsson (33,34). In 1934, P. Rousthoi in Stockholm published a preliminary report in which he coined the word "angiocardiography" to describe the contrast visualization of the heart (35). His experiments were carried out on rabbits, with catheterization of the root of the aorta from the right carotid artery and the injection of thorotrast. His conclusion was that this procedure would become applicable to man as well. Radner, in Lund, Sweden in 1945, based his method on that of Antonio C. Egas Moniz who soon after Forssmann described a method of visualizing the blood vessels in the brain. The question was how to get the contrast material into the coronary arteries. Radner's technique consisted of perforating the sternum and puncturing, under fluoroscopic control, the ascending aorta. This was then followed by an injection of contrast material, which filled the bulb of the aorta and outlined the coronary arteries (36). In 1947, Radner used a less dramatic procedure by catheterization of the aorta from the radial artery (33). He based his studies on those of G.P. Robb and I. Steinberg who had rapidly injected intravenously diodrast solution and x-rayed the structures of the cardiovascualar system at the point of arrival of the contrast material (37). Radner positioned a catheter in the radial artery and introduced the tip into the ascending aorta under fluoroscopic control. In order to get the opaque substance out into the coronary arteries, the injection had to be performed with the catheter inserted far down in the ascending aorta, preferably with the tip close to the semilunar valves (33). Non-selective coronary arteriography was also the method of choice by L. DiGuglielmo and M. Guttadauro (38), of A. Thal (39), and of Charles T. Dotter (40). The latter placed a double lumen catheter into the ascending aorta momentarily occluding that vessel while simultaneously injecting radio-opaque material through the other lumen of the catheter. In retrospect, it is astonishing how many investigators continued direct puncture of the aorta, despite the fact that catheterization through a peripheral artery appeared to be safe and simpler.

All this changed with the advent of selective coronary arteriography by F. Mason Sones and E.K. Shirey, and later by Melvin P. Judkins. The paper by Sones was published in *Modern Concepts of Cardiovascular Disease* in 1962, although the procedure had first been carried out in 1958 (41). In his report, Sones mentions that this procedure was to provide a more objective and precise standard of diagnosis for human coronary artery disease. He mentioned that a direct (selective) coronary catheterization had been used for deliberate selective opacification of individual coronary arteries in more that 1,020 patients. Rather than publishing extensive papers, Sones prepared a film on coronary arteriography which was distributed by the Committee on Professional Education of the American Heart Association. This film did more to introduce coronary arteriography than any large number of articles could have done.

The first deliberate efforts to perform selective coronary arteriography were made by Sones in 1958. In 1959, a special catheter was fabricated at his request. The history of this epochal discovery is described by Litwak in Cardiovascular Clinics 1951 and reprinted by Comroe in his book, *The Retrospectroscope* (23). In 1958, Sones and his colleagues at the Cleveland Clinic were studying a young adult and had withdrawn their catheter from the left ventricle into the supravalvular area in preparation for an aortogram. Their equipment at that time did not allow them to precisely visualize the catheter tip immediately prior to injection of the contrast material. The contrast material was injected; to Sones' horror, the right coronary artery and its distal branch were clearly visualized. Obviously the catheter had accidentally entered the right coronary orifice when the dye was injected. The patient had remained stable throughout the entire procedure. This fortuitous event taught Sones that, contrary to views held at the time concerning electrical instability of the heart, non-oxygen carrying fluid could be injected into a major coronary artery without untoward events. Sones realized that with proper equipment he could reduce the coronary artery injectate by ten-fold and would then be able to sequentially study the entire coronary circulation of man.

Sones career began at the University of Maryland with his M.D. degree and then as a resident at the Henry Ford Hospital in Detroit. He then joined the Cleveland Clinic (Figure 9). Like Forssmann, Sones was an extraordinary personality. He preferred the positive and visible to the theoretical and speculative. Without the work of Sones the efforts in myocardial revascularization could not have been possible. He had a refreshing bluntness that sometimes stunned younger colleagues. When he visited my department

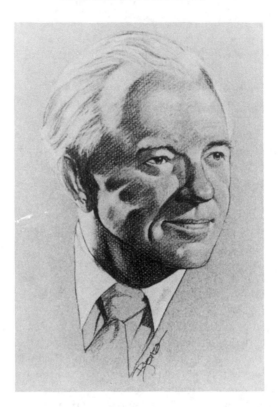

Figure 9.   F. Mason Sones (*Courtesy of the Texas Heart Institute Journal*)

(RJB) at Wayne State University in Detroit as part of a project site visit, and one of my (RJB) young colleagues presented his studies on coincidence counting in the measuring of coronary blood flow, Sones thoroughly startled the poor fellow with his critical remarks. Once I brought a patient to him, a young woman of 22, who had what probably now would be diagnosed as spasm of coronary arteries (syndrome X), but which was at that time considered small vessel disease. To prove his point he performed a myocardial puncture, with an unusual amount of skill and courage. He died in 1985 at the age of 66 from lung cancer.

A seemingly simple idea was instrumental in making coronary artery visualization more accessible: the percutaneous introduction of a catheter as described in 1952 by Sven I. Seldinger from Sweden (42; Figure 10). He described a method which he considered suitable for aortography via the femoral artery. He writes, "There is a simple method of using a catheter in the

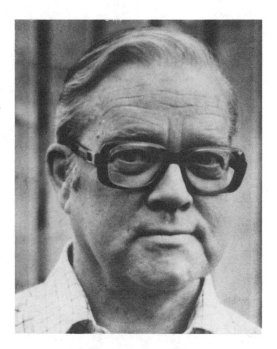

Figure 10.   Sven Ivar Seldinger (*Courtesy of The New York Academy of Medicine*)

same size as the needle and which has been used at Karolinska Sjukhuset since April 1952. The main principle consists in the catheter being introduced over a flexible leader through the puncture hole, after withdrawal of the puncture needle." Sones' technique necessitated incision into the brachial artery and suture of the vessel after the procedure had been terminated, a technique which may be beyond the surgical skill of many cardiologists. Judkins, with a group of investigators of similar interests, made selective coronary arteriography possible by the construction and design of preformed catheters (43; Figure 11). These catheters were preformed to enter the left and/or the right coronary artery. He described results on 100 consecutive patients. In each, both coronary arteries were selectively catheterized from the femoral artery and contrast injections were filmed by direct serial radiography and cinephotofluorography. Here the Seldinger technique was essential.

Judkins was born in Los Angeles and, after military service as Chief of Urology in an American service hospital in Japan, was in family practice for ten years. Following this he took a radiology residency at the University of

D. BAIM AND R.J. BING

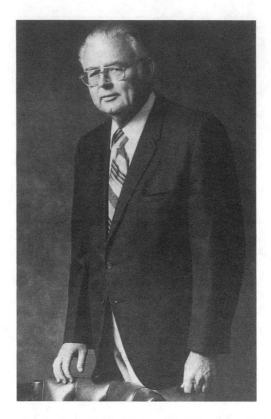

Figure 11. Melvin P. Judkins (*Courtesy of The New York Academy of Medicine*)

Oregon Medical Center followed by fellowships in cardiovascular radiology at the University of Oregon and the University of Lund, Sweden. In 1966, Judkins introduced the method he developed for transfemoral selective coronary arteriography, now known as the Judkins technique. His efforts grew out of a need to reliably and consistently perform high quality coronary arteriography in any patient suspected of having ischemic heart disease. Judkins approach to coronary arteriography was to seek a method of percutaneous catheterization from the large, readily accessible femoral artery to obviate the need for a cutdown and subsequent arterial repair. Up to this time it had been considered virtually impossible to consistently catheterize the coronaries from the femoral approach because of the long distance. Thus he developed left and right coronary-seeking catheters each with

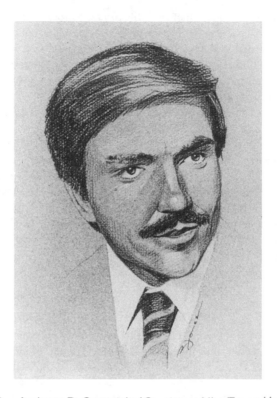

Figure 12. Andreas R. Gruentzig (*Courtesy of the Texas Heart Institute Journal*)

unique configuration, preshaped to conform to the usual anatomy. The shape of both was unconventional but the configurations were the key to consistent catheterization. When the technique was introduced the shapes were completely foreign to the thinking of the day; now they are universally accepted.

One of the most important advances in the field of catheterization was made by Andreas Gruentzig (Figure 12). Cardiology, and with it all mankind, owes Gruentzig a tremendous debt of gratitude. He adopted a technique for treating obstructed coronary arteries mechanically with a catheter (44). His work is based on that of Dotter and Judkins. The principle of Gruentzig's catheter was to dilate an area of hemodynamically important arterial stenosis or recanalize a short arterial occlusion by compressing the soft atheromatous material against the vessel wall. While Dotter used coaxial catheters to dilate the vessel lumen up to size #12 or #14 french catheter, Gruentzig's important addition was the introduction of a double lumen balloon catheter with an inflatable balloon near its tip. Thus with the aide of the balloon, dilatation could be performed to the size of #9 or #10 french catheter with only a #7 catheter. The balloon could be inflated to predetermined diameter and a pressure of about 4 atmospheres could be applied to an atherosclerotic plaque with no risk of overdistension of the vessel.

Gruentzig was born in Dresden, Germany, and studied at the University of Heidelberg, as well as in England, Switzerland and Germany. His pioneering work was done at the University of Zurich, Switzerland, where in 1979 he became Chief of the Department of Cardiology at the University Hospital (45). In a symposium in Germany Gruentzig reported on his method of angioplasty of the coronary arteries on his first group of 40 patients. The technique was successful in about 60% with improved cardiac function. Gruentzig recalled his own reaction, after he performed the first successful percutaneous transluminal coronary angioplasty in a 38-year-old man with 85% stenosis in the left anterior descending artery. "I was surprised and the patient was surprised over how easy it was." Three months after Sones' death on October 27, 1985, he and his wife were the unfortunate victims of a plane crash near Atlanta, Georgia.

As with each of the other cardiac catheterization techniques, the acceptance of Gruentzig's percutaneous transluminal coronary angioplasty (PTCA) was at first limited by the skepticism on the part of the medical community and by the crude nature of the available catheters. Gruentzig's balloon was a two-lumen device in which one lumen was used for inflating and deflating the balloon, and the other was used for pressure monitoring and contrast injection through a small port terminating ahead of the balloon (46). While there was a short segment of flexible guide wire attached to the tip of the balloon to minimize the chance for subintimal passage of the device, this wire could not be steered or manipulated in any way once the balloon had been introduced into the outer "guiding catheter." The combination of this lack of steering control, the large (1.5 mm) deflated diameter of the deflated balloon, and the low balloon rupture pressure (6 atm or 90 psi), made the device suitable for only a select subgroup of patients with proximal, discrete, sub-total, concentric and non-calcified lesions of a single vessel. Such patients were estimated to account for no more than 5-10% of the patients with coronary artery disease requiring catheterization, and even with limitation of this technique to such favorable candidates, the success of PTCA in the original (1979-1981) NHLBI PTCA Registry was only 65% while the incidence of emergency surgery for correction of a PTCA-induced complication was 6% (47).

Despite these short-comings, a number of cardiologists in the United States (Myler, Stertzer, Block, Faxon, Kent, Simpson, among others) persisted in refining the technique of PTCA. One of the most important contributions was made by John B. Simpson, while a cardiology fellow and junior faculty member at Stanford University in the early 1980's. He felt that the use of the second lumen of a coaxial dilatation catheter to carry an independently moveable and shapeable guide wire would allow improved and safer access to lesions located more distally in the coronary tree (48).

Simpson recalls an interesting moment during the early times of the development of this technique when Charles Dotter came to visit his lab on a grant visit at Stanford University. He was so excited to demonstrate the new catheter device that in his enthusiasm the balloon catheter was overinflated; as Dotter took a very close view of the inflated balloon the balloon ruptured spraying contrast medium over his glasses and over a very clean coat.

This concept ultimately led to the present precisely steerable guide wires, over which improved balloon with deflated diameters as small as 0.5 mm and rupture pressures as high as 20 atm, can be advanced. These improvements directly contributed to the increased success (85%) of PTCA in the second (1985-86) NHLBI Registry (49), and allowed pioneering cardiologists like Geoffrey Hartzler of Kansas City to extend the technique to patients with increasingly complex multi-vessel coronary disease (50). In fact by 1987, more than 250,000 PTCA procedures were being performed annually in the United States, accounting for roughly half of the revascularization (bypass surgery being the other half) (51). Angioplasty procedures are now performed in nearly 800 of the country's approximately 2,000 cardiac catheterization laboratories, for a variety of indications ranging from stable angina, to unstable angina, to acute myocardial infarction.

Despite its evident successes, PTCA continued to be faced with four major limitations:

(1)   difficulty in crossing totally occluded arteries,

(2)   difficulty in dilating rigid (calcified) or markedly elastic (eccentric) lesions,

(3)   difficulty in preventing or reliably reversing abrupt closure of the freshly dialated segment due to excessive local trauma by the balloon, and

(4)   restenosis of the dialated segment over subsequent months due to an excessive local healing response.

In the late 1980s it became apparent that little progress was being made against these four limitations of PTCA, and a number of physician inventors began to explore alternative techniques for using the cardiac catheter to enlarge stenotic coronary lumena (52).

This creativity was fostered by an enthusiastic venture capital community which had witnessed the explosive growth of PTCA and the staggering success of companies supplying leading technology. The first of these new approaches to win approval from the Food and Drug Administration was also developed by John Simpson. Directional atherectomy (53) uses a cylindrical steel capsule with an oval window on one side to cross the target lesion. As the window is pressed up against the obstructing plaque by a low pressure balloon mounted on the opposite side of the cylinder, a cup shaped cutter is advanced inside to shave off the protruding plaque and trap it within the catheter. Another still-investigational approach is the placement of several designs of permanent internal armatures (stents) within the coronary segment to maintain a large, round, and smooth lumen (54). Still others are trying to ultilize high energy pulsed laser energy at various wavelengths to ablate obstructing plaques (55).

These developments in the field of coronary intervention have helped to stimulate the development of catheter-based interventions for other forms of heart disease. Balloon catheter dilatation of congenitally stenotic pulmonic, aortic and mitral valves by pediatric cardiologists (notably James Lock of Boston's Children's Hospital) was intended to the treatment of rheumatic mitral stenosis in adult patients, and to the treatment of calcific aortic stenosis in the elderly (56). Balloon mitral valvuloplasty remains a viable option to surgical commissurotomy or valve replacement (57), but balloon aortic valvuloplasty appears to provide too transient an improvement in the elderly patient to be considered in lieu of surgical aortic valve replacement. Other avenues of catheter therapy in congenital heart disease are impressive. Atrial septal defects can be created using a balloon (Rashkind) or blade-tipped catheter, or closed using a double umbrella device developed James Lock patterned after an earlier device for closure of persistent patent ductus arteriosus (58). Unwanted coronary fistulae or collateral vessels can be closed percutaneously using embolizable coils or detachable balloons. At Boston's Children's Hospital, more than 700 interventional catheterization procedures are now performed yearly, providing non-surgical correction for more than 25% of congenital cardiac defects.

With this strong and enthusiastic wave of interventional catheter development has also come a demanding standard for the evaluation of new technology. Tighter oversight by the Food and Drug Administration, the demand by the medical community for randomized trials showing the advantage of these newer techniques over existing medical or surgical options, and increasingly stringent policies of third party payors, will inevitably separate the wheat from the chaff of interventional cardiology.

While the lineage of each of of today's commonplace techniques can indeed be traced back to the innovations of our predecessors, we are frequently less cognizant of the blind alley-ways they tried and abandoned. Before openly accepting the glowing promise of today's innovations, I (DSB) am always reminded of a talk entitled "The Way We Were" given by Kurt Amplatz at a June 1989 meeting of some of the world's most experienced interventional cardiologists, devoted to examining the results of some of today's investigational techniques. During that talk, Dr. Amplatz showed a film from the 1950's about the then promising technique of left heart catheterization via direct cardiac puncture. The statement that "more than 100 cases had been performed, with a mortality of only 1%," made many shift uncomfortably in our seats to think about which of our current techniques would endure, and which would join direct cardiac puncture.

Another new development is invasive electrophysiologic testing combined with therapy in the definition and treatment of arrhythmias. Invasive testing for supraventricular tachycardia, ventricular tachycardia combined with insertion of an automatic defibrillator, cardiac electrosurgery or catheter ablations are becoming useful. Because of the relatively high surgical mortality particularly in patients with poor left ventricular function, insertion of the automatic defibrillator has become increasingly popular. Although there are still complications, the incidence of sudden death is reduced by the insertion of automatic defibrillators. However, there is still some operative mortality, incidence of infection and incidence of inappropriate shocks. Catheter ablation of ventricular tachycardia foci has still a very limited clinical role (59, 60). Whatever the future turns taken by cardiac catheterization a prediction made at a symposium in Leichlingen, Germany by one of us (RJB) in 1978, nearly the fiftieth anniversary of Forssmann's daring experiments, will undoubtedly ring true "There is no doubt in my mind that the cardiac catheter has become of lesser importance for physiological methods and of ever greater interest in clinical and diagnostic cardiology" (61). It has, almost exclusively, become a clinical tool, particularly because of the introduction of coronary arteriography which led to a localization of lesions in the coronary artery, and became essential for the development of coronary artery surgery and for the usage of His bundle recording.

REFERENCES

1. Bernard, C. Leçons sur la Chaleur Animale, sur les Effets de la Chaleur et sur la Fièvre. Paris, Bailliere, 1876.

2. Bernard, C. Leçons de Physiologie Operatoire. Paris, Bailliere, 1879.
3. Grande, F., and M. B. Visscher, eds. Claude Bernard and Experimental Medicine. Collected Papers. Cambridge, Mass., Schenkman, 1967.
4. Chaveau, A., and E. J. Marey. Determination graphique des rapports du choc du coeur avec les mouvements des oreillettes et des ventricles: experience faite a l'aide a un appareil enregistreur (sphygmographe). C. R. Hebd. Acad. Sci., 53:662, 1861.
5. Exposition and Catalogue on Etienne Jules Marey. Medtronics, France, 1–70, 1980.
6. Snellen, H.A. E. J. Marey and Cardiology. Rotterdam, Kooyker, 1980.
7. Handwritten manuscript by Claude Bernard nominating E. J. Marey for the physiology prize of the Fondation Lecaze by the Institut de France, 1875. St. Julien, Rhone, Musee Claude Bernard.
8. Forssmann, W. Selbstversuch: Erinnerungen eines Chirurgen. Duesseldorf, Drost, 1972.
9. Forssmann, W. Die Sondierung des rechten Herzens. Klin. Wochenschr., 8:2085–2087, 1929.
10. Forssmann, W. Ueber Kontrastdarstellung der Hoehlen des lebenden rechten Herzens und der Lungenschlagader. Muench. Med. Wochenschr., 78:489–492, 1931.
11. Klein, O. Zur Bestimmung des zirkulatorischen Minutenvolumens beim Menschen nach dem Fickschen Prinzip. Muench. Med. Wochenschr., 77:1311–1312, 1930.
12. Personal communication: letter from Werner Forssmann to R. J. Bing. September 26, 1978.
13. Schadewaldt, H. Werner Forssmann. Sonderdruck im Jahrbuch der Universitaet Duesseldorf. Duesseldorf, Triltsch, 1978–80, pp. 35–38.
14. Cournand, A. Cardiac catheterization: development of the technique, its contributions to experimental medicine, and its initial applications in man. Acta Med. Scand. Suppl. 579:3–32, 1975. Originally: Jiminez Diaz Memorial Lecture, Fundacion Conchite Rabago de Jiminez Diaz, Madrid, 1970, pp. 47–80.
15. Cournand, A., and H. A. Ranges. Catheterization of the right auricle in man. Proc. Soc. Exp. Biol. Med., 46:462–466, 1941.
16. Snellen, H. A. History and Perspectives of Cardiology. Interview with Andre Cournand at Leiden, Holland, November, 1979. The Hague, Leiden University Press, 1981, pp. 33–37.
17. Cournand, A. Dickinson Woodruff Richards 1895–1973. Trans. Assoc. Am. Physicians, 86:33–38, 1973.
18. Fishman, A. P., and D. W. Richards, eds. Circulation of the Blood: Men and Ideas. New York, Oxford University Press, 1964.
19. Richards, D. W. Medical Priesthoods and Other Essays. Connecticut Printers, 1970.
20. Swan, H. J. Personal communication.
21. Swan, H. J., and W. Ganz. Hemodynamic monitoring: a personal and historical perspective. Can. Med. Assoc. J., 121:868–871, 1979.
22. Ganz, W. Personal communication.
23. Comroe, J. H. Retrospectroscope: Insights into Medical Discovery. Menlo Park, California, Von Gehr, 1977, p. 60.

24. Bing, R. J., L. D. Vandam, F. Gregoire, J. E. Handelsman, W. T. Goodale, and J. E. Eckenhoff. Catheterization of the coronary sinus and the middle cardiac vein in man. Proc. Soc. Exp. Biol. Med., 66:239–240, 1947.
25. Bing, R. J., M. M. Hammon, J. C. Handelsman, S. R. Powers, F. C. Spencer, J. E. Eckenhoff, W. T. Goodale, J. H. Hafkenschiel, and S. Kety. The measurement of coronary blood flow, oxygen consumption, and efficiency of the left ventricle in man. Am. Heart J., 38:1–24, 1949.
26. Bing, R. J. The metabolism of the heart. Harvey Lectures, 50:27–70, 1954–55.
27. Bing, R. J. Cardiac metabolism. Physiol. Rev., 45:171–213, 1965.
28. Himmelstein, A., A. Cournand, and J. S. Baldwin. Cardiac catheterization in congenital heart disease: a clinical and physiological study in infants and children. New York, Commonwealth Fund, 1949.
29. Hellems, H. K., F. W. Haynes, L. Dexter, and T. D. Kinney. Pulmonary capillary pressure in animals estimated by venous and arterial catheterization. Am. J. Physiol., 155:98–105, 1948.
30. Bing, R. J. Physiological methods in the diagnosis of congenital heart disease. Surg. Gynecol. Obstet., 88:399–401, 1949.
31. Griswold, H. E., R. J. Bing, J. C. Handelsman, J. Campbell, and E. LeBrun. Physiological studies in congenital heart disease. VII. Pulmonary arterial hypertension in congenital heart disease. Johns Hopkins Hosp. Bull., 84:76–88, 1949.
32. Bing, R. J., L. D. Vandam, J. C. Handelsman, J. Spencer, J. Campbell, and H. Griswold. Physiological studies in congenital heart disease. VI. Adaptations to anoxia in congenital heart disease with cyanosis. Bull. Johns Hopkins Hosp., 83:439–456, 1948.
33. Radner, S. Thoracic aortography by catheterization from the radial artery. Acta Radiol., 29:178–180, 1948.
34. Broden, B., G. Jonsson, and J. Karnell. Thoracic aortography. Acta Radiol, 32:498–508, 1949.
35. Rousthoi, P. Ueber Angiokardiographie. Acta Radiol., 14:419–423, 1933.
36. Radner, S. An attempt at the roentgenologic visualization of coronary blood vessels in man. Acta Radiol., 26:497–502, 1945.
37. Robb, G. P. and I. Steinberg. Visualization of the chambers of the heart, the pulmonary circulation, and the great blood vessels in man. Am. J. Roentgenol., 41:1–17, 1939.
38. DiGuglielmo, L., and M. Guttadauro. Anatomic variations in the coronary arteries. An arteriographic study in living subjects. Acta Radiol., 41:393–397, 1954.
39. Thal, A. P., L. S. Richards, R. Greenspan, and M. J. Murray. Arteriographic studies of the coronary arteries in ischemic heart disease. JAMA, 168:2104–2109, 1958.
40. Dotter, C. T., and L. H. Frische. Visualization of the coronary circulation by occlusive aortography: a practical method. Radiology, 71:502–523, 1958.
41. Sones, F. M. and E. K. Shirey. Cinecoronary aorteriography. Mod. Concepts Cardiovasc. Dis., 31:735–738, 1962.
42. Seldinger, S. I. Catheter replacement of the needle in percutaneous arteriography: a new technique. Acta Radiol., 39:368–376, 1953.
43. Judkins, M. R. Selective coronary arteriography. Part I: a percutaneous transfemoral technique. Radiology, 89:815–824, 1967.

44. Gruentzig, A. R. Transluminal dilatation of coronary–artery stenosis. Lancet, 1:263, 1978 (letter).
45. Hurst, J. W. Tribute: Andreas Roland Gruentzig (1939–1985): a private perspective. Circulation, 73:606–610, 1986.
46. Gruentzig A. R., A. Senning, W. E. Siegenthaler. Nonoperative dilation of coronary artery stenosis — percutaneous transluminal coronary angioplasty. N Engl J Med 301:61, 1979.
47. Kent K. M., et al. (eds). Proceedings of the National Heart, Lung and Blood Institute workshop on the outcome of percutaneous transluminal angioplasty (June 7–8, 1 1983). Am J Cardiol 53:1C, 1984.
48. Simpson, J. B., D. S. Baim, E. W. Robert and D. C. Harrison. A new catheter system for coronary angioplasty. Am J Cardiol 49:1216, 1982.
49. Detre, K., et al. Percutaneous transluminal coronary angioplasty in 1985–1986 and 1977–1978. The NHLBI Registry. N Engl J Med 318:265, 1988.
50. Hartzler, G.O., et al. "High–risk" percutaneous transluminal coronary angioplasty. Am J. Cardiol 61:33G, 1988.
51. Baim, D.S., E.J. Ignatius. Use of percutaneous transluminal coronary angioplasty: Results of a current survey. Am J Cardiol 61:3G, 1988.
52. Baim, D.S., K. Detre, K. Kent. Problems in the development of new devices for coronary intervention — Possible role for a multicenter registry. J Am Coll Cardiol 14:1389, 1989.
53. Simpson, J. B., et al. Transluminal atherectomy for occlusive peripheral vascular disease. Am J Cardiol 61:96G, 1988.
54. Schatz, R. A. A view of vascular stents. Circulation 79:445, 1989.
55. Litvak, et al. Interventional cardiovascular therapy by laser and termal angioplasty. Circulation 81:IV–109, 1990.
56. Letac, B., L. I. Gerber, R.Koning. Insights on the mechanism of balloon valvuloplasty in aortic stenosis. Am J Cardiol 62:1241, 1988.
57. Palacios, I. F., P. C. Block, G. T. Wilkins, A. E. Weyman. Follow–up of patients undergoing percutaneous mitral balloon valvotomy: analysis of factors determining restenosis. Circulation 79:573, 1989.
58. Lock, J. E., J. T. Cockerham, J. F. Keane, et al. Transcatheter umbrella closure of congenital heart defects. Circulation 75:593, 1987.
59. Scheinman, M. M., Evans–Bell, T., and the Executive Committee of the Percutaneous Cardiac Mapping and Ablation Registry. Catheter ablation of the atrioventricular junction: A report of the Percutaneous Cardiac Mapping and Ablation Registry. Circulation, 70:1024–1029, 1984.
60. Kastor, J. A., L. N. Horowitz, A. H. Harken, et al. Clinical electrophysiology of ventricular tachycardia. N Engl J. Med., 304:1004–1020, 1981.
61. Bing, R. J. History of cardiac catheterization. In: History of Cardiology (Beitraege zur Geschichte der Kardiologie), edited by G. Bluemchen, published by the editor, Monheim, 1979, pp. 165–175.

Chapter 2

Echocardiography And The Doppler Method

P. DOUGLAS AND R.J. BING

The physical principle underlying echocardiography (ultrasound of the heart) is based on piezoelectricity, that is, electricity created by transformation of crystals. These crystals act both as transmitter and receiver of sound pulses. These sound pulses are termed ultrasound because their frequency is much higher than audible soundwaves. As applied to cardiology, they are aimed at a heart valve or the wall of the heart chambers from which the pulses are then reflected, forming an echo. The time delay between emission and detection of reflected sound is displayed graphically as distance from the transducer. The sound beam can either be recorded as a single line, as in M-mode echocardiography, or as a composite of many lines forming a two-dimensional tomographic image. Ultrasound permits simultaneous visualization of a whole sector of the heart, thus making possible the evaluation of cardiac wall motion and the motion of the heart valves.

Echocardiography enables real time, noninvasive imaging of all cardiac and vascular structures. Its impact on the practice of cardiology is immense and the indications for its use so broad as to include the diagnosis and evaluation of all forms of cardiovascular disease. The technique has for example become invaluable in the assessment of the physiology and pathophysiology of the left ventricle, determining regional wall motion and the proportion of blood ejected by the heart during systole (the ejection fraction).

29

The simple reflection of sound from the cardiac walls and valves provides much structural information but does not permit measurement of direction or velocity of blood flow. Doppler ultrasound must be used for such measurements. In this method, an ultrasound beam is directed toward and reflected from blood flow itself. The wavelength of the reflected beam is shifted (Doppler Shift) depending upon the direction of flow and velocity of the moving cells. Doppler flow measurements together with echocardiography are particularly useful, enabling measurement of velocity and flow across a cardiac valve together with imaging of the anatomy of the malformation. Thus, the hemodynamics of valvular lesions can be accurately measured. The technique has become an indispensable tool in the evaluation of patients with congenital, valvular, and coronary heart disease. Blood flow determinations can also be used to calculate pressure gradients across a valve to within 10 percent of those obtained by catheterization of the heart. With the new technology of color flow mapping, Doppler flow measurements have been used as a "non-invasive angiogram."

The principle underlying echocardiography and piezoelectricity was discovered by the brothers Jacques and Pierre Curie (Figure 1). The life of Pierre Curie, husband of Marie, is well known, less is known of Jacques Curie. After graduation, he worked with his brother and Friedel in the laboratory of mineralogy at the Sorbonne. As Marie Curie wrote in the biography of her husband:

> Their experiments led the two young physicists to great success: the discovery of the hitherto unknown phenomenon of piezoelectricity, which consists of an electric polarization produced by the compression or the expansion of crystals in the direction of the axis of symmetry; this was by no means a chance discovery. It was the result of much reflection on the symmetry of crystalline matter, which enabled the brothers to foresee the possibilities of such polarization. With an experimental skill rare at their age, the young men succeeded in making a complete study of the new phenomenon, established the conditions of symmetry necessary, and formulated remarkably simple laws (1).

The technical difficulties of this work, the measurement of minute amounts of deformations of the crystal were described by Marie: "Fortunately, they were provided with a small room adjoining the physics laboratory so that they might proceed successfully with their delicate operations. From these theoretical and experimental researches, Pierre and Jacques Curie immediately deduced a practical application in the form of a new apparatus, a piezoelectric quartz electrometer, which measures in absolute terms small quantities of electricity, as well as electric currents of low intensity. This apparatus has since then rendered great service in experiments on radio-

activity (1)." This statement is no exaggeration if we think of the wide application of piezoelectricity in the field of cardiology alone.

In a paper published in 1879, entitled "Physique Cristallographique,"
Jacques and Pierre Curie presented to the French Academy the experimental
results leading them to "the conclusion that in nonconductive crystals the
surface of the crystal and the production of electricity are related (2)." In a
second report, published in 1880, Jacques and Pierre Curie again reported "a
new way of developing polar electricity in crystals, by putting pressure on
the axis of symmetry (3)." In 1881, they described the converse piezoelectric
effect: when a voltage was applied to the crystal, displacement and
compression occurred. This phenomenon was first theoretically predicted by
M. Lippmann in 1881 (4).

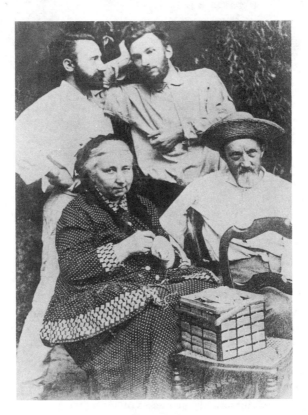

Figure 1. Jacques and Pierre Curie with their parents at a picnic. (*Courtesy of the New York Academy of Medicine*)

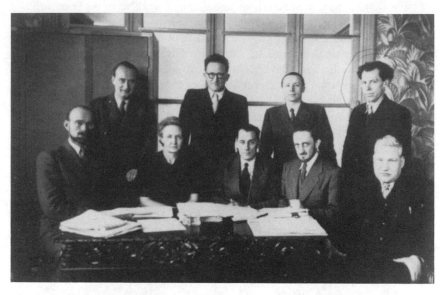

Figure 2. The scientific staff of Irène Joliot-Curie and her husband Fredérick Joliot. Jean Langevin is standing at the upper right. (*Courtesy of the Université Pierre et Marie Curie, Paris, France*)

These pioneering experiments were soon followed by those of other scientists of the late 19th century. Lord Kelvin suggested a molecular theory underlying piezoelectric phenomena and produced a mechanical model of piezoelectricity (5). W. Voight formulated the fundamental piezoelectric principle (6).

The first application of piezoelectricity was made under the duress of World War I. Langevin (Figure 2) at the Curie Institute in Paris in 1917, constructed an ultrasound generator for underwater detection of submarines, thereby originating the modern science and art of ultrasonics. He commented that during these original experiments he felt almost insupportable pain "as if the bones were heated," when he held his hand under water near the transmitter. It was also noted that fish died when they swam into the ultrasound beam. Langevin's device consisted of a mosaic of quartz crystals glued between steel plates (7). When a voltage was applied, the crystal expanded and sent out longitudinal waves. Similarly, when a wave struck the crystal, it would cause the quartz to vibrate and generate a voltage which could be detected by vacuum tubes. In 1921, W. Cady, at Wesleyan University in the USA, demonstrated that quartz crystals could be used to control oscillators and that stable oscillators could be obtained in this fashion (7). This was a forerunner of the wide application of crystals to control the frequency of military communication equipment, which now accounts for the use of more than 30 million crystals in a single year.

In 1946, ultrasound was still used only for industrial purposes, for example, to inspect the interior of solid parts (8). F.M. Firestone, at the University of Michigan, used a quartz crystal which was in contact with the object through a thin film of oil squirted onto the surface. He was the first to measure the reflected rather than transmitted sound waves. As Firestone wrote,

> When an oscillatory voltage is applied between these coatings, the crystal grows thicker and thinner in synchronism with the electrical oscillations. This causes the lower phase of the crystals to vibrate (change shape rapidly) and thereby radiate sound waves through the oil film into the object to be studied. By proper choice of the thickness of the crystal, it will give a thickness resonance and correspondingly increase the strength of the radiated sound waves. This permits determinations of defects in the matter examined.

The first attempt to use ultrasound for medical diagnosis was reported in 1942 by K.T. Dussik (9). In 1950, W.D. Keidel used ultrasound transmitted through the chest to a receiver placed on the back (10). In his article, "On a New Method for the Registration of Volume Changes of the Human Heart," Keidel demonstrated the application of a "field of ultrasound" to register phasic volume changes of the heart. The article was, as could be expected, primarily concerned with technical considerations, but it contained three illustrations comparing ultrasound tracings with phonocardiograms. The technique did record cyclic variations in ultrasound transmission synchronous with the cardiac cycle but was not sufficiently advanced to obtain quantitative measurements of cardiac volume changes.

The greatest advance in the use of ultrasound in cardiology was made in Lund, Sweden, by Inge Edler and C. Hellmuth Hertz, when they applied the unidimensional ultrasound method to examination of the in vivo human heart in 1954 (11). This also represented a tremendous advance in the use of ultrasound in medicine, as the heart was the first organ visualized by this technique. Hertz, a physicist, and Edler, a cardiologist, later received the Lasker Award in Medicine in 1977 for this work (Figures 3 and 4). They obtained echograms with a sound generating crystal applied to the chest wall in the left precordial area. The echo signal varied with the position of the crystal and the direction of the beam. They moved the crystal back and forth along the axis of the heart and recorded the reflected signal on film. They summarized the results by stating that with the ultrasound method, signals from various parts of the human heart can be obtained in vivo, and that the movement of the structures of the heart can be continuously recorded. One of the most signifi-

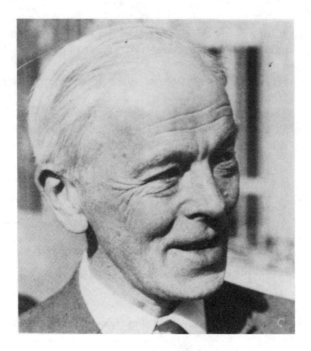

Figure 3.   Inge Edler. (*Courtesy of the New York Academy of Medicine*)

cant advances was the finding that it was possible in the living subject, by means of ultrasound, to produce real time reflections from identifiable cardiac structures. At first, Edler and Hertz were only able to visualize the posterior left ventricular wall. With improvements in instrumentation, the anterior leaflet of the mitral valve was visualized. They and others originally thought it represented the anterior surface of the left atrium, in part because it was not clear that cardiac valve tissue could actually reflect ultrasound. Thus, several years passed before the origin of this echo was properly identified by anatomic correlation (*see below*), and its significance fully appreciated. Once this structure was identified, Edler's work focused on the abnormal motion pattern of the mitral valve and he was able to identify the restricted movement characteristic of mitral stenosis. The ability to make this diagnosis by ultrasound sparked the interest of a number of other investigators and provided the stimulus for growth of the technique in the late 1950s.

In part because of early difficulty in identifying the site of reflection of cardiac echoes in man, Edler and Hertz based their results on experimental

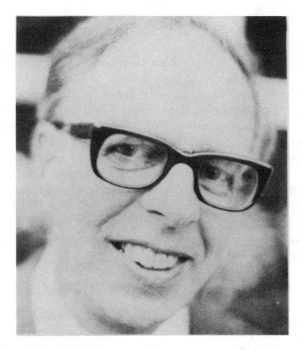

Figure 4. Carl Hellmuth Hertz. (*Courtesy of the New York Academy of Medicine*)

data on animals. In 1953 and 1954, they used the isolated heart of calves and cows suspended in the upright position, creating artificial valve movements by induced phasic left ventricular pressure changes. A sequence of photographs of the manipulated anatomic specimen was then compared frame by frame with the ultrasonic record. The direction of the ultrasonic beam was further verified by needle puncture, giving them the opportunity to define the structures encountered. In this way, Edler and colleagues were able to visualize and identify most of the cardiac structures now recognized by M-mode echocardiography. Through this in vitro work, Hertz and Edler demonstrated the potential for in vivo imaging of wall thickness, thrombi, and cavity and vascular sizes. One of several important observations was that ultrasound was reflected from both internal and external surfaces of the heart, as well as the cardiac valves.

Further work in the 1950s led to in vivo recognition of the tricuspid valve echogram and aortic regurgitation by Edler et al and of a left atrial tumor and thrombus in 1959 by a German group working under Effert (12). Edler et al went on to present a movie at the Third European Congress of Cardiology in 1960 demonstrating the echocardiographic appearances of mitral and aortic stenosis, mixed mitral disease, left atrial masses, and exudative pericarditis. Their subsequent review, published in 1961 in the Acta Medica Scandanavica (13) remained the most comprehensive available until 1972.

The first echocardiograms were performed in the United States in 1957 by J.J. Wild in an excised heart (14). One of Wild's co-workers, an engineer named John Reid, joined with Claude Joyner at the University of Pennsylvania and reported imaging of the in vivo human heart in 1962 (15). In a presentation to the American Heart Association's National Meeting, Joyner summarized his experience with "echo ultrasound cardiograms" in man. Some 260 patients had been scanned. Joyner describes "a characteristic echo...which appears to represent motion at the mitral valve" and compares the motion of this echo in normals, and in patients with atrial fibrillation, mitral regurgitation and mitral stenosis, before and after commissurotomy. The authors quickly recognized the usefulness of ultrasound in decision making and assessment of prognosis, publishing a study on the preoperative evaluation of mitral stenosis in 1965 (16).

Harvey Feigenbaum has significantly contributed to the development of echocardiography. His textbook has been used by virtually every cardiology fellow since its publication in 1972 as the first book on the topic (17). Feigenbaum trained scores of academic and clinical cardiologists, founded the American Society of Echocardiography in 1975, and continues to contribute substantially to the echocardiographic literature. It is interesting to consider Feigenbaum's early experiences with the technique. In his own words, he "became interested in echocardiography in the latter part of 1963, while operating a hemodynamic laboratory and becoming frustrated with the limitations of cardiac catheterization and angiography (17)." Although he was originally intrigued by the prospect of measuring cardiac chamber sizes, his first achievement was the detection of posterior pericardial effusions in 1965 (18). While this discovery provided much of the initial impetus for the growth of echocardiography in the United States, it really arose from the limitations of the equipment employed--a borrowed system intended only for echo encephalography. Attention was directed toward the posterior left ventricular wall by default, "principally because our gain settings were low, and this was the only echo that we could reasonably record. We were afraid to turn up the gain because we then recorded so many echoes that we became totally confused (17)." Feigenbaum, Popp, and co-workers soon obtained more suitable equipment and rapidly described measurement of posterior wall thickness, pericardial effusion, and left ventricle and right ventricle volumes and stroke volumes (19,20,21,22), proving that left ventricular structure and function could be assessed noninvasively. While these early, pioneering efforts produced remarkable results, they were not always accurate. For example, in 1967, Feigenbaum et al, described a technique for ultrasound measurement of stroke volume (19). In it the most anterior cardiac echo was incorrectly ascribed to the left ventricular free wall rather then the right ventricular free wall since it was not known that the ultrasound beam must first pass through the anteriorly located right ventricle before arriving at the left ventricle, and because septal echoes had not yet been identified. In addition, a posterior wall echo was wrongly attributed to the mitral ring. The difference between these two misidentified structures was taken to be representative of left ventricular diameter. However, rather than measuring systolic and diastolic volumes directly, stroke volume was calculated by multiplying the distance between the left ventricular anterior and posterior echoes by the maximal excursion of the echo ascribed to the mitral ring. By incorporating a measure of left ventricular size and one of systolic function, the method yielded results which correlated closely (r = .97) with Fick determinations of stroke volume.

Two years later a report was published recognizing septal echos, stating that: "A new group of echoes was found (22)." This was not strictly accurate, however, since Hertz and Edler had noted echoes between the tricuspid and mitral valves in the 1950s but had failed to identify them. The previous error in anatomic orientation of the cardiac chambers relative to the chest wall was however corrected.

The identification of an increasing variety of structures and diseases by echocardiographers in the late 1960s owed much to refinement of image display. Initial instrumentation provided only an unidimensional oscilloscopic display, to which the element of time was added by delayed exposure of polaroid film. Strip chart recorders eliminated the need to capture brief echoes and enabled continuous hard copy recordings of the left heart from apex to left atrium (sector scan). Coupled with the introduction of beam focusing, this advance paved the way to more detailed imaging and enabled the use of ultrasound in older patients in whom adequate images could not previously be obtained.

For the first fifteen years, echocardiograms were used primarily to diagnose valvular and pericardial disease by means of M-mode echocardiography. M-mode echocardiogarphy is a uni-dimensional record of sound waves reflected from cardiac structures—an "ice pick" view. The signal is displayed over time, often on paper, to give a linear recording of the motion of a valve or wall throughout several cardiac cycles. The method was not initially used to address coronary artery disease in part because of the technical limitations noted above; in addition, coronary disease held a much less central position in those early years of coronary care units (first implemented in 1963) selective angiography (1958) and coronary revascularization (1964). Indeed the first echocardiographic description of the segmental wall motion abnormalities characteristic of acute myocardial infarction appeared as recently as 1971 (23,24). In one of these early reports, Inoue et al described a decrease in the amplitude of posterior wall excursion and systolic thickening velocity in coronary artery disease. His "gold standard" for comparison was the apexcardiogram since normal values for these echocardiographic parameters had been defined only one year before, by Kraunz and Kennedy (25).

In 1972, Stefan and Bing published experimental work correlating the appearance of echocardiographic and mechanical evidence of myocardial infarction, confirming the importance of echocardiography in the diagnosis of coronary artery disease (26).

The growth of echocardiography can also be gauged by its acceptance in medical science. Echocardiography was first included as a subtitle in the Index Medicus in 1973. The American Society of Echocardiography was formed in 1975 to "promote, maintain, and pursue excellence in the ultrasonic examination of the heart." Surveys taken by the new organization revealed that 21% of cardiology departments had echocardiographic equipment in 1975, rising rapidly to 57% in 1979 and 65% in 1981 (27).

APPLICATION TO CONGENITAL HEART DISEASE

Given the limited field of view of M-mode echocardiography and early instrumentation, congenital heart disease generally proved much more difficult to diagnose than mitral stenosis or pericardial effusion. The complexity of congenital heart disease delayed the appreciation of the true usefulness of echocardiography. Early echocardiographic diagnosis relied chiefly on the appearance of right ventricular volume overload in the diagnosis of atrial septal defect and was otherwise limited to detection of an atretic valve or chamber. One of the first reports of direct diagnosis of congenital heart disease was a description of hypoplastic right and left heart syndromes published by Chestler et al in 1970 (28). He went on to describe a variety of other abnormalities, and along with Lundstrom and the still active Edler, wrote the first reviews on the subject in 1971 (29,30). In 1972 the first echocardiography text published devoted only 10 pages and 9 figures to congenital heart disease and cited but 12 references (17). Given this limited experience, it is not surprising that the 1972 edition of Alexander Nadas' classic text *Pediatric Cardiology* devoted 31 pages to vector- and phonocardiography, but did not even mention ultrasound (31). The value of echocardiography in young patients was quickly recognized over the next few years, aided by the introduction of two-dimensional imaging. Sahn et al published the first descriptions of two-dimensional dimensional imaging in cyanotic congenital heart disease in 1973 and noted its usefulness in defining great artery and chamber orientation and outflow tract anatomy (32). The second edition of Feigenbaum's text published in 1976, devoted 38 pages to congenital heart disease and included 33 figures, 10 of which were two dimensional echograms (33). More importantly, even at this early date, echocardiography was already beginning to be considered as a replacement to angiography, "In many situations, catheterization may be eliminated and in others, the catheterization can be markedly limited, thus reducing the risk of the invasive procedure (33)." In many instances, intrauterine echocardiography now furnishes the diagnosis of complicated congenital cardiac malformations before birth.

TWO-DIMENSIONAL ECHOCARIOGRAPHY

Two-dimensional echocardiography records reflected sound waves from a pie-shaped slice of the heart, thereby providing information about structures across an entire plane (tomographic imaging). Two-dimensional echocardiograms are recorded on video tape so that cardiac motion may be seen in a real time format. Two dimensional echo allows visualization of much more of the heart than does M-mode echo.

In addition to pioneering work with M-mode echocardiography, Wild and Reid built the first two dimensional scanner in 1952 (34). Using this single crystal, mechanical "echoscope," they first directed their attention to tissue characterization of human breast malignancy and later, in 1957, obtained cross sectional images of the excised human heart, including recordings of a myocardial scar, the left coronary artery and the aorta (14). Other investigators were experimenting with similar equipment, including Howrey and Bliss in 1952 (35). Japanese investigators played an important role in developing the technique, with in vivo human two dimensional echocardiography first described in Japan in 1962 by Nagayama et al at Kagoshira University (36). The technique was further refined by other investigators in Japan during the next ten years (37,38). The technique was variously termed "ultrasonic cardiokymography" and "ultrasonotonography" to reflect its unique ability to provide cross sectional images. Ebina et al first began clinical studies in 1965 with a mechanically rotating single crystal device and published a large series in 1967 (37). The transducer used was extremely bulky as it contained its own water bath within which the transducer moved. Ebina instituted the significant advancement of a simultaneously displayed electrocardiogram, providing a reference for timing during the cardiac cycle, and noted that the motion of cardiac contraction occurred most prominently in the minor rather than the major axis.

N. Bom, a Dutch engineer, described the first practical real-time multiscan ultrasonograph in 1971 (39), and published his experience with a series of 150 patients in 1973 (40). This machine provided rapid electronic activation of an array of crystals thereby achieving accurate reproduction of cardiac motion. Prototype instruments were built nearly simultaneously in the United States at the National Institute of Health (41), Indiana University (42), and Duke University (43), and by McDicken in Scotland (44), and elsewhere. Hertz was a pioneer with this method as well as with M-mode and noted some of the problems common to these early scanners--limited frame rate and bulky transducers (45). Engineers and cardiologists were soon debating the relative merits of linear or phased array and mechanical techniques (46) and commercially made systems rapidly became available. Two- dimensional echocardiography represented a tremendous advance over the unidimensional M-mode technique, to the extent that M-mode strip chart recording has been rendered an anachronism in some clinical laboratories two-dimensional imaging continues to improve with refinements in instrumentation, especially transducers and image processing techniques.

NEW VIEWS ON ECHOCARDIOGRAPHY

Several new methods have recently been developed using gastroscope and catheter mounted two-dimensional transducers such that echocardiography now is capable of imaging previously inaccessible or unresolvable cardiac anatomy. One of these, transesophageal echocardiography, was first attempted in man nearly simultaneously by Japanese and American investigators in the mid 1970's (47,48,49,50,51). Impetus for these developments came from the difficulty of obtaining adequate images in obese or barrel chested patients or those with chronic lung disease and, for the Japanese, in the specific hope that the anterior left ventricular free wall could be better visualized (48). In addition to the discomfort of swallowing the transducer, the vibrations created by some early mechanical probes were severe enough to limit examinations. Refinements eliminated this problem and instrumentation progressed rapidly from a rigid M-mode transducer to one mounted on a flexible shaft to mechanical and then phased array, steerable two dimensional systems. Introduction of the currently available phased array systems was slower, since such instrumentation was thought to be too bulky. In fact Hisanaga et al, the first to use a mechanical two dimensional system, stated in 1980 that phased array was "probably not suited for transesophageal scanning because of the proximity of the esophageal transducer to cardiac structures and because of the difficulty of swallowing a linear array of transducers with many coaxial cables (49)." Nevertheless, phased array systems have proven to be eminently feasible. The ability to angle as well as rotate the transducer and pulsed Doppler and biplane capabilities also followed, and the first commercially made probe became available in 1987.

Most initial studies were performed in the awake patient, but widespread acceptance of the new methodology in the U.S. followed clear demonstration of its usefulness as a monitoring as well as diagnostic tool during cardiac and vascular surgery. Anesthesiologists and, to a lesser extent, surgeons have therefore played an important role in popularizing transesophageal echo and demonstrating its value in detecting regional and global left ventricular dysfunction and assessing the adequacy of valve repairs and of corrections of congenital abnormalities (52,53,54,55,56). These new indications have taken echo out of the hands of radiologists and cardiologists for the first time, and promise substantial further development.

In a very short time, transesophageal echo has become widely available in both academic and community hospitals. The technique has proven very useful in the evaluation of prosthetic valves, endocarditis, cardiac masses and clots, aortic dissection and septal defects (57). These current indications for its use were accurately predicted by Hisanaga et al, who, in 1980 in the first report of the use of a mechanical two dimensional probe, noted that detection of left atrial thrombus, wall motion abnormalities, and atrio-ventricular valve abnormalities should be counted among the potential uses of transesophageal echo, and that for visualization of the atrial septum, the "transesophageal view is essential--it cannot be replaced by other views (49)." Indeed, in a remarkably short time, this technique has become an essential part of the echocardiographers, surgeons, and anesthesiologists armamentarium.

Intravascular echocardiography, another new approach to cardiac ultrasound imaging, remains in its infancy. Following early work by Martin and Watkins in 1980 (58), Paul Yock and David Linker, Americans from the University of California at San Francisco, working with Norwegian investigators from the University of Trondheim, published the first reports of clinically useful intravascular echocardiography (59). At this writing, no such catheter is yet approved for routine use although several companies are conducting clinical trials. The high frequency (20 and 30 MHz) miniaturized transducers currently under investigation are mounted on catheters and can be used to visualize arteries and veins, limited only by the size of the catheter. They are capable of providing high resolution images of peripheral arteries as well as coronary vessels, and may prove immensely useful in characterizing local vessel and plaque anatomy as well as guiding interventional procedures. This technique holds great promise in providing "direct vision" guidance of rapidly developing interventional techniques including angioplasty, atherectomy, stent placement, laser angioplasty, etc. Other potential applications of this new technique include diagnosis of vascular pathology, determination of vessel lumen size, wall and plaque architecture and vascular distensibility. Intravascular methods are also being investigated for use in the pulmonary and peripheral circulations (60).

APPLICATION OF THE DOPPLER PRINCIPLE TO CARDIOLOGY

In 1842, Johann Christian Doppler called attention to the fact that "the color of luminous bodies, just like the pitch of a sounding body, changes with motion of the body to and from the observer." Doppler was born in Salzburg, Austria, on November, 19, 1803 and died in Venice, Italy on March 17, 1853 (Figure 5). The son of a noted master stonemason in Salzburg, Doppler showed exceptional gifts for this craft. But his poor health led his father to plan a career in business for him. Doppler's mathematical abilities were soon recognized by the astronomer Simon Stampfer who suggested that Doppler attend the Polytechnic Institute in Vienna. Doppler found this experience dull and returned to Salzburg in 1825 where he pursued his studies privately. After finishing the high school courses in philosophy in a short time and after tutoring in mathematics and physics, he moved to Vienna in 1829 where he was employed for three years as a mathematical assistant. In Vienna he wrote his first paper on mathematics and electricity. In 1835 he was on the verge of emigrating to America going as far as selling his possessions and reaching Munich, when he was informed that he had obtained a position as Professor of Mathematics and Accounting at a secondary school in Prague. In 1841, he became full Professor of Elementary Mathematics and Practical Geometry at the technical academy in Prague; it was here that he enunciated his famous principle. In 1847, Doppler moved to a mining academy in Schemnitz, Bohemia as a Professor of Mathematics and Physics. In 1848, he returned to Vienna where, in 1850, he became Professor of Experimental Physics at the Royal Imperial University of Vienna. In 1853, he sought a cure for a lung ailment, probably tuberculosis, dying during a trip to Venice (61).

It is a fascinating facet of Doppler's life that he gave private instruction to a twenty year old Augustinian monk, Johann Gregor Mendel, who failed the oral examination in physics. As Doppler wrote "his essay (Mendel's) makes it clear the candidate is formally well educated, but in the physical sciences, he has not progressed beyond the elementary stage." Mendel finally passed the course to become the founder of modern genetics.

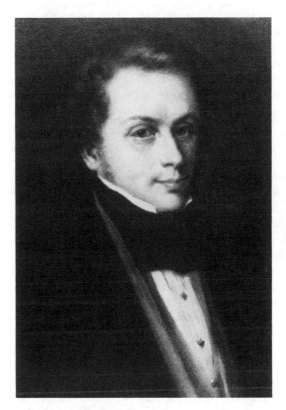

Figure 5. Johann Christian Doppler. (*With permission from the Christian Doppler Institute, Salzburg, Austria*)

Doppler was interested in applying his principle first to astronomy. In his article published in 1842, "Ueber das farbige Licht der Doppelsterne und einiger anderen Gestirne des Himmels," he argued that all stars emitted white light and that the color of some of the stars was due to their motion toward us, or away from us (62). This was an erroneous conclusion: the approach of a star would simply produce a slight shift, and no change in color would take place. But the principle is correct: an apparent shift in the frequency of waves received by an observer depends on the relative motion between the observer and the source of the waves. This principle applied to all wave phenomena. The most spectacular application was in astronomy. In 1929, E.P. Hubble examined the frequency shift of light from distant galaxies. He found that the light was red shifted (its frequency decreased), as he looked at the increasingly distant galaxies; he thus verified that the galaxies are receding from us with relative velocities that increase in the proportion to the distance. This knowledge led to the concept of an origin of the universe, commonly referred to as the "Big Bang."

Buys Ballot, a Dutch student who was working for his doctorate at the University of Utrecht, did not believe Doppler's theory. He was able to persuade the Dutch government to place at his disposal the railroad between Utrecht and Amsterdam, together with a locomotive capable of obtaining a speed of fifty miles per hour and a flat-car (63). In the Winter of 1845, Ballot had horn-players posted along the track and on the railway car. But it was so cold that the musicians were unable to blow their instruments. In June of the same year, the experiment was repeated involving teams of musicians with previously calibrated instruments, musically trained observers, and Ballot himself riding on the foot plate of the locomotive. It was observed that as the locomotive passed the players stationed on each side of the track, the note blown by the musicians on the train was perceived one-half a tone higher as it approached and one-half a tone lower as it receded. Thus, the Doppler effect for sound waves was confirmed in a curious way.

Doppler's concept also encountered criticism from Petzval (61). Petzval's opposition to Doppler's theory was based partly on its simplicity: "Without the application of differential equations, it is not possible to enter the realms of great science." In addition, Petzval confused two completely different situations: one in which there is relative movement between the sound source and the listener, and the other in which the medium is in motion, but the sound source and listener are stationary. In this latter case, the Doppler principle agrees that there would be no change in tone. In the bitter controversy between Petzval and Doppler, the latter was backed by his pupils von Ettingshausen and Mach.

At the time of the unveiling of the bust of Doppler in the colonnades of Vienna University in 1901, Egon von Oppolzer referred to the argument between Petzval and Doppler as:

His opponent bandied with such expressions as 'great science' and 'small science' in the Academy of Sciences, being of the opinion that great truths could not be found in a few lines and through an equation with only one unknown, and that at least one differential equation is necessary—and in this way he believes to have shown the incorrectness of the Doppler principle. Whoever probes somewhat deeper will find in these attacks, not a purely scientific motive, but a more personal goal. It is the old contradiction between genius and talent, which must lead to a struggle when, on the side of the talent there is no understanding of intuitive action and individual brilliance. For Doppler surveying his principle, it is of clear certainty, and for him—a true natural researcher—the attack on a law which has already been confirmed through experiments is completely incomprehensible (61).

The potential usefulness of the Doppler principle in cardiovascular diagnosis was first recognized in 1954 by Kalmus who devised an intravascular acoustic flow meter which measured the differences in frequency between sound transmitted across upstream and downstream flow (64). Doppler's principle was first utilized in cardiology by S. Satomura in 1956 (65) to detect cardiac motion and time the opening and closing of the cardiac valves. He used a continuous ultrasound beam transmitted through the chest wall to the heart and reflected from the heart structures, which underwent a frequency shift, or Doppler effect, of the transmitted sound whose magnitude and direction was based on the speed and direction of the movement of the heart. The frequency of the reflected sound was proportional to the velocity of components of the target. Satomura noted the superiority of this method over conventional phonocardiography but did not appreciate that sound could be reflected from blood cells as well as cardiac structures—that flow could be detected. Indeed he mentions "Doppler heart noises" as occurring only in diseased hearts "when the reflecting object of the ultrasound, such as the ventricular wall, suffers an irregular vibration of small amplitude (66)." Nevertheless, the ability of this application of Doppler's theory to detect valve motion was subsequently found to be of value in measuring isovolumic relaxation time and therefore diastolic function in a variety of disease states (67).

Simultaneously, an appreciation of the potential value of Doppler based ultrasound measurements of blood flow velocity in the aorta was gained in animal experiments which used a pair of implanted crystals to record velocity shifts in sound transmitted obliquely across flow (68). This method was adapted to use in man by measurement of the frequency shift of reflected rather than transmitted sound. Once the velocity of blood flow in the ascending aorta could be recorded, the technique was adapted for measurement of cardiac output (69,70,71). Appreciation of the difficulties involved and of potential sources for error have contributed to the failure of Doppler measurements of cardiac output to be included in routine clinical practice. However, the concept of measurement of volume flow by integration of the Doppler velocity curve is routinely applied in the echocardiographic laboratory for calculation of pulmonary to systemic flow ratios in cardiac shunts and aortic valve area among other uses. Early on, investigators noted that the pattern of flow in the ascending aorta was characteristically altered in some disease states. Joyner and colleagues noted diastolic flow reversal in aortic regurgitation in 1970 (72) and mid systolic notching in idiopathic hyper-trophic subaortic stenosis in 1971 (73).

By far the most important development in cardiac Doppler analysis was range-gating or pulsed wave Doppler by Baker et al at the University of Washington in 1970 (74). This method allows localization of flow velocity measurements to specific valves and chambers. It is based upon the principle that blood flow in a small area within the heart can be recorded by the use of intermittent pulses of transmitted sound. The receiver then "listens" for re-flected sound only at the end of the time interval required for the pulse to travel from the transducer to the area of interest and back. Sound reflected from both nearer and more distant structure is thereby excluded. Coupled with localization of the signal, the ability of the technique to distinguish be-tween laminar and turbulent flow enabled accurate identification of cardiac murmurs. They correctly noted its potential usefulness in murmur localiza-tion, determination of orifice size from jet diameter and measurement of pul-monary flow. Unfortunately the concept of murmur localization caused confusion between the new Doppler technique and the then currently popu-lar, and far less useful, electronic stethoscopy.

The development of pulsed Doppler resulted from a close collaboration between industry and academia which benefitted both. Baker's group worked closely with Astengo and colleagues at Advanced Technologies Laboratory (ATL) in the initial development of the pulsed wave Doppler technique. The first commercial system was introduced in 1975 by ATL, a mere two years after publication of the first report of its use in man. Industry contributed further with the introduction of fast Fourier analysis of the pulsed Doppler signal by Gessert and Taylor at Honeywell. This allowed lin-ear signal processing and two-dimensional visualization of the area from which flow velocity was recorded.

Soon after the introduction of pulsed Doppler, Holen et al (75) demon-strated the correlation between measured Doppler flow velocities and pres-sure gradients, forming the basis for assessments of valvular and vascular stenosis, prosthetic valves and estimation of chamber pressures using regur-gitant or shunt jet velocities. Two years later, in 1976, Holen et al (76) and Hatle et al (77) simultaneously published methods for estimating mitral ori-fice area. Publication of methods for calculation of mitral valve area by the pressure half time method, and measurement of pulmonary artery pressure and aortic stenosis gradients soon followed (78,79,80). The ability to quan-tify stenosis by continuous wave methods and detect turbulent flow due to regurgitation or shunts by pulsed methods combined to make Doppler an immensely important and widely adopted addition to the echocardiographic laboratory in the early 1980's.

Another group at the University of Washington, Brandestini and colleagues, developed a multi-gated or multichannel Doppler system which allowed determination of velocity in several areas of interest simultaneously (81). This digitally processed system displayed velocity by color coding superimposed on a conventional M-mode echocardiogram. The first report of its clinical use in abstract form in 1982 (82) coincided with a preliminary report by Bommer et al at the University of California at Davis, of "real time, two dimensional color flow Doppler (83)." The Japanese investigators Kitabatake, Namekawa, et al (84,85) were also developing "blood-flow imaging" based on color-coded blood flow mapping on two dimensional echoes, including the development of the auto-correlation method capable of the rapid data analysis required (85). Indeed the first book on color Doppler and the first commercially available machine were introduced in 1982 (86), both in Japan.

Current instrumentation allows for superimposition of color coded velocity on the tomographic image. While, in theory, color Doppler's ability to detect flow is identical to that of pulsed Doppler, the display format substantially enhances both the sensitivity and specificity of the technique. Small or eccentric jets are more easily detected and the origin of abnormal flow more easily identified. Color Dopppler is also extremely useful for describing the direction of a jet, so that the continuous wave beam may be more accurately oriented to high velocity flow. Finally, color flow substantially decreases the time necessary to perform the echocardiographic exam.

It has taken nearly a hundred and fifty years for the clinical importance of the Doppler effect to be widely appreciated in cardiac diagnosis and almost a hundred years for the Curies' early experiments with piezoelectricity to be applied to cardiac imaging in routine practice. The developments which have enabled translation of their work into useable format occurred in the 1950s and 60s for both Doppler and conventional imaging echocardiography--long before the clinical significance of this work was appreciated by most cardiologists. The development of echocardiography has been a truly international effort, with major contributions by investigators in Europe, Japan, and the United States, and has frequently depended on contributions from industrial as well as academic research. Few techniques have so profoundly altered the approach to cardiovascular diagnosis. Ultrasound, at its best, can provide information otherwise unobtainable by the physical examination or invasive pressure monitoring, and angiography combined. Ultrasound also provides much valuable information regarding both cardiac structure and function.

REFERENCES

1. Curie, M. Pierre Curie. New York, Macmillan, 1923.
2. Curie, J., and P. Curie. Physique cristallographique sur l'électricité polaire dans les hemièdres à faces inclines. C. R. Hebd. Sci., 9:383–387, 1880.
3. Curie, J., and P. Curie. Lois du dégagement de l'électricite par pression dans l'armedine. C. R. Hebd. Acad Sci., 92:186–188, 1881.
4. Lippman, M. Principes de la conservation de l'électricite. Ann. Chim. Phys., 145, 1881.
5. Kelvin, L. On the piezoelectric property of quartz. Philos. Mag., 36:1–99, 1890.
6. Voight, W. Lehrbuch der Kristallphysik. Leipzig, Teubner, 1910.
7. Cady, W. G. Piezoelectricity. New York, Dover, 19644.
8. Firestone, F. M. The supersonic reflectoscope, an instrument for inspecting solid parts by means of sound waves. J. Acoust. Soc. Am., 17:287–299, 1946.
9. Dussik, K. T. Ueber die Moeglichkeit hochfrequente mechanische Schwindungen als diagnostiches Hilfsmittel zu verwenden. Z. Gesamte Neurol. Psychiatr., 174:153–165, 1942.
10. Keidel, W. D. Ueber eine neue Methode zur Registrierung der Volumenaenderungen des Herzens am Menschen. Z. Kreislauf., 39:257–271, 1950.
11. Edler, I. and C.H. Hertz. Use of ultrasonic reflectoscope for continuous recording of movements of heart walls. Kungl Fysiogr Sallsk (Lund) Forhandl, 24:5–40, 1954.
12. Effert, S. and E. Domanig. The diagnosis of intra-atrial tumor and thrombi by the ultrasonic echo method. Germ. Med. Mth., 4:1, 1959.
13. Edler. I, A. Gustafson, T. Karlefors, and B. Christensson. Mitral and aortic valve movements recorded by an ultra-sonic echo method. An experimental study. Acta. Med. Scand., (Suppl. 370):67–82, 1961.
14. Wild, J.J., H.D. Crawford, and J.M. Reid. Visualization of the excised human heart by means of reflected ultrasound or echography. Am. Heart J., 54:903–906, 1957.
15. Joyner, C.R., J.M. Reid, and J.P. Bond. Reflected ultrasound in the assessment of mitral valve disease. Circulation, 27:503–511, 1963.
16. Joyner, C.R. and J.M. Reid. Ultrasound cardiogram in the selection of patients for mitral valve surgery. Ann. NY Acad. Sci, 118:512–524, 1965.
17. Feigenbaum, H. and S. Chang. Echocardiography. Philadelphia: Lea & Febiger, 1972.
18. Feigenbaum, H., J.A. Waldhausen, and L.P. Hyde. Ultrasound diagnosis of pericardial effusion. JAMA, 191:711–717, 1965.
19. Feigenbaum, H., A. Zaky, and W.K. Nasser. Use of ultrasound to measure left ventricular stroke volume. Circulation, 35:1092–1099, 1967.
20. Feigenbaum, H., R.L. Popp, J.N. Chip, and C.L. Haine. Left ventricular wall thickness measured by ultrasound. Arch. Int. Med., 121:391–395, 1968.

21. Feigenbaum, H., S.B. Wolfe, R.L. Popp, C.L. Haine, and H.T. Dodge. Correlation of ultrasound with angiocardiography in measuring left ventricular diastolic volume. Am. J. Cardiol., 23:111, 1969.
22. Popp, R.L., S.B. Wolfe, T. Hirata, and H. Feigenbaum. Estimation of right and left ventricular size by ultrasound. A study of the echoes from the interventricular septum. Am. J. Cardiol., 24:523–530, 1969.
23. Inoue, K., H. Smulyan, S. Mookherjee, and R.H. Eich. Ultrasonic measurement of left ventricular wall motion in acute myocardial infarction. Circulation, 43:778–785, 1971.
24. Ratchin, R.A. C.E. Rackley, and R.O. Russell. Serial evaluation of left ventricular volumes and posterior wall movement in the acute phase of myocardial infarction using diagnostic ultrasound. (Abstr.) Am. J. Cardiol, 29:286, 1972.
25. Kraunz, R.F. and J.W. Kennedy. Ultrasonic determination of left ventricular wall motion in normal man. Am. Heart J., 79:36–43, 1970.
26. Stefan, G. and R.J. Bing. Echocardiographic findings in experimental myocardial infarction of the posterior left ventricular wall. Amer. J. Cardiol, 30:629–639, 1972.
27. American Society of Echocardiography White Paper: Echocardiography: 1986 and Beyond, March, ASE.
28. Chestler, E., H.S. Jaffe, R. Vecht, W. Beck and V. Shrire.. Ultrasound cardiography in single ventricle and hypoplastic left and right heart syndromes. Circulation, 42:123–129, 1970.
29. Chestler, E., H.S. Joffe, W. Beck, and V. Schrire. Echocardiography in the diagnosis of congenital heart disease. Pediat. Clin. N. Am., 18:1163–1190, 1971.
30. Lundstrom, N.R. and I. Edler. Ultrasoundcardiography in infants and children. Acta. Pacdiat. Scand., 60:117–128, 1971.
31. Nadas, A.S. and D.C. Fyler. Pediatric Cardiology, 3rd Ed. Philadephia:. W.B. Saunders, 1972.
32. Sahn, D.J., R. Terry, R. O'Rourke, G. Leopold, and W.F. Friedman. Multiple crystal cross-sectional echocardiography in the diagnosis of cyanotic congenital heart disease. Circulation, 50:230–238, 1974.
33. Feigenbaum, H. Echocardiography, 2nd Edition. Lea & Febiger, 1976.
34. Wild, J.J. and J.M. Reid. Application of echo-ranging techniques to the determination of structure of biological tissues. Science, 115:226–230 1952.
35. Howry, D.H., and W.R. Bliss. Ultrasonic visualization of soft tissue structures of the body. J. Lab. Clin. Med., 40:579–592, 1952.
36. Nagayama, T., S. Nakamura, K. Hayakawa, and Y. Komo. Ultrasonic cardiokymogram. Acta. Med. Univ. Kagoshima, 4:229, 1962.
37. Ebina, T., S. Oka, M. Tanaka, S. Kosaka, Y. Terasawa, K. Unno, D. Kikuchi, and R. Uchida. The ultrasono-tomography for the heart and great vessels in living human subjects by means of the ultrasonic reflection technique. Jap. Heart J., 8:331–353, 1967.
38. Uchida, R., Y. Hagiwara, and T. Irie. Electroscanning ultrasonic diagnostic equipment. Jap. Med. Elec., 58, 1971/1972.
39. Bom, N., C.T. Lancee, J. Honkoop, and P.G. Hugenholtz. Ultrasonic viewer for cross-sectional analyses of moving cardiac structures. Bio-Medical Eng., 6:500, 1971.

40. Bom, N., C.T. Lancee, G. Van Zwieten, F.E. Kloster, and J. Roelandt. Multiscan echocardiography. I. Technical description. Circulation, 48:1066–1074, 1973.
41. Griffith, J. M. and W. L. Henry. A sector scanner for real time two-dimensional echocardiography. Circulation, 49:1147–1152, 1974.
42. Eggleton, R.C., J.C. Dillion,H.C. Feigenbaum, K.W. Johnston, and S. Chang. Visualization of cardiac dynamics with real time B-mode ultrasonic scanner (abstr). Circulation, 49/50 (Suppl. III):27, 1974.
43. Von Ramm, O.T., and F.L. Thurstone. Cardiac imaging using a phased array ultrasound system. I. system design. Circulation, 53:258, 1976.
44. McDicken, W.M., K. Bruff, and J. Patton. An ultrasonic instrument for rapid B-scanning of the heart. Ultrasonics, 12:269–272, 1974.
45. Hertz, C.H. and K. Lundstrom. A fast ultrasonic scanning system for heart investigation. 3rd international conference on medical physics. August, 1972, Gottenburg, Sweden.
46. Eggleton, R.C. and K.W. Johnston. Real time mechanical scanning system compared with array techniques. IEEE, Proc. Sonics Ultrasonics, Catalog No. 74-CH 0896–1, p.16, 1974.
47. Frazin, L., J.V. Talano, L. Stephanides, H.S. Loeb, L. Kopel, and R. Gunnar. Esophageal echocardiography. Circulation, 54:102–108, 1976.
48. Matsuzaki, M., Y. Matsuda, Y. Ikee, Y. Takahashi, T. Saskai, Y. Toma, K. Ishida, T. Yorozu, T. Kumada, and R. Kusukawa. Esophageal echocardiographic left venticular anterolateral wall motion in normal subjects and patients with coronary artery disease. Circulation, 63:1085–1092, 1981.
49. Hisanaga, K., A. Hisanaga, N. Hibi, K. Nishimura, and T. Kambe. High speed rotating scanner for transesophageal cross-sectional echocardiography. Am. J. Cardiol, 46:837–842, 1980.
50. Hisanaga, K., A. Hisanaga, K. Nagata, and Y. Ichie. Transesophageal cross-sectional echocardiography. Am. Heart J., 100:605–609, 1980.
51. Hisanaga, K., A. Hisanaga, Y. Ichie, K. Nishimura, N. Hibi, Y. Fukui, and T. Kambe. Transesophageal pulsed doppler echocardiography. (Abstr.) Lancet, 1:53–54, 1979.
52. Schlueter, M., B.A. Langenstein, and J.A. Polster, et al. Transesophageal cross-sectional echocardiography with a phased array transducer system. Technique and initial clinical results. Br. Heart J., 48:67–72, 1982.
53. Kremer, P., M. Cahalan, and P. Beaupre, N.S. Schiller and P. Hanrath. Intraoperative myocardial ischemia detected by transesophageal two-dimensional echocardiography. (Abstr.) Circulation, 68(suppl. III):332, 1983.
54. Pandian, N.G., M. England, J. Hudson, et al. Continuous monitoring of cardiac function by two-dimensional echocardiography using precordial and esophageal transducers. Ultrasonic Imaging, 6:225, 1984.
55. Topol, E.J., J.L. Weiss, P.A. Guzman, et al. Immediate improvement of dysfunctional myocardial segments after coronary revascularization: detection by intraoperative transesophageal echocardiography. J. Am. Coll. Cardiol, 4:1123–1134, 1984.
56. Spotnitz, H.M., C.Y.H. Young, and A.J. Spotnitz, et al. Intra-operative left ventricular performance evaluated by two-dimensional ultra-sound. Circulation, 62:329, 1980.

57. Seward, J.B., B.K. Khandheria, J.K. Oh, M.D. Abel, R.W. Hughes Jr., W.D. Edwards, B.A. Nichols, W.K. Freeman, and A.J. Tajik. Transesophageal Echocardiography: Technique, anatomic correlations, implementation, and clinical applications. Mayo Clin. Proc., 63:649–680, 1988.
58. Martin, R.W. and D.W. Watkins. An ultrasonic catheter for intravascular measurement of blood flow: Technical details. IEEE Trans. Sonics Ultrasound, 27:277–278, 1980.
59. Yock, P.G., E.L. Johnson, and D.T. Linker. Intravascular ultrasound: Development and clinical potential. Am. J. Cardiac Imaging, 2:185–193, 1988.
60. Pandian, N.G., A. Weintraub, A. Kreis, S.L. Schwartz, M.A. Konstam, and D.N. Salem. Intracardiac, intravascular, two-dimensional, high-frequency ultrasound imaging of pulmonary artery and its branches in humans and animals. Circulation, 81:2007–2012, 1990.
61. Eden, A. Christian Doppler, Thinker and Benefactor. Salzburg, Austria, The Christian Doppler Institute for Science and Technology, 1988.
62. Doppler, C. Ueber das farbige Licht der Doppelsterne und einiger anderen Gestirne des Himmels. Abhandl. Koenigl. Boehmisch. Gesellsch. Wissensch., 2:465–482, 1842.
63. Doppler, J. C. Dictionary of Scientific Biography, 4:167, 1971.
64. Kalmus, H.P. Electronic flowmeter system. Rev. Sci. Instr., 25:201–206, 1954.
65. Satomura, S., T. Yoshida, M. Mori, Y. Nimura, M.Okimura, G. Hikita and K. Nakanishi. Studies on cardiac function test by ultrasonic Doppler method (Abstr.) Jpn. Circ. J., 20:227–228 1956.
66. Satomura, S. Ultrasonic Doppler Method for the inspection of cardiac function. J. Acoustical Soc. Am, 29:1181–1185, 1957.
67. Yoshida, T., M. Mori, Y. Nimura, G. Hikita, S. Takagishi, K. Nakanishi, and S. Satomura. Analysis of heart motion with ultrasonic Doppler method and its clinical application. Am. Heart J., 61:61-75, 1961.
68. Franklin, D.L., R.M. Ellis, and R.F. Rushmer. Aortic blood flow in dogs during treadmill exercise. J. Appl. Phys., 14:809, 1959.
69. Light, L.H. Transcutaneous observation of blood velocity in the ascending aorta in man. Biol. Cardio., 26:214, 1969.
70. Light, L.H., G. Gross, and P.L. Hansen. Non-invasive measurement of blood velocity in the major thoracic vessels. Proc. Roy. Soc. Med., 67:142–143, 1974.
71. Huntsman, L.L, E. Gams, C.C. Johnson, and E. Fairbanks. Transcutaneous determination of aortic blood-flow velocities in man. Am. Heart J., 89:605–612, 1975.
72. Thompson, P.D., R.G. Mennel, H. Mac Vaugh, and C.R. Joyner. Evaluation of aortic insufficiency in humans with a transcutaneous Doppler velocity probe. (Abstr.) Ann. Intern. Med., 72:781, 1970.
73. Joyner, C.R., F.S. Harrison, Jr., and J.W. Gruber. Diagnosis of hypertrophic subaortic stenosis with a Doppler velocity flow detector. Ann. Inter. Med., 74:692–696, 1971.
74. Baker, D.W. Pulsed ultrasonic Doppler blood-flow sensing. IEEE Trans. Sonic Ultrasonics, SU-17:3, 1970.
75. Holen, J., R. Aaslid, K. Landmark, and S. Somonsen. Determination of pressure gradient in mitral stenosis with a noninvasive ultrasound Doppler technique. Acta. Med. Scand., 199:455–460, 1976.

76. Holen, J. and S. Nitter-Hauge. Evaluation of obstructive characteristics of mitral disc valve implants with ultrasound Doppler techniques. Acta. Med. Scand., 201:429–434, 1977.
77. Hatle, L., A. Brubakk, A. Tromsdal, and B. Angelsen. Noninvasive assessment of pressure drop in mitral stenosis by Doppler ultrasound. Br. Heart J., 40:131–140, 1978.
78. Hatle, L. Noninvasive assessment and differentiation of left ventricular outflow obstruction by Doppler ultrasound. Circulation, 64:381–387, 1981.
79. Hatle, L., B.A. Angelsen, and A. Tromsdal. Noninvasive estimation of pulmonary artery systolic pressure with Doppler ultrasound. Br. Heart J., 45:157–165, 1981.
80. Hatle, L., B.A.J. Angelsen, and A. Tromsdal. Noninvasive assessment of atrioventricular pressure half-time by Doppler ultrasound. Circulation, 60:1096–1104, 1979.
81. Brandestini, M.A., M.K. Eyer, and J.G. Stevenson. M/Q-mode echocardiography: the synthesis of conventional echo with digital multigate Doppler. In: Echocardiology, edited by C.T. Lancee, The Hague, Martinus Nijhoff, 1979.
82. Stevenson, G., I. Kawabori, and M. Brandestini. Color-coded Doppler visualization of flow within ventricular septal defects: Implications for peak pulmonary artery pressure (Abstr.) Am. J. Cardiol., 49:944, 1982.
83. Bommer, W. and L. Miller. Real-time two-dimensional color flow Doppler: enhanced Doppler flow imaging in the diagnosis of cardiovascular disease (abstr.). Am. J. Cardiol., 49:944, 1982.
84. Kitabatake, A., M. Inoue, and M. Asao, et al. Non-invasive visualization of intracardiac blood flow in human heart using computer-aided pulsed Doppler technique. Clinical Hemorheology, 1:85, 1982.
85. Namekawa, K., C. Kasai, M. Tsukamoto, and A. Koyano. Realtime bloodflow imaging system utilizing auto-correlation techniques. Ultrasound Med. Biol., 8:Suppl 2203–208, 1982.
86. Omoto, R. Color atlas of real-time two-dimensional Doppler echocardiograpy. 1st Ed. Tokoyo, Shindan-to-Chiryo, 1984; 2nd Ed. 1987.

Chapter 3

Cardiopulmonary Bypass, Perfusion Of The Heart And Cardiac Metabolism

R. DEWALL AND R.J. BING

PERFUSION OF THE HEART AND CARDIAC METABOLISM

Perfusion systems of several different types are used in medicine and physiology: cardiopulmonary bypass; perfusion of isolated hearts (Langendorff and supported heart preparation); Perfusion of isolated organs (Carrel-Lindbergh System); and heart-lung preparation.

In cardiopulmonary bypass, the whole body with the exception of the heart and lung is perfused. In perfusion of the heart in vitro, the perfusion fluid either enters the aorta and coronary arteries by gravity (Langendorff Preparation) or is pumped into the left atrium; the left ventricle then ejects against a variable resistance (supported heart preparation). In perfusion of an isolated organ, a pumping system directs perfusion fluid into that organ, which is maintained in vitro. Pulsation rate and pressures are adjustable and sterility can be observed (e.g. Carrel-Lindbergh perfusion system). In the heart-lung preparation of Starling, the heart pumps blood through the lung for oxygenation, and the perfusate is returned to the heart.

The Langendorff Preparation was first described in 1885 (1). Langendorff himself devised several variations. In 1903, in the Munich Medical Journal, he defended the priority of his discovery against the American workers Martin, Applegarth, and Porter (2). "I feel obliged, even though it goes against my grain to fight for priorities, to defend my publications in the most decisive terms and to protest against giving credit to authors who neither deserve nor claim it." He gives credit to Martin who attempted to nourish the isolated mammalian heart through an isolated blood supply. But Martin, so says Langendorff, did not work with the completely isolated heart. Langendorff stated, "In Martin's case, coronary flow depended on activity of the left ventricle." He continued, "It is therefore not permissible, as it has happened, to write of the method of Martin *and* Langendorff, particularly since independent of Martin and without knowledge of his publications I was able to finally conclude my procedure (2)."

Major controversies toward the end of the 19th century and the early 20th concerned oxygen usage by the heart, the importance of glucose and lactic acid in cardiac metabolism, and particularly the role of inorganic material in the initiation and maintenance of cardiac rhythm. It was the time of Clark in Edinburgh (3), Loewi in Graz (4), Langendorff in Rostock (1), Lussana in Bologna (5), Howell in Baltimore (6), Ringer in London (7), Vernon in Oxford (8), Starling in London (9), Martin in Baltimore (10), Evans and Locke from London (11,12), Rohde from Heidelberg (13), and many others, all of them perfusing isolated hearts.

Perfusion of the heart was the only method for the study of cardiac metabolism in the 19th and the beginning of the 20th century. Tigerstedt summarized these studies in an admirable way in his "Physiology of Circulation (14)." The twelfth chapter in his book is titled "The chemical conditions for the beating heart." The first portions of this chapter are devoted to the perfusion and metabolism of the heart of cold-blooded animals. The remainder deals with the perfusion and metabolism of warm-blooded animals. Both sections review the subject thoroughly. Without perfusion of the isolated heart none of the early studies on cardiac metabolism would have been possible. Many of the findings on the isolated perfused organ, particularly on the utilization of food stuffs by the perfused heart, were later confirmed on the human heart in situ (15). Utilization of "fat" by the perfused frog heart is one example. On the occasion of Tigerstedt's 100th birthday, Liljestrand wrote an article summarizing his life and accomplishments (16). Tigerstedt served as professor of physiology at the Karolinska Institute in Stockholm and in the same capacity in Helsingfors, in his native Finland. Aside from his general interest in the circulation, Tigerstedt was particularly interested in the kidney. This led to the discovery of renin, arrived at by extracting kidney homogenates with saline and injecting the extract into rabbits. He determined that the resulting elevation in blood pressure was derived from the re-

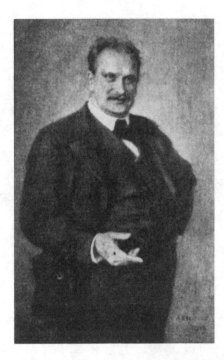

Figure 1.   Robert A. Tigerstedt (*Courtesy of The New York Academy of Medicine*)

nal cortex. Tigerstedt and Bergman pointed out that the newly discovered substance, which they called renin, may be active in producing cardiac hypertrophy in patients with renal disease. Tigerstedt's name should be prominently mentioned whenever the history of hypertension and cardiac metabolism is discussed (Figure 1).

The Carrel-Lindbergh System maintains an organ outside the body at any desired "pulse rate" and perfusion pressure (17). How did Charles A. Lindbergh, who was the first to fly over the Atlantic Ocean, become interested in a subject that appears to be far removed from his chosen field of aviation (Fig. 2)? Like many factors that redirect our lives, the occasion here was one that came about by chance. In 1929, Lindbergh's wife's oldest sister was found to have rheumatic heart disease. When an operation of the heart was ruled out by the physician because, "The heart could not be stopped long enough for surgeons to work on it," Lindbergh asked why a mechanical pump could not be substituted until the arrested heart could be repaired

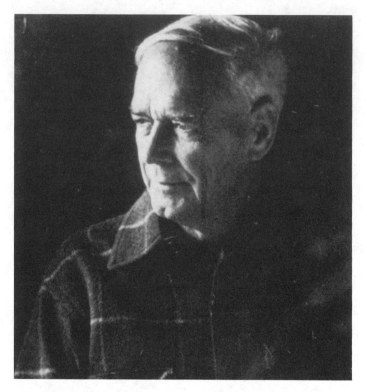

Figure 2.   Charles Lindbergh (*Collection of R.J. Bing*)

(18,19). Lindbergh therefore made up his mind to design a pump capable of circulating blood through the body while the heart was being repaired. This farsighted idea was discouraged by Alexis Carrel of the Rockefeller Institute who, well aware of the extreme difficulties of oxygenating the blood in such a system, believed that it was easier and more promising to design a pump for the "culture" of whole organs. Carrel, an ingenious surgeon, had previously worked on a new method of suturing blood vessels and on the culture of cells introduced by Ross Harrison. Carrel now was interested in extending his ideas to studying the interplay between perfusion fluid and organ in sterile perfusion experiments lasting days or weeks. By using artificial fluids, Carrel felt that he could examine individually and separately the influence of each constituent of the perfusate on the integrity and behavior of the isolated organ which was being perfused. Actually, this was a big step into the future, as the last thirty years have demonstrated. During my (RJB) years of cooperation with Lindbergh and Carrel, I never heard them refer to the original idea of Lindbergh—that of devising a pump for cardiopulmonary bypass. Lindbergh had been way ahead of his time!

Starling, a distinguished professor of physiology at University College, London, used the heart-lung preparation to study the relation between muscle fiber and length and strength of contraction—the basis of the subsequent Starling's law (9). Previous work by Otto Frank a well trained mathematician and physicist, also dealt with the relationship between length of muscle fibers and strength of contraction (20).

Frank used a small, simple yet elegant preparation of the whole frog heart, perfused with diluted ox blood. He was able to fill or empty the heart chambers and make continuous records throughout the cardiac cycle of pressures in various parts of the systems, volumes in the heart chamber (filling), and volume output. Frank wrote, "I discovered the following law concerning the dependence of the form of the isometric pressure curve on the initial tension: the peaks (maxima) of the isometric pressure curve rise with increasing initial length (filling). I call this part of the family of curves the first part. Beyond a certain level of filling, the pressure peaks decline (second part of the family of curves)." Starling expressed his final conclusion in a similar vein: "The law of the heart is therefore the same as that of skeleton muscle, namely that the mechanical energy set free on passage from the resting to the contracted states depends on the area of chemically active surface, i.e., on the length of the muscle fiber. This simple formula serves to explain the whole behavior of the isolated mammalian heart (9)." The law of the heart is now referred to as the Frank-Starling Law.

The heart-lung preparation represented a milestone in the development of our knowledge of cardiac metabolism. In a seminal paper in Recent Advances in Physiology of 1939, Evans wrote a chapter on the metabolism of cardiac muscle, in which he described the gaseous metabolism of heart muscle, oxygen usage of the mammalian heart, mechanical efficiency of the heart, the influence of diastolic volume on myocardial oxygen usage, influences of heart rate, and foremost, myocardial usage of foodstuffs for example, fat and carbohydrates (11). He also added a paragraph on the changes in cardiac metabolism during lack of oxygen. Most of the work described was done on the heart-lung preparation. Evans presented formulae on the mechanical efficiency of the heart and he demonstrated the influence of Starling's law of the heart on the oxygen utilization of the heart. He found a connection between diastolic volume and myocardial oxygen utilization. He predicted, from the low respiratory quotient of 0.7, that the heart uses "fat."

He determined that glucose utilization by the heart was a function of glucose concentration in the blood, and confirmed that the heart utilizes lactic acid.

These studies represented the basis for future work by Bing on metabolism of the human heart as carried out by coronary sinus catheterization, and still further gave impetus to other biochemical observations on the human heart (15).

CARDIOPULMONARY BYPASS

Many inspired contributors advanced the development of heart surgery and heart-lung bypass techniques. The work in both areas served to build the foundation of successful open-heart surgery that we know today.

Successful cardiopulmonary bypass became a reality in the early 1950's. While it seemed a new idea at the time, the foundations were in fact prepared over many preceding decades. The success of open-heart surgery required resolution of two primary problems: the first was developing the perfusion equipment and understanding how to use it; the second was integrating the knowledge of cardiac surgical problems with an understanding of cardiopulmonary bypass techniques. Unfortunately, in the early days of bypass surgery, difficulties were experienced initiating successful open-heart surgical programs (21-24). These continued to exist for two decades or more after the beginnings of open-heart surgery (25, 26).

Problems in the design of an effective cardiopulmonary bypass machine are manifold. Cardiopulmonary bypass is accomplished by means of a device, a heart-lung machine or pump-oxygenator. A heart-lung machine is used to support a patient's total blood circulatory system, freeing the body's need for its own heart and lung function. This permits the opening of the patient's heart for surgical repairs. Due to the anatomic relationship of heart to lungs, circulation must be diverted for surgical repair on the heart.

Two basic components comprise the heart-lung machine. The first is the pump (heart substitute) that serves to maintain the patient's circulation through the pump-oxygenator circuit. The second is the oxygenator (lung substitute) that adds oxygen and removes excess carbon dioxide from the blood. In the development of pump- oxygenator systems, providing a suitable blood pump was easily accomplished as serviceable pumps had been in existence for decades.

All oxygenators have a common theme: a respiratory gas mixture must be placed in close relationship to blood. The reaction time between hemoglobin and oxygen is less than one-hundredth of a second (27, 28). The limiting factor in the oxygenation of blood is the passage of the respiratory gas through the alveolar membrane (lung tissue), through the blood plasma, and through the red blood cell wall to reach the hemoglobin within the red blood cell.

For oxygenation, the blood must be delivered from a pool (the pulmonary artery in the human case) or from a reservoir or collecting chamber (artificial oxygenator) and spread in a thin film to minimize the distance through which the respiratory gasses must diffuse to reach the hemoglobin within the red blood cell. In the biologic sense, this is the thin film created by passage of blood through the pulmonary capillaries. In mechanical oxygenators, the blood must be distributed in a thin film. This filming is accomplished by pouring the blood to cover a large two-dimensional surface, such as spreading it over a screen, or casting it in a thin film over bubbles of a respiratory gas. More recent oxygenator innovations pass the blood through gas-permeable, tiny plastic tubes that mimic the normal lung.

Another necessary factor in oxygenator function is the respiratory gas to which the blood is exposed. The normal air we breathe is composed of approximately 78% nitrogen and 21% oxygen with the balance made up of lesser gasses. Water vapor (humidity) in the respiratory gas is of lesser importance for the oxygenating process. The thickness of the blood film and the length of time the blood film is exposed to the respiratory gas are other variables in the blood-oxygenation process. As hemoglobin absorbs oxygen, carbon dioxide is released.

The respiratory gas is generally exposed to the blood film at one atmosphere of pressure—760 mm Hg. at sea level. The oxygenation process depends upon the altitude at which the oxygenator is expected to function. For example, Denver's altitude of 5,000 feet affects the oxygenation process differently than altitudes at sea level. For example people may even experience high-altitude mountain sickness due to the low atmospheric pressure at higher altitudes (29). Conversely, if the respiratory gas and blood film were exposed to more than one atmosphere of pressure, the thickness of the blood film could be increased, and the time of exposure decreased. This would be similar to the effect upon an individual exposed to a hyperbaric situation, i.e. deep-sea scuba diving.

For the development of successful extracorporeal circulation, it was necessary to have a mechanism to keep the blood from clotting outside the body in a mechanical pump-oxygenator system. The essential component required was an anticoagulant the body would tolerate.

Anticoagulation

The success of extracorporeal circulation depends upon proper anticoagulation. In early studies (30, 31, 32), defibrination was the method used to prevent blood from clotting. In 1903, Brodie introduced hirudine, a leach extract, and sodium citrate as anticoagulants (33). None of the agents was suitable for cardiopulmonary-bypass activities in laboratory experiments seeking animal survival.

The discovery of heparin by Jay McLean was necessary to enable practical extracorporeal circulation (34). In 1915, McLean arrived at Johns Hopkins University as a second-year medical student. He immediately began working in the laboratory of William Henry Howell (35, 36) who was investigating which body tissues contained clot-promoting agents. McLean stated in his primary paper that he was assigned to "determine, if possible, whether the thromboplastic effect (of tissue extracts) may be attributed to an impurity, or as a property of cephalin itself" (34). In addition he wrote, "The cuorin (from ox heart) on the contrary when purified by repeated precipitation in alcohol at 60 degrees, has no thromboplastic effect, indeed it possesses an anticoagulating power." This was McLean's only reference to a natural anticoagulant that he incidentally observed while working on other substances. McLean did not use the name heparin for his newly discovered agent. After this primary effort in the study of blood clotting mechanisms, his attention was directed to other areas, and he left Howell's laboratory.

Howell and his associates continued work on the purification of the newly discovered anticoagulant and named the substance heparin since the extract was derived from the liver following McLean's departure (35,36). Commercial-, but not clinical-, grade heparin was first available in 1922 through the Baltimore firm of Hynson, Westcott, and Dunning (37).

In 1929, the development of heparin moved from Baltimore to the Toronto laboratories of Charles H. Best, of insulin fame (37). Best, working at the Connaught Laboratories, experienced difficulties with the clotting of glass cannulas. He persuaded two organic chemists, Arthur Charles and David Scott, to pursue the purification of heparin. Their work was published in 1936 (38), and purified heparin became available by 1937. It was from Toronto that John Gibbon was able to obtain a supply of heparin for his first successful experiments with a heart- lung machine that resulted in animal survival (39).

While the availability of heparin was necessary for the development of extracorporeal circulation, the practical applicability of heparin was enhanced by the observation in 1937 that protamine was a heparin antagonist (40). This discovery permitted a time-limited application of heparin, desirable for successful extracorporeal circulation.

During the 1930s, heparin purification was achieved in Denmark (41) and Sweden (42,43,44). Craafoord's familiarity with heparin in Sweden in 1937

(45) laid the foundation for Björk's successful perfusion experiments in 1948 (46).

Instrumentation

As early as 1812, Le Gallois wrote, "If one could at least substitute for the heart a kind of injection of arterial blood, either natural or artificially made, one would succeed easily in maintaining alive indefinitely, any part of the body whatsoever" (47). Dozens of systems for pumping and oxygenation of blood outside the body have been described since 1812.

John Gibbon's work ushered in the modern era of extracorporeal circulation that was made possible by the availability of heparin.

John Gibbon

John Gibbon, a fourth-generation physician, was born in 1903 (Fig. 3). He seriously considered dropping out of medical school after the first semester because he was unhappy with the heavy load of memorization that normally accompanies the first two years of medical school. Gibbon had developed an interest in poetry and had actually considered becoming a poet. As he writes,

> During my days at Princeton, I entertained the idea of becoming a poet. The courses I enjoyed most were advanced composition and two courses in 16th Century French—one poetry, the other prose. And I loved English poetry. But my father pointed out, like thousands of fathers before him, that poetry is a rather uncertain mode of livelihood. I was also smitten with painting, and to this day I put in considerable time in front of the easel. However, bowing to the goddess of necessity, I enrolled at Jefferson Medical College in Philadelphia, where my father was a professor of surgery. The first year in medical school was, frankly, boring as hell—all the needless memorization. But when I told my father that I liked (sic) to quit he replied that he did not care if I did not wind up practicing medicine, but that when a person starts something, he should finish it. I agreed to continue and after that things got interesting anyway (48).

Gibbon writes that his passion for research stems from his internship at Pennsylvania Hospital. At that time, he was comparing the effects of potassium chloride with those of sodium chloride in the diet of a hypertensive patient who did not know which kind of salt was being served him. Gibbon was supposed to keep track of the patient's blood pressure. "What the results were I cannot recall, but I do remember my excitement at realizing that such controlled experimentation could add to the store of human knowledge" (48, 49).

Gibbon served on the surgical service of Edward D. Churchill at the Massachusetts General Hospital, Harvard Medical School, from 1930 to 1931.

During 1931, Churchill operated upon a female patient to remove her gall-bladder. The operation seemed to go well, but several days later all the signs and symptoms of a pulmonary embolism developed. In 1931, the only possible cure for a pulmonary embolism was the Trendelenburg operation that involved rapidly opening the patient's chest, localizing the thrombus in the pulmonary artery, and incising the artery and removing the thrombus. Unfortunately, rapid was not fast enough, and the mortality rate of the Trendelenburg operation was forbidding. For these reasons, Churchill decided to wait until the patient appeared to be in the last stages of the disease before attempting to remove the embolus. Gibbon observed the patient's vital signs all night. After ten hours, her blood pressure began to decrease, and her condition became critical. Churchill was able to remove the embolus and clamp the incision in the pulmonary artery in six and one-half minutes, but the patient died (48, 49).

Assisting Churchill and waiting with the mortally ill patient during this stressful night, Gibbon began to think about some sort of device that might

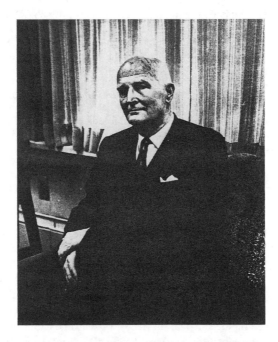

Figure 3.   John H. Gibbon, Jr. (*Courtesy of The New York Academy of Medicine*)

prevent a fatal outcome for those suffering pulmonary embolus. As he said later, "The thought occurred to me that the patient's life might be saved if some of the blue blood in her veins could be continuously withdrawn into an extracorporeal blood circuit, exposed to an atmosphere of oxygen and then returned to the patient by way of a systemic artery in the central direction" (48, 49). The same thought occurred to Lindbergh (17), but Gibbon was surgically trained and, therefore, better qualified for the difficult task of devising a treatment for pulmonary embolism.

Mary Hopkins, Gibbon's wife and a trained surgical technician aided his endeavor. Although Gibbon worked on various problems, he never abandoned the idea of developing a heart-lung bypass. He often mentioned his ideas to his surgical colleagues, but rarely met an enthusiastic response. He said, "Nobody encouraged me." When Gibbon approached the head of the department of Medicine at the Massachusetts General Hospital concerning his ideas of making a heart-lung bypass, he was strongly advised to spend his time on more promising projects if he wanted to succeed in academic medicine (49).

Churchill, while skeptical of Gibbon's ideas, agreed to grant him a year-long fellowship. He also provided him with a laboratory and money to hire a technician, who was Gibbon's wife. In 1934, Gibbon and his wife studied the possibility of building a heart-lung machine. As Gibbon writes, "So my wife and I, now with two children, returned to Boston in the autumn of 1934 to spend a year working on the first temporary artificial heart-lung blood circuit" (48).

At that time, Gibbon's research took some bizarre forms. He writes,

My wife and I experimented on ourselves and on friends. For instance, to find out how vasoconstriction and vasodilatation in the extremities could be caused by a slight shift in body temperature, we used to sit in the bathroom with thermal couplers attached to our toes and with our hands and forearms immersed in hot water. Also, and I know this sounds odd, my wife would stick a highly sensitive thermometer into my rectum, after which I would swallow a stomach tube. We then poured ice water down the tube and measured the effect of this on temperature. We also tried such things as injecting an ice-cold solution into a vein of my forearm (48).

After his year of research in Boston, Gibbon returned to Philadelphia where he noted that he learned a great deal about research techniques through his association with Eugene Landis. He writes, "It was this man (Landis) who gave me unwavering encouragement in what had by now become a principle ambition, to build an extracorporeal-blood circuit capable of temporarily taking over the cardiorespiratory functions" (49, 50).

Gibbon first used a Dale-Schuster finger-cot pump (51, 52). Gibbon added the internal valves that he had constructed from solid rubber stoppers. The blood oxygenator was the main problem. In systematic fashion, Gibbon read the literature and consulted engineers, but engineers dealt with fluids other than blood and did not consider the relationship of oxygen to hemoglobin. Blood foaming also became an obstacle. Blood foam cannot be returned to the systemic circulation and must be removed from the oxygenator. Gibbon decided to use cats as experimental animals since they were small and less expensive than dogs. The cats' size fitted the technical resources available at the time. Of all the oxygenator models tried, Gibbon decided that a revolving vertical cylinder with blood distributed over the interior surface by centrifugal force would be the most effective approach. Such a model was built after the method Hooker devised in 1915 (53). The problem with this system was hemolysis and the difficulty preserving a thin film of blood on the interior surface of the revolving cylinder.

Gibbon initially primed his pump with saline solution and gum acacia, the latter to give it more colloidal-osmotic pressure. In the beginning, the animals survived only for the immediate period following the procedure. By reducing the priming volume, the traumatic effect of extracorporeal circulation on the blood, such as hemolysis, was reduced.

Later, the finger-cot pump was replaced by a roller pump and primed with donor cat blood. Using this approach, Gibbon was able to occlude the pulmonary artery of cats for at least ten minutes, followed by survival of the cats for several hours.

Issekutz introduced the roller pump in 1927 (54), and DeBakey modified it in 1934 (55). A roller pump uses a flexible hollow conduit placed within a rigid circular channel. The ingress and egress of the conduit are connected by long tubes to conduct fluids from patient to pump-oxygenator and back. The conduit is stroked within its channel by a roller attached to the end of a bar. The end of the bar opposite the roller is attached to a motorized axle located at the center of the circle defined by the arc of the channel. The bar is driven in one direction with the roller adjusted to nearly occlude the flexible conduit forcing fluid through the conduit. The roller bar's speed of rotation governs the fluid's rate of flow. The roller- pump principle served as the major pumping mechanism for heart-lung machines during the first several decades of open-heart surgery.

Gibbon's work on the heart-lung machine was interrupted by four years of Army service beginning in 1942. In 1946, he returned to Philadelphia as professor of surgery and Head of Surgical Research at the Jefferson Medical College (48, 49). An important development occurred. Executives of International Business Machines (IBM) offered to help modify his pre-war apparatus. Both IBM and Gibbon agreed that neither party would profit commercially from the arrangement. The engineers from IBM transformed Gibbon's pre-war apparatus into an elaborate machine that was completed in 1949. The new instrumentation permitted the use of dogs which introduced other problems, particulate embolization that necessitated use of a filter placed between the arterial pump of the extra-corporeal circuit and the arterial cannula of the recipient dog.

The first clinical use of the Gibbon heart-lung machine occurred in April of 1952. Unfortunately, this patient was misdiagnosed (as atrial septal defect, not found at the operation), and the baby died soon after. An autopsy revealed that the child had a patent ductus arteriosus. Success was achieved on May 6, 1953 when the second intracardiac prodecure using a heart-lung machine was accomplished. This time an atrial septal defect was found and successfully repaired. The procedure progressed without complications (48). This was the first successful surgical correction of an intracardiac defect using a heart-lung machine, and marked the beginning of a new era in cardiac surgery.

Gibbon's records show that the patient was connected to the heart-lung apparatus for a total of 45 minutes. For 27 of those minutes, her cardiorespiratory functions were maintained by the machine alone. With the patient's atrium opened, Gibbon closed the defect using a continuous silk suture. Cecilia, the patient, recovered uneventfully. Later, cardiac catherization showed the defect had been completely closed.

The publicity surrounding that operation disturbed the patient at first; later she shed her shyness and in 1963 made appearances as the American Heart Association's National Queen. Gibbon writes, "For me the experience was emotionally draining. In fact, I think that operation was the only time in my career that I did not personally dictate or write the operative procedure. I guess the tension of the event was too much to relive immediately afterwards" (48).

Gibbon attempted intracardiac surgical repair of congenital heart defects in two children, but the results were not encouraging. He continued experimental work on dogs for several years. His article on the repair of an atrial septal defect was published in 1954 (56); it was the last paper from Gibbon's research laboratory.

The Swedish Influence

Efforts to purify heparin took place in Denmark (41) and Sweden (42, 43, 44) simultaneously with the developments in Toronto. Crafoord, from the

Karolinska Institutet in Stockholm wrote in 1936 of his experience with the clinical use of heparin as a post-operative treatment for the prevention of thrombosis (45). Crafoord influenced the work of Björk (46) at the Karolinska who, in 1948, published his work involving a rotating-disc oxygenator that resulted in successful animal perfusion.

The rotating-disc oxygenator, as described by Björk, was formed of many metallic discs, separated by thin spacers and mounted on a centrally located axle. The disc assembly, contained in a horizontal glass cylinder, rotated on its central axis in a pool of venous blood several centimeters deep. A thin film of blood collected on each rotating disc and was elevated into a respiratory gas mixture. Venous blood was pumped into one end of the rotating-disc oxygenator. The thin film of blood on each rotating disc absorbed oxygen as it released its excess carbon dioxide. Becoming oxygenated as it flowed through the oxygenator reservoir, the blood was then pumped out the opposite end as arterialized blood.

Melrose developed some variations in the geometry of the Björk system, reporting them in 1953 (57).

Fredrick Cross, who received his surgical education at the University of Minnesota in Owen Wangensteen's department, adapted the Björk rotating-disc oxygenator concept (58), improving its design and efficiency to accomplish important clinical success. The Cross concept achieved acceptance in many of the world's open-heart surgical centers. Cross's adaptation employed 60-120 plastic-coated, stainless-steel discs, 12 centimeters in diameter. Flow rates could be increased or decreased, depending upon the number of discs used; likewise, the rotational speed of the discs could be altered. There was a practical limit to the rotational speed used, as foaming could develop at higher rates of speed. The Cross system had three basic advantages: it worked well, it was simple to use, and it was relatively inexpensive. The disadvantages included being labor intensive and requiring a large priming volume. The rotating-discs systems were constructed of a great many parts, and all blood proteins had to be cleaned after each use; then the system needed reassembly. This preparation was burdensome.

A variation of the disc-filming technique was developed and used by Crafoord in 1957 (59). It consisted of six cylinders rotating in a basin of venous blood while being exposed to a respiratory gas. At higher flow rates this system was inefficient, and, as a consequence, incorporated a bubbling device on the venous inlet as a preoxygenator. The Crafoord cylinder system achieved some regional popularity (in Europe). It had the same advantages and disadvantages as the Cross disc oxygenator.

University of Minnesota Contributions

The pacesetting and driving spirit for the development of open- heart surgery occurred at Minneapolis and Rochester, Minnesota, following World War II, due to the cooperation of gifted men. First of all, Owen H. Wangensteen headed the Department of Surgery at the University from 1930 to 1967. Wangensteen was characterized by Lillehei as follows:

> Wangensteen was a truly visionary surgeon. His lifelong recognition of the relevance of basic science, and the insight to be derived from research in the training of young surgeons created the milieu and opportunities for great achievements by many of his pupils. Proverbial was Dr. Wangensteen's ability to spot talent and capabilities in his younger men whose aptitudes were not all obvious to others, often not even themselves, and then he would proceed to develop those assets by blending his material assistance with intellectual stimulation and encouragement (60).

Maurice Visscher, a renowned cardiovascular physiologist, was also on the faculty of the University serving as chairman of the Department of Physiology from 1936 to 1968. Working together, these two educators were great inspirational leaders for several decades (61).

During the late 1940s, Clarence Dennis at the University of Minnesota became interested in the development of cardiopulmonary bypass. His expertise was in both physiology and surgery. Dennis continued pump-oxygenator studies at the Downstate Medical Center of the State University of New York where he was Chairman of Surgery. While still in Minnesota, Dennis tried various ideas on oxygenators and ultimately developed a filming system in which venous blood was delivered to the center of multiple, 50 cm. diameter rotating circular screens (62, 63). The Dennis screen oxygenator was used as cardiopulmonary support during the repair of a child's atrial septal defect on April 5, 1951 (64). Unfortunately, due to technical considerations, the patient died. Later, Dennis and his group concluded that air embolization was a major problem. Perfusion rates approximating normal cardiac output were used by Dennis (65).

On September 2, 1952, at the University of Minnesota Hospital, F. John Lewis became the first person to close an intracardiac defect under direct vision using inflow stasis and moderate hypothermia (66) without circulatory support. Lewis and Bigelow's work (67) described much of the physiology of hypothermia that would later be used with hypothermic perfusions.

Azygos Flow Principle

Until the early 1950s, concepts of extracorporeal circulation did not include using perfusion rates less than a normal cardiac output. This development of oxygenators was required to process a greater quantity of blood than would be necessary if significantly lower flow rates would suffice.

In a new discovery, Andreason and Watson in 1952 published their work describing the ability of dogs to withstand 30 minutes of complete vena-caval occlusion, provided the flow through the azygos vein into the heart was maintained (68). They determined that an animal could survive without noticeable harm for short periods of time with a total blood flow to its body considerably reduced from its resting cardiac output. Until these experiments were reported, it was generally considered that a resting cardiac output (90-150 ml/Kg/Min.) must be supplied to an animal for successful total cardiopulmonary bypass.

Andreason and Watson described cross-circulation experiments in 1953, one year after their description of the azygos-flow principle (69). Cross-circulation experiments made use of a donor animal as an oxygenator. Arterial blood was pumped from the donor animal to a recipient animal while the recipient had the blood supply bypassed to its heart and lungs. Venous blood was returned from the recipient animal in amounts equal to the arterial blood taken from the donor. The results of Andreason and Watson's cross-circulation experiments were unpredictable, probably because the blood exchange between the two animals was not well controlled.

Cohen, in 1952, independently of Andreason and Watson, also demonstrated the validity of the azygos flow concept in 1952 while working in C. Walton Lillehei's laboratory (70). Cohen further proceeded to quantify this flow as 8-14 ml/Kg body weight/min. With this information, Cohen was able to show that an animal would survive without noticeable harm for thirty minutes at normothernic conditions with a blood supply of only 10% of normal cardiac output (71). The realization that a dramatically reduced flow of blood to a patient was sufficient furnished the key Lillehei and his associates needed to open the age of repeatable, successful open-heart surgery.

Controlled Cross Circulation

In 1897, Theodor Billroth noted that the limits of surgery stopped at the walls of the heart since it would never be possible to perform surgery on such a vital organ (72). Billroth's admonition seemed to hold true into the early 1950s. Progress towards successful open-heart surgery appeared stalled due to a number of unsuccessful attempts with the perfusion systems available at that time. A feeling prevailed that a sick human heart would never tolerate surgical intervention with the necessary cutting and sewing required to the heart muscle (73).

Lillehei distanced himself from these gloomy prospects by pursuing new ideas to overcome the obstacles. Years later, John Kirklin of the Mayo Clinic characterized Lillehei as "one of the most talented cardiac surgeons ever to work in this field" (73). In the same forum, Denton Cooley of the Texas Heart Institute observed Lillehei as "a talented investigator and pioneer surgeon who provided the can opener for the largest picnic thoracic surgeons will ever know" (73). Lillehei thoroughly earned these and many more accolades that came to him over the years (see Chapter 10, Valvular Surgery, Fig. 7).

With the new awareness that successful cardiopulmonary bypass aided open-heart surgery and was possible with reduced perfusion rates, C. W. Lillehei and two surgical fellows, Morley Cohen and Herbert Warden, envisioned a solution to the problems of extracorporeal circulation. A small portion of a donor animal's arterial blood supply could be withdrawn through a precisely regulated pump. This blood was perfused (pumped) to a smaller animal while simultaneously returning from the smaller animal an equal amount. Open-heart surgery could then be accomplished on the smaller animal while its blood flow and metabolic needs were supplied by the larger animal. After dozens of successful laboratory experiments, controlled cross circulation was deemed safe for clinical application (74, 75, 76). The key to its success was the precise regulation of blood exchange between the donor and recipient animal through well-calibrated pumps (Fig. 4).

Clinical application of controlled cross circulation raised some ethical problems, uppermost being the donor risks. These risks included: potential problems of a general anesthetic, mixing blood from two individuals in spite of its being well matched, and the possibility of a pumping mishap. Against these donor risks, the alternative was the inevitable early death of the patient if left untreated. Before proceeding with the clinical application, all of these considerations were reviewed with Dr. Wangensteen and other members of the surgical department. Also of great importance to the project was the approval and participation of the pediatric cardiology department, particularly Paul Adams and Raymond Anderson (77).

In 1954, with all concerned parties in concurrence, the first successful correction of a ventricular septal defect was accomplished on March 26, 1954. Over the next 16 months 45 patients had surgical corrections of congenital heart defects with the aid of controlled cross circulation. One non-fatal donor complication was followed by complete recovery (73).

Successful open-heart surgery by Lillehei and his associates immediately attracted world attention that stimulated renewed interest in the use of extracorporeal circulation at the world's major heart centers.

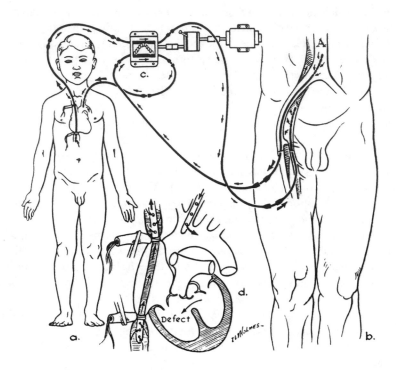

Figure 4. Cross circulation arrangement used by C. Walton Lillehei. (*Courtesy of the Journal of the American Medical Association 75:928–945, copyright 1957*)

In 1955, a year following his initial success, Lillehei presented a paper on the first total repair of tetralogy of Fallot defects (78). Alfred Blalock in a discussion of this paper said,

> I must say that I never thought I would live to see the day when this type of operative procedure could be performed. It is my guess that the ultimate answer will be the artificial heart-lung as developed by our president, Dr. Gibbon, and as it is being used now by more and more people. Dr. Gibbon has used it successfully for intracardiac surgery. I have heard that Dr. Kirklin of the Mayo Clinic, has now used it successfully in closing several ventricular septal defects (78).

Clarence Dennis and his associates' interest in extracorporeal circulation filtered down to the medical students on the surgical services at the University of Minnesota. Richard DeWall was among these students. Finishing medical school in 1952, DeWall spent a year of internship in the United States Public Health Service in New York before returning to general practice in Minnesota.

DeWall was interested in laboratory medicine and expressed this interest to Richard Varco, the head of heart surgery at the University under Wangensteen. Varco offered DeWall an opportunity to work in C. W. Lillehei's laboratory where Lillehei and his personnel were in the midst of experiments with Controlled Cross Circulation. DeWall was hired as an animal attendant and began work in Lillehei's laboratory on March 1, 1954, the month of the first clinical Controlled Cross Circulation operations. DeWall had the benefit of Wangensteen's educational philosophy of giving young aspirants the chance to prove themselves.

The controlled cross circulation experiments on dogs served as an excellent learning experience in perfusion physiology. DeWall gained significant experience in laboratory methods and perfusion physiology due to Lillehei, Cohen, and Warden's shared knowledge. DeWall served as the perfusionist for most of the clinical Controlled Cross Circulation operations. The donor for the operations provided an excellent physiologic oxygenator as well as continuously maintaining metabolic and blood homeostasis of both donor and patient. From the beginning, Lillehei had recognized the obvious disadvantages of using donors, namely donor risk and size limitation of the patient. Thus, during the early course of cross-circulation clinical activities, Lillehei asked DeWall if he would be interested in directing his efforts toward the development of an oxygenator system to replace the donor. In early 1954, no generally recognized oxygenator existed. DeWall accepted the challenge.

Bubble Oxygenators

Clark and associates' work (79) in 1950 marked the opening of the modern era of the bubble oxygenator. In their system, venous blood was bubbled by oxygen introduced through a microporous glass filter that produced pin-head sized bubbles. Clark introduced silicone defoaming agents to bubble-oxygenator design. The silicone agents removed excess bubbles from the blood and coated surfaces the blood might contact. Silicone-coated surfaces were gentler to blood than glass or metal surfaces. The Clark system was tested clinically by Hellmsworth (80, 81) with disappointing clinical results, possibly due to air embolism. Other bubble systems described at this time did not advance the application of perfusion systems. Bubble systems for extracorporeal oxygenation remained suspect.

DeWall decided to pursue concepts not previously studied in oxygenator systems. Since a hyperbaric approach had not been investigated, this seemed a logical course to follow. For materials, Lillehei suggested that DeWall explore the use of a large-bore polyvinyl hose. The hose was inexpensive, used in the food processing industry, and readily available. Polyvinyl proved to be more compatible to blood than metal or glass containers. DeWall's hyperbaric concept involved exposing a thick film of venous blood to three atmospheres of oxygen pressure. He anticipated that a thick blood film would be easier to manage than spreading a thin layer over a large area. The arterial venous oxygen difference is six volumes percent (82). Six volumes percent of oxygen could be transferred to blood plasma in the absence of hemoglobin; at three atmospheres pressure, it would supply the total oxygen requirement to oxygenate normal venous blood without elaborate filming or bubbling techniques.

The hyperbaric apparatus used a four foot polyvinyl hose. Venous blood streamed down the hose placed in a helical coil on its vertical axis. The lower quarter of the tube, filled with blood, served as a reservoir. Half-way down the hose, an oxygen inlet put oxygen into the system under three atmospheres pressure. At the top of the helix, a valve regulated pressure within the tube. Exposed to the high oxygen pressure, blood flowing down the tube became arterialized and accumulated in the reservoir. However, bubbles developed in the reservoir blood and in the blood after decompression. It was then observed that bubbles remaining in the reservoir of the helix would layer on top of the oxygenated blood, becoming trapped, and would not be evacuated with the arterialized blood.

Previous oxygenator literature indicated problems with bubble or foam formation. Using these observations, DeWall decided to accept bubbles and learn how to master them. In reviewing methods for the oxygenation of blood, the direct introduction of oxygen into the venous blood seemed the simplest and most economical approach to blood oxygenation. It also appeared that if the bubbles were kept large, there would still be sufficient blood gas interface for the exchange of oxygen and carbon dioxide; yet the coalescence and removal of the bubbles could be simplified.

Clark's bubble oxygenator used a microporous glass filter for oxygen dispersion causing the formation of bubbles, one mm or less in size, that were difficult to remove from the arterialized blood. Such small bubbles also did not adequately transfer the excess carbon dioxide from the blood into the respiratory gas mixture for elimination from the system (79). DeWall chose to make a gas-dispersion system forming large bubbles, 5 to 10 mm in diameter. This was accomplished by means of multiple size 22 hypodermic needles inserted through a rubber stopper and placed at the bottom of a 1.5 inch diameter polyvinyl hose. The length of the tube carrying the bubble mixture was altered depending upon the time desired for the blood-oxygen contact and the expected perfusion rate. Venous blood was introduced over the top of the oxygen-dispersion needles. With these variables, the size of the oxygenator could be changed depending upon the patient's size and optimize the amount of blood necessary for priming the system.

Silicone, as described by Clark (79), was used to coat the top of the bubble chamber. The blood's contact with the silicone-coated surfaces served to coalesce the flowing bubble mass, but it did not eliminate all of the smallest bubbles. The blood was arterialized by the bubble contact and after the bubbles were eliminated, the arterialized blood was introduced from the oxygenation hose into the top of a vertically positioned coiled (helix) hose, 1 inch in diameter and 150-250 inches long. The hose length varied with individual patient needs. About this time, Norman Shumway, working with F. J. Lewis at the University of Minnesota, confirmed that larger bubbles dispersed more easily than small, foam-sized bubbles (83).

A safe blood debubbling system evolved using information from DeWall's hyperbaric-oxygenator experiments which demonstrated that bubbles could be removed from a bubble blood mixture by being trapped in a helically coiled hose. It was apparent that blood containing bubbles had a lesser density than blood free of bubbles. Blood containing bubbles from a blood, respiratory-gas mixing chamber, as described above, flowed into the top of a coiled-hose helix 18 inches high filled with blood. This blood was continuously removed from the bottom end of the hose through a blood filter and returned to the patient. As the mixed blood progressed down the tube, lighter bubbled blood layered above normal blood becoming trapped against the upper wall of the hose, allowing heavier bubble-free blood to slide beneath. Hydrostatic pressure increased as the blood passed down the tube. The bubbles in bubble-containing blood coalesce under increasing hydrostatic pressure as the blood flows down the tube. The coalesced bubbles release their excess oxygen and carbon dioxide that pass up and out of the tube.

DeWall with the encouragement, support, and input of Lillehei, had the helical-reservoir blood oxygenator ready for use in open-heart surgery by Lillehei and his team within nine months after starting the project (84, 85).

The simple, disposable helical-resevoir oxygenator was first used May 13, 1955 (85,86) on a small child with a ventricular septal defect. Dr. Lillehei was the operating surgeon. The appeal of the helical-reservoir system was that it was efficient, heat sterilized, easy to assemble, inexpensive, disposable after a one-time use, and had no moving parts. The system fulfilled its purpose when used by knowledgeable surgeons.

A number of surgical groups were unsuccessful at that time using the helical-reservoir system (as well as other systems) and in the process, condemned it (22, 23, 24). Their lack of success could be attributed to two factors, first, success in the early days of open-heart surgery required the union of two disciplines, understanding of perfusion physiology and competence with the perfusion equipment, and surgical acumen was needed in the new surgical specialty of open-heart surgery. As the helical- reservoir oxygenator appeared to be a jerry-built apparatus, some observers thought they could improve upon it without understanding the principles involved. They were unwilling to spend the time and effort in research laboratories and teaching clinics to learn their craft.

The helical-reservoir pump oxygenator system came into wide use in the United States and abroad (87, 88, 89, 90). The pump used with the helical-reservoir system was a finger-cam pump (Sigmamoter Inc. Middleport, NY) readily available at the time as a laboratory pump for fluids. This was also the pump used for all controlled cross-circulation circulation experiments and clinical cases. The principle of this pump was that a flexible conduit was placed between a compression plate and serially compressed by metal fingers. Each finger's base was adapted to a cam shaft, activating each finger a few degrees out of phase with the preceding finger. In this manner, fluid (blood) was pushed in one direction.

The inexpensive, disposable helical-reservoir, bubble-oxygenator system soon evolved into commercially available units constructed with polyvinyl sheet material (91). Thorough animal laboratory work tested the commercial design and animal safety preceded the approval for this oxygenator's manufacture for clinical application. The commercial oxygenators had one especially important characteristic. They were constructed using set measurements that eliminated the tendency for inquiring yet often unprepared minds to tinker with design.

The Rygg-Kyvsgaard oxygenator system (92), similar in many respects to the plastic-sheet oxygenator (91), became popular towards the end of the 1950's, especially in Europe. In the early 1960s, a disposable rigid-bubble oxygenator made of polycarbonate (92,93) became available. Several manufacturers provided such rigid, simple systems that replaced the use of filming oxygenators. Bubble oxygenator systems remained in general use until the introduction of membrane oxygenators in the early 1980s.

Three comprehensive books were published in the years 1960, 1962, and 1981, reflecting the status of extracorporeal circulation, its related physiology, and equipment (22, 94, 95).

Mayo Clinic Contributions

In 1948, John Kirklin developed his interest in congenital heart disease while working with children at the Boston Children's Hospital, during a six-month tutelage, following his surgical residency at the Mayo Clinic.

Upon returning to the Mayo Clinic from Boston, Kirklin mentioned that his renewed interest in intracardiac surgery had been stimulated by an operation on a patient with pulmonary valvular stenosis. The autopsy on the patient who died two days later revealed that the patient suffered from a severe secondary subvalvular obstruction that thwarted the attempt to relieve the right ventricular obstruction by a closed valvotomy. Kirklin studied the autopsy specimen with Jesse Edwards, a cardiac pathologist, and Earl Wood, a cardiac physiologist, and concluded that an open technique would have been necessary for successful surgery (96).

Kirklin and his associates decided to develop an extracorporeal-circulatory system of the Gibbon-IBM type (97). After two and one-half years of intensive work in Mayo's engineering shops and animal laboratories, a Mayo-Gibbon pump-oxygenator was produced (98, 99). At the Mayo Clinic on March 22, 1955, one year after Lillehei's success in Minneapolis with controlled cross circulation, John Kirklin successfully repaired a child's ventricular septal using the Mayo-Gibbon heart-lung machine (100).

Kirklin developed a thorough knowledge of the pathophysiology and surgical problems represented by congenital heart disease. This, combined with diligent effort in the research laboratories in perfecting their heart-lung machine, enabled him and his team to be masters of open-heart surgery early on. Kirklin effectively coordinated two new and difficult disciplines. as Lillehei had done. Following his first success, Kirklin soon operated upon seven other patients, promptly reporting these cases (96, 100). This clinical success immediately attracted worldwide attention.

The Mayo-Gibbon pump-oxygenator was costly to produce and expensive to maintain and clean. Consequently, it never achieved widespread usage once the simple, inexpensive, and disposable systems became available in the late 1950s.

For the first two years of open-heart surgery, only two centers in the world performed these operations: The University of Minnesota, Minneapolis, and the Mayo Clinic in Rochester; the fact that the two cities were only ninety miles apart made it convenient for heart surgeons from all over the world to visit both places on the same trip. At the University of Minnesota, they saw what appeared to be simple techniques, using a primitive-appearing apparatus. Although appealing, due to affordability and seemingly easy duplication, was it too simple? Could it be trusted? At the Mayo Clinic, they saw a beautifully engineered and sophisticated Mayo-Gibbon machine with its gleaming, stainless-steel appearance, but it was very costly. This presented a real dilemma for most visitors.

Membrane Oxygenators

Original concepts usually undergo refinements and continuous improvement. Such was the case with pump-oxygenator systems. The first successful oxygenators had employed a direct exposure of a respiratory gas to blood filmed over discs, screens, or bubbles. If an ideal oxygenator had been possible, it would have separated the blood from the respiratory gas by means of a membrane. Efficient and well understood gas-permeable membranes were not available during most of the 1950s The belief that blood-membrane-gas interface creates less blood trauma than direct blood-gas interface rationalized the pursuit of a membrane oxygenator.

Clowes experienced difficulties with bubble oxygenators (21); consequently, he directed his attention from 1955 to 1960 to the development of a membrane oxygenator system. The gas permeability of a number of membranes was one of his studies that he reported in 1960.(94) Galletti expanded this list of potentially suitable membranes (22). Clowes developed a parallel-plate oxygenator using two membranes, polyethylene and ethylcellulose. The parallel-plate concept involved layering multiple sheets of membrane, 0.5 sq. meters in size, that were supported and sealed at the edges by a frame. Venous blood and respiratory gas were directed into alternate layers of the membrane plates and removed from the opposite end. The oxygenator was positioned on its horizontal axis. The Clowes membrane oxygenator worked clinically (94), but it was cumbersome to manage and difficult to assemble. It could not compete with the simplicity of filmers and bubblers. Clowes's work helped lay the foundation for future membrane-oxygenator development.

Bramson initiated the next stage in membrane oxygenation in 1965, summarizing his work in 1981 (95). The Bramson membrane oxygenator used a reinforced silicone rubber membrane that was more efficient than the membranes available to Clowes. The Bramson oxygenator was a parallel-plate design in a circular, rather than rectangular shape and accessed by a complicated manifold introduced into its core. The membranes however were disposable in this system and the apparatus required arduous hand assembly.

By 1980, the stage was set and the time right for an efficient, commercially produced membrane oxygenator. Such systems could provide circulatory support for days at a time. Filmers and bubblers had been unable to do this because of their destructive impact on blood when used over long periods of time.

Three configurations evolved. One geometry employed the use of hollow fibers or tiny tubes as small as 200 microns in diameter, grouped in parallel. Venous blood was directed through the tubes with the respiratory gas outside. DeWall described such an oxygenator in 1958 (101), but, this work predated the availability of materials and technology for commercial development. In the 1980s, systems built to the hollow-fiber configuration became available. A second-type membrane oxygenator, made available in the 1980s, was a parallel-plate oxygenator with the plates folded as an accordion bellows. The third design took the form of a large sheet of reinforced silicone rubber. The sheet was rolled into a spiral with separate pathways for the venous blood and respiratory gas, as described by Kolobow (102). Membrane-oxygenator history and performance are found in several books relating to extracorporeal circulation (22, 94, 95, 103).

Membrane oxygenators are now used in most perfusions in the United States. A partial list of membrane-oxygenator manufacturers includes: Bentley, Bos-CM40 Capillary Membrane Oxygenator, American Bentley-American Hospital Supply; Cobe Membrane Lung (CML EXCEL) Cobe Labs, Lakewood, CO (Parallel Plate, folded membrane); and Sci-Med Spiral Membrane Oxygenator, Minneapolis, MN. One can expect technology and perfusion equipment to be refined and further developed in the future.

Hemodilution

Extracorporeal circulation implies blood circulation by means of an apparatus outside the body. To begin circulation, the apparatus must be primed, or filled with a fluid. In the early days of open-heart surgery, surgeons only considered blood as the priming fluid. Due to preservatives used, stored blood was highly acidic; it also lost its ability to clot. Because of this, fresh blood, drawn the day of surgery and preserved in a non- acidic heparin mixture, was the standard priming fluid of the times. Blood volumes required for priming was up to 1,800 cc for bubble oxygenators and 3,000 for film oxygenators (22).

In addition, surgical blood loss had to be replaced. The blood-banking system became severely strained. Early in the morning prior to surgery, blood types between donors and patients had to be matched. Using many different blood sources increased the risk of hepatitis. Logistic problems limited the number of patients that could be accommodated for surgery. By the late 1950s, the introduction of low-prime, commercially available bubble-oxygenator systems (91,92,93, and others) began to replace the filming systems.

In 1961, Foote, Trede, and Maloney recommended the use of standard ACD (acid-citrate-dextrose) preserved-bank blood as acceptable for priming an extracorporeal circuit (104). They showed that the natural body-blood buffer system compensated for the acid state of the bank blood. The use of ordinary, stored bank blood as a prime for perfusion systems eased procurement problems; however, surgeons continued to search for alternative priming solutions.

Hemodilution is the dilution of blood with non-blood agents. Cooley (105, 106), Zuhdi (107), and Greer (108) introduced a major movement using hemodilution techniques for priming an extracorporeal circuit. Cooley's discovery of hemodilution resulted from emergency surgery on a patient with a pulmonary embolism. Since there was insufficient time to obtain blood for a prime, he used 5% dextrose and water in place of a blood prime. The patient did well in spite of a significant dilution of blood. These surgeons noted the patient's exceptional recovery following perfusions using a hemodilution prime.

The patient's hematocrit was reduced from the normal value of 40% to 20-25% following a perfusion using hemodilution prime. Because of hemodilution, the patient's urinary output during the operation was excellent. With such good urinary output during the perfusion, circulating blood volume dropped. To compensate for this drop, an additional amount of diluting solution was returned to the oxygenator system, to equal the urinary loss. When the procedure ended, the pump-oxygenator contents were returned to the patient, as needed.

Surgeons continued to investigate a variety of priming solutions (109, 110). They hoped to find a perfusate more physiologic than 5% dextrose and water. Some tried adding blood plasma and albumin thinking their greater osmotic pressure would be advantageous. These agents, however, were expensive and still carried the hepatitis risk. Many groups added a variety of electrolytes and buffers to priming solutions. The hope was to offset the hyponatremia caused by the non-electrolyte containing 5% dextrose in water. Today, balanced-electrolyte solutions, commercially prepared, serve as priming agents.

Hemodilution techniques, combined with improved perfusion equipment, have reduced blood needs for the average open-heart surgical case by over fifty percent. In some circumstances, open-heart surgical procedures can be accomplished totally without using blood.

Hypothermia

Decreasing a patient's temperature (hypothermia) is an important adjunct to open-heart surgery. A body's metabolic rate increases or decreases with temperature, as does the rate of all chemical rections. A person with a normal body temperature can tolerate about four minutes of complete circulatory arrest without experiencing cerebral damage. As the body temperature decreases, the brain can tolerate longer periods of time without blood flow.

In 1950, Bigelow (67) wrote of his experiments using moderate hypothermia in dogs. This work studied the animals' physiologic responses to a body temperature drop of eight to ten degrees Farenheit. Bigelow accomplished this by wrapping the subject in temperature-controlling blankets that could cool or warm. The experiments' purpose was to develop techniques permitting surgery inside a dog's heart for up to eight minutes with temporary inflow occlusion and circulatory arrest. Inflow occlusion involved the blockage of blood flow to the heart. No extracorporeal circulatory support was used.

Lewis (66) also studied the effects of moderate hypothermia and applied it clinically, becoming the first man to repair a defect inside the heart under direct vision. This occurred on September 2, 1952 when he repaired an atrial septal defect in a five-year-old child.

Unfortunately, the repair of some intracardiac defects requires more than eight minutes, and some defects can only be approached by an incision through the ventricle. The heart can tolerate an incision through the atrium at temperatures of moderate hypothermia without disturbing heart function. However, at such temperatures, the ventricle becomes irritable from an incision and fibrillates, or loses an effective beat. Operating at moderate hypothermic temperatures requires that the patient maintain a regular heart beat even if slower than normal. The cold, fibrillating heart is difficult to restart, compromising the patient's recovery. These factors limited the usefulness of moderate hypothermia for open-heart surgery. Without an extracorporeal-circulation method to rewarm the patient, trans-ventricular surgery is hazardous.

During the earliest open-heart operations, attempts were made to maintain body temperatures at normo-thermic levels by placing the patient on heated blankets. Cool operating rooms and large surfaces of the exposed open chests created significant heat loss, and, as a consequence, heating elements were incorporated into extracorporeal circulatory circuits. Adverse metabolic changes in the patient that came as a result of increasingly long and difficult operations became apparent. The lessons of moderate hypothermia, which reduced metabolic demands and resulted from lowered body temperatures, led to the introduction of combined blood cooling and warming systems to extracorporeal blood-circulation circuits. This occurred by the late 1950's and has since been incorporated into all extracorporeal-blood circuits.

Metabolic Homeostasis

General anesthesia compromises a patient's metabolic normalcy. Extracorporeal circulation contributes to this compromise and interferes with normal cardio-vascular reflexes. A patient's survival depends upon maintaining a normal metabolic balance; therefore, an extracorporeal circulation system must be monitored for the patient's metabolic responses during perfusion. In the early years of perfusion-supported surgery, blood samples were removed from the circuit for periodic checks of the patient's metabolic and blood responses. Blood content was checked for hematocrit, oxygen content, acid-base balance, and electrolyte values. Additional constituents of the blood were also occasionally tested.

Anesthesia, hypothermia, extracorporeal circulation, and duration of the surgery can cause many rapid changes in the important metabolic factors in the blood, making intermittent spot checks inadequate. From the beginning of open-heart surgery, efforts have been directed toward the development of rapid monitoring systems of metabolic balance. Many systems, now incorporated directly in the extracorporeal-blood circuit, provide continuous data for the patient's safety.

Advances in the treatment of heart disease during the last 20 years would not have been posible without the cardiopulmonary bypass. It took many years of hard work before its first clinical use. Many more years later it became generally available throughout the world. Each individual step (anticoagulation, oxygenators, hemodilution, metabolic homeostasis, azygos flow principle) had its own tortuous road to success. It is to be expected that this development will continue, making open heart surgery even more accessible and successful.

REFERENCES

1. Langendorff, O. Untersuchungen ueberlebender Säugetierherzen. Arch. Gesamten Physiol., 61:291–338, 1895.
2. Langendorff, O. Geschichtliche Bemerkungen zur Methode des Ueberlebenden Warmblueterherzens. Muench. Med. Wochenschr., 50(1):508–509, 1903.
3. Clark, A.J. The action of ions and lipoids upon the frog's heart. J. Physiol., 47:66–107, 1913.

4. Loewi, O. and O. Weselko. Ueber den Kohlehydratumsatz des isolierten Herzens normaler und diabetischer Tiere. Pfluegers Arch. Gesamte Physiol., 158:155–188, 1914.
5. Lussana, F. Action de l'Alanine sur le coeur isole de tortue. Arch. Int. Physiol., 9:393–406, 1910.
6. Howell, W.H. On the relation of the blood to the automaticity and sequence of the heart beat. Am. J. Physiol., 2:47–81, 1899.
7. Ringer, S. Concerning the influence exerted by each of the constitutents of the blood on the contraction of the ventricle. J. Physiol., 3:380–393, 1882.
8. Vernon, H.N. The respiration of the tortoise heart in relation to functional activity. J. Physiol., 40:295–316, 1910.
9. Starling, E.H. The Linacre lecture on the development of the heart given at Cambridge, 1915. London, Longmans Green, 1918.
10. Martin, H., and E.C. Applegarth. On the temperature limits of the vitality of the mammalian heart. Studies from the Biology Laboratory, Johns Hopkins University, 4:285, 1890.
11. Evans, C.A. The metabolism of the cardiac muscle. Recent Advances in Physiology. 6th ed. London, Churchill, 1939, pp. 157–215.
12. Locke, F.S. and O. Rosenheim. The disappearance of dextrose when perfused through the isolated mammalian heart. J. Physiol., 31:xiv, 1904.
13. Rohde, E. Stoffwechseluntersuchungen am ueberlebenden Warmblueterherzen: zur Physiologie des Herzstoffwechsels. Hoppe-Seyler's Z. Physiol. Chem., 68:181–235, 1910.
14. Tigerstedt, R.A. Physiologie des Kreislaufes. 2nd ed. Berlin, DeGreyter, 1921, vol. 1, pp. 334.
15. Bing, R.J. The metabolism of the heart. Harvey Lectures, 50:27–70, 1954–1955.
16. Liljestrand, G. Zum hundertsten Geburtstage Robert Tigerstedts. Acta Physiol. Scand. Suppl., 31:9–29, 1954.
17. Carrel, A. and C. Lindbergh. The culture of organs. New York, Hoeber, 1938.
18. Bing, R.J. Lindbergh and the biological sciences. Texas Heart Inst. J. 14:231, 1987.
19. Malinin, T.I. Surgery and Life: The extraordinary career of Alexis Carrel. New York, Harcourt, Brace, Jovanovitch, 1979.
20. Frank, O. Zur Dynamik des Herzmuskels. Z. Biol. 14:370–439, 1895.
21. Clowes, G.H.A. Jr., W.E. Neville, A. Hopkins, J. Anzola, and F.A. Simeone. Factors contributing to success or failure in the use of a pump-oxygenator for complete by-pass of the heart and lungs, Experimental and Clinical Surg. 36:557–559, 1954.
22. Galletti, P.M. and G.H. Brecher. Editors, Heart-Lung Bypass: Principles and techniques of extracorporeal circulation. Grune and Stratton, New York, 1962.
23. Diesh, G., S.A. Flynn, D. Marable, D.G. Mulder, K.J. Schmutzer, W.P. Longmire, Jr., and J.V. Maloney, Jr. Comparison of low flow (azygos) and high flow principles of extracorporeal circulation employing a bubble oxygenator. Surg. 42:67, 1957.
24. Abrams, L.D. F. Ashton, E.J. Charles, A.L. D'Abreu, J. Fejfar, E.J. Hamley, W.A. Hudson, R.E. Lee, R. Lightwood and E.T. Matthews,. Total cardiopulmonary bypass in the laboratory. Lancet 2:239, 1958.
25. Showstack, J.A., K.E. Rosenfeld, D.W. Garnick, H.S. Luft, R.W. Schaffarzick,

and J. Fowles. Association of volume with outcome of coronary artery bypass graft surgery. Scheduled vs. nonscheduled operations. JAMA, 257(6):785 and 257(18):2438, 1987.

26. Kaiser, G.C.: Institutional variation of coronary artery bypass graft surgery: emphasis on myocardial protection. Circ. 65:85–89, 1982.

27. Hartridge, H., and F.J.W. Roughton,. The kinetics of haemoglobin II. The velocity with which oxygen dissociates from its combination with haemoglobin. Proc. Roy. Soc. 104:395, 1923.

28. Hartridge, H., and F.J.W. Roughton. The rate of distribution of dissolved gases between the red blood corpuscle and its fluid environment. J. Physiol. 62:232–242, 1927.

29. Houston, C.S.: Going higher, the story of man and altitude. Little, Brown and Co., 1987.

30. DeWall, R.A., T.B. Grage, A.S. McFee, and M.A. Chiechi. Theme and variations on blood oxygenators. I. Bubble oxygenators. Surg. 50:931–940, 1962.

31. DeWall, R.A., Grage, T.B., McFee, A.S. and Chiechi, M.A.: Theme and variations on blood oxygenators. II. Film oxygenators. Surg. 51:251, 1962.

32. DeWall, R.A. and Grage, T.S.: The evolution of blood bubble oxygenators. In congenital heart disease. F.A. Davis Co., Philadelphia pp. 133–148, 1962.

33. Brodie, T.G.: The perfusion of surviving organs. J. Physiol. 29:266–275, 1903.

34. McLean, J.: The thromboplastic action of cephalin. Am. J. Physiol. 41:250–257, 1916.

35. Howell, W.H. E. Holt. Two new factors in blood coagulation, heparin and pro-antithrombin. Am. J. Physiol. 47:328, 1918.

36. Fry, W.B. Heparin: The contributions of William Henry Howell. Circ. 69:1198, 1984.

37. Baird, J. Presidential address: "Give us the tools..." The story of heparin as told by sketches from the lives of William Howell, Jay McLean, Charles Best and Gordon Murry. J. Vasc. Surg. 11:4, 1990.

38. Charles, A.F. and D.A. Scott. Studies on heparin: IV. Observations on the chemistry of heparin. Biochem. J. 30:1926, 1936.

39. Gibbon, J.H., Jr. Artificial maintenance of circulation during experimental occlusion of pulmonary artery. Arch. Surg. 34:1105–1131, 1937.

40. Chargaff, E. and K. Olson. Studies on the chemistry of blood coagulation, studies on the action of heparin and other anticoagulants. The influence of protamine on the anticoagulant effect in vivo. J. Biol. Chem. 122:153–167, 1937.

41. Schmitz, F. and A. Fisher. Über die chemiche Natur des Heparins: II. Die Reindarstellung des Heparins. Ztschr. f. Physiol. Chem. 216:264–273, 1933.

42. Jorpes, J.E. The chemistry of heparin. Biochem. J. 29:1817, 1936. 1) On heparin, its chemical nautre and properties. 427–433

43. Jorpes, J.E. Heparin its chemistry, physiology and application in medicine. London, Oxford Press,218–229, 1939.

44. Jorpes, J.E. The origin and physiology of heparin: The specific therapy in thrombosis. Ann. Inter. Med. 27:361–370, 1947.

45. Crafoord, C.: Preliminary report on post-operative treatment with heparin as a preventative of thrombosis. Acta. Chir. Scand. 29:1817, 1937.

46. Björk, V.O.: Brain perfusions in dogs with artificially oxygenated blood. Acta. Chir. Scand. 96:1–122, 1948.
47. LeGallois, J.J.C. (1770-1814) Quoted and illustrated by Griffenhagen, G.B. and C.H. Hughes, in: The history of the mechanical heart. "Smithsonian Report for 1955, pp 339–356. Publication #4241.
48. Gibbon, J.H., Jr.: Medicine's living history. Medical World News. 13:47, 1972.
49. Gibbon, J.H., Jr.. The development of the heart-lung apparatus. Rev. Surg. 27:231, 1970.
50. Hill, J.D. and J.H. Gibbon, Jr. The development of the first successful heart-lung machine. Ann. Thorac. Surg. 34:337–341, 1982.
51. Finnegan, M.O.: The development of the heart-lung for intracardiac surgery 1930-1957. *Thesis* (B.A.) Princeton, NJ. Princeton University. 1983.
52. Dale, H.H. and E.H. Schuster,. A double perfusion pump. J. Physiol. 64:356–364, 1928.
53. Hooker, D.R.: The perfusion of the mammalian medulla: The effect of calcium and of potassium on the respiratory and cardiac centers. Am. J. Physiol. 38:200–208, 1915.
54. Issekutz, V.B. Beitraege zur wirkung des Insulins. Biochem. Ztschr. 183:283, 1927.
55. DeBakey, M.E. Simple continuous-flow blood transfusion instrument. New Orleans M & SJ 87:386–389, 1934.
56. Gibbon, J.H., Jr. Application of a mechanical heart and lung apparatus to cardiac surgery. Minn. Med. 37:171, 1954.
57. Melrose, D.G.: A mechanical heart-lung for use in man. Brit. Med. J. 2:57, 1953.
58. Cross, F.S., R.M. Berne, U. Horose, E.B. Kay, and R.D. Jones,. Evaluation of rotating disc type of reservoir-oxygenator. Proc. Soc. Exper. Biol. and Med. 93:210, 1956.
59. Crafoord, C., B. Norberg, and A. Senning, A.. Clinical studies in extracorporeal circulation with a heart-lung machine. Acta. Chir. Scand. 112:220, 1957.
60. Lillehei, C.W.. A personalized history of extracorporeal circulation. Trans. Am. Soc. Artif. Int. Org. 28:5, 1982.
61. Wangensteen O.H. and S.D. Wangensteen. The rise of surgery, University of Minnesota Press, Minneapolis, 1978.
62. Karlson, K.E., C. Dennis, D. Westover, and D. Sanderson, D. Pump oxygenator to support the heart and lungs for brief periods. I. Evaluation of oxygenator techniques. Surg. 29:678, 1951.
63. Dennis, C., K.E. Karlson, W.P. Eder, R.M. Nelson, F.D. Eddy, and D. Sanderson. Pump oxygenator to supplant the heart and lungs for brief periods. II. A method applicable to dogs. Surg. 29:697, 1951.
64. Dennis, C., D.S. Spreng, Jr., G.E. Nelson, K.E. Karlson, R.M. Nelson, J.V. Thomas W.P. Eder, R.L. Varco. Development of a pump oxygenator to replace the heart and lungs. An apparatus applicable to human patients and applied to 1 case. Ann. Surg. 134:709, 1951.
65. Newman, M.H., J.H. Stuckey, B.S. Levowitz, L.A. Young, C. Dennis, C. Fries, E.J. Gorayeb, M. Zuhdi, K. Karlson, S. Adler, and M. Gliedman. Complete and partial perfusion of animal and human subjects with the pump-oxygenator. Surg. 38:30, 1955.

66. Lewis, F.J., and M. Taufic. Closure of atrial septal defects with aid of hypothermia: experimental accomplishments and the report of one successful case. Surg. 33:52, 1953.
67. Bigelow, W.G., J.C. Callaghan, J.A. Hopps. General hypothermia for experimental intracardiac surgery. Ann. Surg. 132:531, 1950.
68. Andreason, A.T. and F. Watson. Experimental cardiovascular surgery. "The Azygos Factor". Brit. J. Surg. 39:548, 1952.
69. Andreason, A.T. and F. Watson. Experimental cardiovascular surgery. Brit. J. Surg. 41:195, 1953.
70. Cohen, M., R.W. Hammerstrom, W. Spellman, R.L. Varco, and C.W. Lillehei. The tolerance of the canine heart to temporary complete vena caval occlusion. Surg. Forum 3:172, 1952.
71. Cohen, M. and C.W. Lillehei. A quantitative study of the "Azygos Factor" during vena cava occlusion in dog. Surg. Gyn. and Obst. 98:225, 1954.
72. Billroth, T.: Cited by Löwenbach, G.: Beitrag zur Kenntniss der Geschwülste der submaxillar-speicheldrüse. Virchow's Arch. (Path. Anat.) 150:73-111, 1897.
73. Lillehei, C.W., R.L. Varco, M. Cohen, H.E. Warden, C. Patton, and J.H. Moller, J.H. The first open-heart repairs of ventricular septal defect, atrio-ventricular communis, and tetraology of fallot using extracorporeal circulation by cross circulation: A thirty year follow-up. Ann. Thorac. Surg. 41:4, 1986.
74. Warden, H.E., M. Cohen, R.C. Read, and C.W. Lillehei. Controlled cross circulation for open intracardiac surgery. J. Thorac. Surg. 28:33, 1954.
75. Warden, H.E., M. Cohen, R.A. DeWall, E. Schultz, J.J. Buckely, R.C. Read, and C.W. Lillehei,. Experimental closure of intraventricular septal defects and further physiological studies on controlled cross circulation. Surgical Forum, American College of Surgeons. 1954, Philadelphia: W.B. Saunders Company, 1955, pp 22–26.
76. Lillehei, C.W., M. Cohen, H.W. Warden, and R.I. Varco,. The direct vision intracardiac correction of congenital anomalies by controlled cross circulation. Surgery 38:11, 1955.
77. Adams, P., R.L. Anderson, C.W. Lillehei, and N. Meyne. Reversibility of pulmonary hypertension following closure of ventricular septal defects. AMA Am. Dis. Child. 98:558, 1955.
78. Lillehei, C.W., M. Cohen, J.E. Warden, R.C. Read, J.B. Aust, and R.L. Varco,. Direct vision intracardiac surgical correction of the tetralogy of Fallot, pentalogy of Fallot, and pulmonary atresia defects. Report of first ten cases. Ann. Surg. 142:418, 1955.
79. Clark, L.C. Jr., F. Gollan, and B. Vishwa. The oxygenization of blood by gas dispersion. Science 111:85, 1950.
80. Helmsworth, J.A., L.C. Clark, Jr., S. Kaplan, R.T. Sherman, and T. Largen,. Artificial oxygenization and circulation during complete bypass of the heart. J. Thorac. Surg. 34:117, 1952.
81. Helmsworth, J.A., L.C. Clark, Jr., S. Kaplan, R.T. Sherman,. An oxygenator pump for use in total by-pass of the heart and lungs. J. Thorac. Surg. 26:617, 1953.
82. Gibbs, E.L., W.G. Lennox, L.F. Nims, and F.A. Gibbs. Arterial and cerebral venous blood: arterial-venous differences in man. J. Biol. Chem. 144:325, 1942.

83. Shumway, N.E., M.L. Gliedman, and F.J. Lewis,. A mechanical pump oxygenator for successful cardiopulmonary by-pass surgery. 40:831, 1956.
84. Lillehei, C.W., R.A. DeWall, V.L. Gott, and R.L. Varco,. The direct vision correction of calcific aortic stenosis by means of a pump-oxygenator and retrograde coronary sinus perfusion. Dis. Chest. 30:133, 1956.
85. DeWall, R.A., H.E. Warden, R.C. Read, V.L.Gott, N.R. Ziegler, R.L. Varco, and C.W. Lillihei. A simple expendable artificial oxygenator for open heart surgery. Surg. Clin. N. Amer. Philadelphia, W.B. Saunders Co., pp. 1025–1034, 1956.
86. Lillehei, C.W., R.A. DeWall, R.C. Read, H.E. Warden, and R.L. Varco. Direct vision intracardiac surgery in man using a simple disposable artificial oxygenator. Dis. Chest. 29:1–8, 1956.
87. Cooley, D.A., B.A. Belmont, J.R. Latson, and J.R. Pierce. Bubble diffusion oxygentaor for cardiopulmonary bypass. J. Thorac. Surg. 35:131, 1958.
88. Cooley, D.A. H.A. Collins, J.W. Giacobine, G.C. Morris, Jr., L.R. Soltero-Harrington, and F.J. Harberg. The pump oxygenator in cardiovascular surgery: observations based upon 450 cases. Amer. Surgeon 24:870, 1958.
89. Dubost, C., G. Nahas, C. Lenfant, J. Pasetcq, J. Guery, J. Rauanet, M. Weiss, and R. Heim de Balsac. Chirurgie a coeur ouvert sous circulation extracorporeal: Ensemble pompe-oxygenateur de Lillehei-DeWall. Poumon-Coeur 12:641, 1956.
90. Dubost, C. R. Heim der Balsac, R.A. DeWall, C. Lenfant, J. Guery, J. Passelcq, M. Weiss, and J. Rounet. Extracorporeal circulation and heart surgery. Brit. Heart J. 19:67, 1957.
91. Gott, V.L., R.A. DeWall, M. Paneth, M. Zuhdi, W. Weirich, R.L. Varco, and C.W. Lillehei. A self contained disposable oxygenator of plastic sheet for intracardiac surgery. Thorax 12:1, 1957.
92. Rygg, I.H. and E. Kvisgaard, E. A disposable polyethylene oxygenator system applied in a heart-lung machine. Acta. Chir. Scand. 112:433, 1956.
93. DeWall, R.A., H. Najafi, D.J. Bentley, and T. Roden,. A hard shell temperature controlling disposable blood oxygenator. JAMA 197:1065, 1966.
94. Allen, J.G. Editor: Extracorporeal Circulation. Charles C. Thomas, Publisher, Springfield, Ill. Second printing 1960.
95. Ionescu, M.I. Editor: Techniques in Extracorporeal Circulation. Second Edition, Butterworths, London 1981.
96. Kirklin, J.W.: Open-Heart surgery at the Mayo Clinic. The 25th anniversary. Mayo Clin. Proc. 55:339, 1980.
97. Miller, B.J., J.H. Gibbon, Jr. and C. Fineberg. An improved mechanical heart and lung apparatus: its use during open cardiotomy in experimental animals. Med. Clin. North A. pp 1603–1624, 1953.
98. Donald, D.E., H.G. Harshbarger, P.S. Hetzel, R.T. Patric, E.H. Wood, and J.W. Kirklin, J.W. Experience with a heart-lung bypass (Gibbon type) in the experimental laboaratory: preliminary report. Proc. Meet. Mayo Clin. 30:113, 1955.
99. Jones, R.E., D.E. Donald, H.J.C. Swan, H.G. Harshbarger, J.W. Kirklin, and E.H. Wood. Apparatus of Gibbin type for mechanical bypass of the heart and lungs: preliminary report. Proc. Staff Meet. Mayo Clinic 30:105, 1955.
100. Kirklin, J.W., J.W. DeShane, J.W., R.T. Patric, D.E. Donald, P.S. Hetzel, H.G. Harshbarger, and E.H. Wood. Intracardiac surgery with the aid of a mechanical

pump oxygenator (Gibbon type): report of eight cases. Proc. Staff Meet. Mayo Clin. 30:201, 1955.
101. DeWall patent—Capillary oxygenator #2,972,349, 1958.
102. Kolobow, T., and W.M. Zapol. Partial and total extracorporeal respiratory gas exchange with the spiral membrane lung. Editors Bartlett, R.H., P.A. Drinker, and P.M. Galletti,. Mechanical Devices for cardiopulmonary assistance, Vol. 6, pp 112, S. Karger, Basel, 1971.
103. Austin, B.A., and D.L. Harner,. The heart-lung machine. Phoenix Medical Communications. Phoenix, AZ 1986.
104. Foote, A.V., M. Trede, and J.V. Maloney, Jr.. An experimental and clinical study of the use of acid-citrate-dextrose (ACD) blood for extracorporeal circulation. J. Thorac. Cardio. Surg. 42:93, 1961.
105. Cooley, D.A., A.C. Beall, Jr. and J.K. Alexander. Acute massive pulmonary embolism: successful treatment using temporary cardiopulmonary bypass: J. Am. Med. Assoc. 177:283, 1961.
106. Cooley, D.A., A.C. Beall, Jr., and P. Grondid. Open-heart operations with disposable oxygenators, dextrose prime and normothermia. Surg. 51:713, 1962.
107. Zuhdi, N., B. McCollough, J. Carey, C. Krieger, and A. Greer. Hypothermic perfusion for open-heart surgical procedure. J. Int. Col. Surg. 35:379, 1961.
108. Greer, A.E., J.M. Carey, and N. Zuhdi. Haemodilution principle of hypothermic perfusion: a concept obviating blood priming. J. Thorac. Cardiovasc. Surg. 43:640, 1966.
109. Long, D.E., V.B. Todd, R.A. Indeglia, R.L. Varco, and C.W. Lillehei. Clinical use of dextran-40 in extracorporeal circulation. A summary of 5 years experience. Transfusion 6:401, 166.
110. Vasco, K.A., A.M. Riley, and R.A. DeWall. Poloxalkol (Pluronic F-68): A priming solution for cardiopulmonary bypass. Trans. Am. Soc. Art. Int. Org. 28:526, 1972.

Chapter 4

Congenital Heart Disease

A. NADAS AND R.J. BING

The 16th and 17th centuries were exciting eras in the anatomical sciences. Anatomists were then what molecular biologists are today, heroes on the frontiers of medical science. One man stands out as a pioneer in the field of anatomy, Niels Stensen, of Copenhagen (Figure 1). Stensen, a wide-ranging, restless, and inquisitive intellect, became the victim of his own restless genius and of his attempt to reconcile it with the world about him. In 1671, Stensen (also referred as to Steensen, or as Steno), described the cardiopathology of a stillborn fetus with a cardiac malformation which now bears Fallot's name (1). Erik Warburg published a Danish translation of the original report (2). An excellent biography of Stensen was published in Danish in 1979 (3). In 1913, William S. Miller wrote a thorough history of Stensen in English followed by F.A. Willius in 1948 (4,5).

The stillborn fetus described by Stensen was a boy with a cleft palate, which was ascribed to the mother's predilection for rabbit meat. The sternum was made of cartilage and was split in the middle. Other congenital malformations were apparently present. Stensen first believed that the embryo was male, since there was a very prominent clitoris; external genitalia and the presence of a uterus however suggested that the fetus was a female. Stensen was particularly impressed by the unusual heart. On the first glance, the pulmonary artery appeared to be much smaller than the aorta. "As I opened the pulmonary artery from the right ventricle, it was immediately clear that the

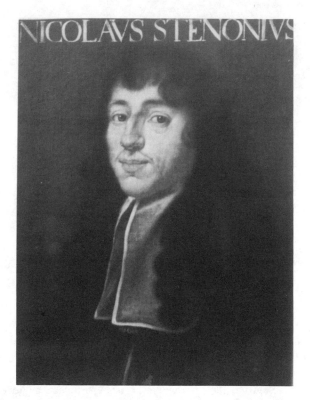

Figure 1. Nicholas Stensen (*Courtesy of The New York Academy of Medicine*)

canal which leads from the pulmonary artery to the aorta and which is quite evident in every embryo, was not to be found. When I subsequently opened the right ventricle, the probe passed along the septum into the aorta, and with the same ease into the left ventricle. Therefore, the right ventricle had three openings, one from the atrium, and two into the large arteries. The aorta had a common origin in both ventricles." Stensen also speculated on the physiological consequences of this anatomical malformation. "The blood must pass equally into both arteries from the right ventricle (6)." He was not certain whether the blood originating in the right ventricle was shunted first into the pulmonary artery and then through a canal (ductus) into the aorta, or whether the aorta received blood primarily from the right ventricle. He emphasized that in this embryo, the patent ductus arteriosus, or as he calls it the "canal," was closed. He compared this to the normal newborn in which the ductus first conducted blood from the pulmonary artery to the aorta.

Stensen was born in 1638 to Steen Pedersen, who was a goldsmith in Copenhagen. Since his father died early and his mother married again, he lived with his grandparents. He was a sickly child and had a lot of contact with older people and little companionship with children of his own age. The conversations to which he listened were largely concerned with religious matters and he apparently heard a great deal of Martin Luther's teachings (4). In 1656, at the age of 18, Stensen entered the University of Copenhagen and selected a mentor, Thomas Bartholin, as was customary at that time. Bartholin was an outstanding anatomist of his time and brought to the University of Copenhagen a fame which extended over all Europe. Stensen not only studied anatomy under Bartholin, but also pursued mathematics and languages—Hebrew, French, German, and later Italian. It has been said that he was able to make such progress in Hebrew that in later life he could easily read the Bible in that language.

These were difficult times for Denmark. Denmark was at war with Sweden; in 1658, the Swedes invaded Denmark and besieged Copenhagen. Stensen was assigned to a regiment composed of students, who were to repair the fortifications and repel the attacks of the foe. Despite this, Stensen found time to attend lectures and perform anatomical dissections with Bartholin. During this period, Stensen also read the great books of his times, such as Descartes, Kepler, and Galileo.

In 1659, Stensen traveled to Amsterdam with a letter of recommendation to Gerhard Blasius. Blasius had taught medicine in Copenhagen and was a friend of Bartholin. In Amsterdam, Stensen discovered the salivary duct, which now bears his name, Stensen's duct or the duct of Steno. As is often the case then as it is now, the fight for priority was a bitter one. A controversy arose between Stensen and Blasius concerning priority for this discovery. Blasius was enraged that Stensen should claim the discovery which he claimed for himself. He called Stensen a liar, blasphemer, and a malevolent person inflated with envy. Stensen replied in a letter to Bartholin that, "Blasius had never looked for the salivary duct; for he does not give to it either the proper point of beginning or ending, and assigns to the parotid gland so unworthy a function, that of furnishing warmth for the ear, that were I not right in having shown him the duct, I should be tempted to assert that he had never seen it (4)."

This bitter experience with Blasius was enough to cut short Stensen's stay in Amsterdam. In 1661, he moved to Leiden to work with the great anatomist, Sylvius. But the controversy followed him. Blasius still claimed the discovery for himself and wrote a letter to Bartholin, who answered, "Your conscience will tell you who is right in this matter . . . farewell and control yourself."

In 1664, Stensen returned to Copenhagen where he published his revolutionary concept of the heart as a muscle. "The heart has been considered the seat of natural warmth, as the throne of the soul and even as the soul itself. Some have greeted the heart as the sun, others as the king: but if you examine it more closely, one finds it to be nothing more than muscle." This simple statement caused consternation and controversy (4). The celebrated Swiss physiologist, Haller, writing in 1774, pronounced Stensen's publication a "golden book which contains the rich seed for new discovery." De Hedoville wrote in 1665, "This simple observation overthrew a system to which medicine clung most tenaciously." It is noteworthy that while in Leiden, Stensen met the philosopher Spinoza who had been excommunicated by his local synagogue and had fled to Leiden. Stensen and Spinoza remained lifelong friends (3).

Since no position was available in Copenhagen, Stensen returned to Holland in 1664 and thence to Paris where he obtained his Doctor's degree. A lecture which he gave in Paris on the structure of the brain attracted much attention. Stensen wrote:

> All you can say is that you find these two different substances, the one gray, the one white in the brain; that the white substance is continued into the nerves which are distributed through the entire body; that the gray substance serves in some places as an envelope for the white, in other places it separates the white fibers from each other (3,4).

From France, Stensen travelled to Italy and, in 1666, he journeyed to Florence, which became of pivotal importance in his life. In Florence, even at the end of the 17th century, the court of the Medici was still the central focus for scientists and artists. Through the influence of his friends, particularly Viviani, the pupil and companion of Galileo, he was appointed personal physician to the Grand Duke, who bestowed on him a pension and a residence. He also received an appointment at the hospital Santa Maria Nuova, which had been founded in 1288 by Portinari, the father of Dante's Beatrice and which still exists today. It was in Florence that Stensen, a Lutheran, converted to Catholicism. This was not in line with his previous philosophy. His friends were either Lutherans or Calvinists—such as Glauber, Borch, Thevenot, Sylvius, Willis (one of the founders of the Royal Society), Lister, Croone—a Pantheist like Spinoza. The fact that he was Lutheran in a high position at a Catholic Institute may have contributed to his conversion; later the position was reversed when as a Catholic he occupied a position at the Lutheran Institutes, the University of Copenhagen (2–5).

In Florence, Stensen received a letter from the Danish King offering him a professorship at Copenhagen. His inaugural address is worth quoting:

> What one sees is beautiful; more beautiful is what one knows; but by far the most beautiful things are beyond our knowledge. For who can contemplate the wonderful structure of the human organism without asking the question: who is its author?

The stay in Copenhagen was not to be a long one. Again he became involved in a controversy, possibly because of his position as a Catholic professor in a Lutheran University. In May 1674, he resigned his position and returned to Florence, where he took charge of the education of the son of the Grand Duke Cosimo III. In 1675, Stensen became a priest and the Pope consecrated him bishop of Titiopolis. He then went to Braunschweig where the Pope appointed him "Apostolic Vicar for the Northern Missions." He moved to Schwerin, in Northern Germany, where he died in 1686 at the age of 48. The end of this saga came when the Grand Duke of Tuscany, hearing of his death, sent for his body and had it transported to Florence, where he was entombed with the Grand Dukes in the cathedral of San Lorenzo.

Stensen also was an outstanding geologist. He was prophetic in his concepts of formation of mountains, citing examples of local earth crust formation, showing how individual strata might remain horizontal, while some might be tilted or even thrown into a perpendicular position, and others might be bent in the form of arches. Mountains, he said, might also originate from the upward action of the volcanic forces on the earth's crust (2–5).

Stensen was one of the least known but brilliant and imaginative scientists of the Baroque era.

In 1777 more than 100 years later, after Stensen's report, Sandifort described the same cardiac malformation, which he called "a very rare disease of the heart." This Dutch physician was born in Dortrecht, in 1742, and received his doctor of medicine degree from Frederik Bernhard Albinus. His life and his description of what was later to be called the Tetralogy of Fallot has been reported in detail by Lydia Russell Bennett (7). The report by Sandifort, when compared to Stensen's, illustrates the progress made in medicine over one hundred years. While Stensen was primarily concerned with basic anatomic features, Sandifort was also interested in the clinical symptoms. While Stensen observed the cardiac pathologic anatomy on an embryo, Sandifort's observations were based on a patient who lived until childhood giving him the opportunity to observe the clinical progress. Following the teachings of Boerhaave, Sandifort took very careful clinical records. Like Stensen, Sandifort taught in Leiden, where he founded the Leiden Museum of Pathology, became president of the College of Surgeons, and was made president of the College of Pharmacology (7). One of Sandifort's statements is particularly noteworthy, "Oh, how difficult it is to cure diseases within the breast! Oh, how much more difficult to recognize them, and to give sure diagnosis about them! (7)."

Sandifort's description of the cardiac malformation which bears Fallot's name was made in the "Observationes Anatomico-Pathologicae," written from 1777 until 1781. Book 1, Chapter 1 of the "Observationes" is entitled "Concerning a very rare disease of the heart." In describing this malformation, he followed the example of the great Leiden physician, Boerhaave, who became the spiritual father of Viennese medicine which flourished during the 19th century. The chapter has 23 pages and numerous beautiful illustrations. He had the opportunity to describe the clinical symptoms as well as the pathological finding in a child whom he called "Blue Boy." He describes the child as being normal during the first year of life, but during the second year "the beginnings of terrible symptoms appeared, which afterward sorely burdened the poor child. In fact, a bluish color of the fingers, even the nails, not continuous, but now more and now less evident, attracted the attention of the parents, particularly when it could be ascribed to no tightness of clothing." The symptoms which he described in this child were "catarrh," blue color of the lips and tongue which often verged toward black, a dry cough, sinking spells, pressing pain in the head, swelling of jugular veins, and "an agitation or a throbbing in the jugular veins." Toward the end stage of the disease, Sandifort observed swelling of the feet and face. Therapy was concerned with venesection, mild laxatives, and leeches which, at the beginning, seemed to have some effect, but later were to no avail. He makes special mention that this child was a "clever boy." Sandifort very carefully searched the literature and quotes Vieussen, Morgagni, Meckel, and others (7).

At autopsy, he found that the foramen ovale was widely patent. He wrote,

> How great was the surprise of the onlookers, how great equally was my own surprise, when we saw the point of the finger to stretch into the aorta, which is not at all accustomed to maintain communications with the right ventricle, in conformity with otherwise constant laws of nature! Thus, the arterial aorta was springing from both ventricles, and had to receive all the blood from both.

He found the pulmonary artery to be very small, almost rigid, and blocked by a certain granular substance. Sandifort came to the conclusion that he dealt with a truly congenital malformation. Scientist and historian that he was, he quoted Stensen. He mentioned that Stensen also had been able to push a probe upward next to the septum directly into the aorta from the right ventricle (7).

Not much changed in the field of congenital heart disease until the middle of the 19th century. In 1858, Thomas B. Peacock published a book on malformations of the heart. The book is based on lectures delivered to medical students in 1854 at the St. Thomas's Hospital in London (8). Peacock carefully describes anatomical studies on congenital heart disease by Burns, Corvisart (Napolean's physician), Berthis, Laennec, Boilland, and Hope. The book contains beautiful illustrations of various congenital malformations such as ventricular septal defects and pulmonary stenosis, with and without foremen ovale. He discusses transposition of the aorta and pulmonary artery described by Baillie in 1797. Peacock's biography was briefly featured in the London Medical and Provincial Directory, 1858 (9), which was advertised as "the only cheap medical journal, instructive in its matter, independent in its policy, and honest in its purpose." (Few journals nowadays can make this claim.) Peacock received his medical degree in Edinburgh in 1852, became a Fellow of the Royal College of Physicians in 1850, assistant physician at St. Thomas's Hospital, physician to the City of London, and medical superintendent and pathologist at the Royal Infirmary in Edinburgh (9).

In 1921, A. Spitzer published a book on congenital heart disease which was very different from that of Peacock (10). He was particularly interested in the origin of the malformations, assuming that many congenital malformations were due to arrested development of the heart and could be explained by an arrested state through which the evolutionary process of the species was carried out. The evolution for the species, therefore, appears to him to be reflected in the formation of the individual, and malformations are explained on an evolutionary basis. To make this theory clear, he repeatedly tried to explain the Cor Triatriatum, by comparing it with the reptile heart. He mentions that in the reptile, the aorta originates from the right ventricle, since in the reptile, when there is enough oxygen available, blood can be shunted directly into the body. According to Spitzer, the force and capacity of the right ventricle is "temporarily placed in service of the larger circulation, when there is no particular need for the pulmonary circulation. The dextraposed aorta converts the right chamber into an auxiliary pump of the larger circulation (10)."

Wilhelm Ebstein (1836-1912) was the discoverer of a malformation which bears his name (11). He was professor of medicine and director of the medical clinic at Goettingen, and he studied at the Universities of Breslau and Berlin. This was Berlin's greatest period in the medical sciences, with Von Graefe, Traube, DuBois-Reymond, Langenbeck, Romberg, Schoenlein, and Virchow. In 1898, Ebstein published an article in which he grouped obesity, gout, and diabetes mellitus as inheritable cellular metabolic diseases. On the basis of this, he was called "the forgotten founder of biochemical genetics (12)." One of Ebstein's often cited observations, which lead to the eponym Pel-Ebstein's fever was his description, in 1887, of the periodic fever of lymphoma (13). Today, the major source of Ebstein's fame is his work on congenital heart disease carried out early in his career and largely ignored until after his death. In 1864, he performed an autopsy on a patient in whom he described three cardiac anomalies: severe malformation of the tricuspid valve, absence of the pulmonary valve, and patent foramen ovale (14). A. Arnstein published his case in 1927, fifteen years after Ebstein's death, and named it "Ebsteinsche Krankheit" (Ebstein's disease) (15).

A Canadian physician, Maude Abbott, forms the connection to today's diagnosis of congenital heart disease (Figure 2). Abbott graduated in Arts from McGill University in Montreal, in 1890, with the third class of women. She was elected President of her class and was the valedictorian. She wrote sometime later that she was "in love with McGill (16)." This passionate affection was clearly not reciprocated. The medical school, in spite of pressures from

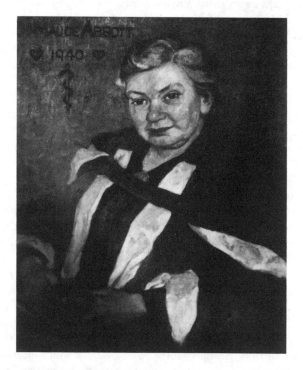

Figure 2.   Maude Abbott (*Courtesy of The New York Academy of Medicine*)

faculty, public agitation, and headlines in the press, refused to consider her because she was a woman. The professor of surgery said he would resign if women were allowed to take the medical course. And this was only 100 years ago.

Since the doors of her beloved McGill Medical School were shut tightly at that time (and did not open to women until 1918), Abbott accepted an offer from the University of Bishops College, in Montreal. She graduated from this small school as the only woman in her class, in 1894. After graduation from medical school, she undertook the required pilgrimage to the European centers of learning—from London to Vienna. Abbott returned to Montreal after three years in Europe and opened an office for the practice of medicine in 1897. She apparently was not comfortable with the requirements of private practice and dealing with patients, so she obtained an appointment as an assistant curator of the medical museum the next year. This is how she became acquainted with the Osler Collection, described the Holmes heart, and devoted all of her life to the study of congenital heart disease.

It was customary until the middle of the 20th century, to collect pathologic specimens in museums. William Osler, when at McGill University in Montreal, had started such a collection. Abbott met Osler in Baltimore in 1898, and he mentioned to her his collection at McGill, which was later referred to as the Osler Collection (17). He saw the teaching possibilities of such a museum, calling the collection: "pictures of life and death together." Abbott wrote, "And thus he gently dropped a seed that dominated all my future work. This is but an illustration of how his influence worked in many lives." When she returned to Montreal, she gave herself entirely to the work at this museum. "The work was very demanding," she wrote, "and it seemed at first a dreary and unpromising drudgery; but as Dr. Osler had prophesied, it blossomed into wonderful things. I shall never forget him as I saw him walking down the old museum toward me, with his great, dark, burning eyes fixed fully upon me (17)."

Abbott's interest in congenital heart disease began at that time. She traces her original interest in congenital heart disease to her work in this museum. Probably Osler's help in identifying some of the specimens focused her attention on the subject, but what made her devote herself to it completely was having been asked by Osler to write the section on congenital heart disease in his "System of Medicine" of 1907 (17). She asked Osler how to approach writing this chapter and his answer was: "Statistically." Thus, she analyzed all the initial cases in large charts arranged according to the special features and symptoms. Finally, she had a large quantity of facts and figures from which she could draw conclusions, with illustrations of many of the type of conditions drawn from the museum specimens. She completed this atlas in

1907. Osler was delighted. He wrote her, "This is by far and away the best thing ever written on the subject in English — possibly in any language." And he added, "I have but one regret, that Rokitansky and Peacock are not alive to see it." Thus, Osler gave direction and intensity to her work.

In Osler's book, *The Principle and Practice of Medicine*, published in 1892, eleven years prior to Abbott's publication, he commenced his chapter on congenital heart disease: "These (congenital affections of the heart) have only limited clinical interest, as in a large proportion of the cases the anomaly is not compatible with life, and in others nothing can be done to remedy the defect or even to relieve the symptoms (18)." Within the next eleven years, thanks largely to Abbott, our knowledge of congenital heart disease increased. The advances of cardiac surgery and pediatric cardiology would not have been possible without her contribution.

In the 1940s, congenital heart disease grew from a field of limited clinical interest into one of considerable practical importance. This progress was to a large extent the result of the development of cardiac surgery and of new diagnostic tools. Robert E. Gross in Boston, Clarence Crafoord in Stockholm, and Alfred Blalock in Baltimore were the pioneers.

August 26, 1938, may be identified as the time when surgery of congenital heart disease was born. Gross, at 33, Chief Resident in Surgery at The Children's Hospital of Boston, successfully ligated the patent ductus arteriosus of a 7 year old girl. There were previous attempts to obliterate the ductus arteriosus; a patient of John Strieder, at Boston University, survived the operation, but succumbed to postoperative infection. Gross, having worked for years in the pathology laboratory and the dog lab of the Children's Hospital and of the Peter Bent Brigham, was intellectually prepared for the undertaking. He was skillful with his hands, knew where he was going, and was lucky. His colleagues, to put it mildly, were not totally supportive of his vision. It was surely no coincidence that the daring tour de force was attempted during the month when his chief, William E. Ladd, was away on vacation. Legend has it that after the little girl seemed to have come through surgery without complications, Gross and his group of young people went to celebrate the success by attending one of the Longwood tennis matches, where they met Ladd. The chief asked Gross after the tennis game, according to the story, "Anything new, Bob?" The chief resident said, "Nothing much," or some such thing. In fact, cardiac surgery was born.

The medical cardiologists, as expected, were no more courageous than the surgical community. At that time, Green and Emerson ran the congenital heart clinic at The Children's Hospital every Thursday afternoon. Neither of their names appeared on Gross' original publication (19). Instead, the coauthor was John Hubbard, who ran the rheumatic fever clinic. How the head of the rheumatic fever clinic had access to a patient with patent ductus arteriosus remains a mystery, but it certainly happened and is another example of Gross' firm determination, skill, and good luck.

Gross was born in Baltimore, Maryland. After graduating from high school, he went to Carleton College, in Minnesota. As an undergraduate, he received a scholarship to the University of Wisconsin for postgraduate studies in Chemistry. During summer vacation, however, he read Harvey Cushing's biography of Sir William Osler (the Osler influence once again), and decided to go to medical school. He chose, and was admitted to, the Harvard Medical School, where Cushing was Professor of Surgery (Note the difference between the career opportunities for men and women, such as Maude Abbott and Helen Taussig).

Having graduated from Harvard in 1931, Gross had training in Pathology under S. Burt Wolbach, Surgery under Elliot Cutler at Peter Brigham, and Ladd at The Children's Hospital. These three people had major influences on his career. Eventually he became the second Ladd Professor of Children's Surgery at the Harvard Medical School. Clearly, surgery was to be his career, but he carried a strong conviction to the very end that thorough training in pathology and the experimental laboratory were indispensable parts of academic surgical training.

Gross' surgical career had two distinct and separate but overlapping, chapters. The first was that of pediatric surgery; the text "Abdominal Surgery of Infancy and Childhood," by Ladd and Gross, bears witness to his seminal contributions to the field (20). Gross repaired the first diaphragmatic hernia in a newborn, resected lobar emphysema, and performed the first successful pneumonectomy in an infant. He contributed significantly to the diagnosis and treatment of Wilms tumors. He learned to manage atresias of the GI tract and choledochal cysts (21). Not only did Gross contribute significantly to the techniques in pediatric surgery, and really established the discipline, but, in addition, most of the heads of pediatric surgical departments in the United States today are either children or grandchildren of the Gross training program.

The second chapter, which overlapped the first, was the start of cardiac surgery. There is no question that Gross opened the field with his ligation of the patent ductus arteriosus in 1938. There is some argument about the first treatment of coarctation of the aorta. The first report of successful surgical treatment appeared in 1945, and was authored by Crafoord (22). Gross always maintained, although seldom articulated, that Crafoord visited his laboratory, learned his end-to-end anastomosis technique there, and beat him to the first report. With Edward Neuhauser, head of Radiology at Children's Hospital, Gross worked out the diagnosis and treatment of vascular rings. He

designed an ingenious approach to atrial septal defect surgery through suturing of a rubber sleeve to the anterior wall of the right atrium allowing the
blood to rise in the sleeve through the atriotomy, to the level of right atrial
pressure (usually low in secundum atrial defects). He then sewed blindly, but
highly successfully, through the blood with a needle attached to a long hemo-
stat. The procedure worked in hundreds of cases and other surgeons have
continued to use it even after he abandoned the technique, using the pump
oxygenator.

Gross was an ingenious, meticulous, and inventive person. He and Savage,
from the machine shop at The Children's Hospital (who formerly worked in
the Springfield Armory on machine guns before he retired to come to Children's) constructed their own pump oxygenator. He would not use "store-
bought stuff." He was clearly a do-it-yourself, independent person. He
wanted to make everything simple. There was (and maybe still is) a sign in
The Children's Hospital operating room saying, "If an operation is difficult,
you are not doing it properly." He did not tolerate "messy" things. He never
took to the hypothermia technique of Henry Swan. To put an anesthetized
child in a tub of ice water just offended his sense of aesthetics. At catheterization conferences, he barely would listen to the complex physiologic data presented and barely looked at the angiograms. He wanted to know what the
final diagnosis was, and mainly, how old the child was and how much he
weighed. Just the facts. Indicative of his dual careers Gross was Surgeon in
Chief at The Children's from 1947-1967 and he acted as Cardiovascular Surgeon in Chief from 1967-1972.

Alfred Blalock was the second in this constellation of cardiac surgeons.
By the time Blalock came to Hopkins from Vanderbilt University, he was
superbly prepared for the surgical work which was to challenge him. He had
already excelled in research on shock which was surely his greatest contribution (the role of the depletion in plasma volume), and later on the role of the
thymus in myasthenia gravis (23,24).

Longmire in an authoritative book on Alfred Blalock concisely stated the
relative role of Blalock and Taussig in the initiation of the shunt operation
(24a).

> Taussig's role on the tetralogy event has been the subject of some controversy
> and has been enlarged or diminished, in part, depending upon whether the nar-
> rator is a surgeon or a cardiologist. The view that I obtained from working with
> Alfred Blalock, and from hearing his comments, was, of course, that he had
> originally performed the subclavian pulmonary anastomosis while working in
> the experimental laboratory at Vanderbilt during a period when he was inter-
> ested in the general subject of hypertension. His object at that time was to cre-
> ate pulmonary hypertension, and he was somewhat disappointed in the

procedure when, due to the low resistance in the pulmonary circulation, such an anastomosis did not immediately produce increased tension in the pulmonary artery. Obviously his experimental animals were not followed long enough, or he would have seen some element of hypertension develop. In any event, he had developed the technique of the anastomosis... When the first three operations were reported in the Journal of the American Medical Association, and in the general conversation in the operating room with early visitors, and others, I recall that Blalock adopted his usual gracious—some would say—overly-generous attitude toward his associates and colleagues, including Helen Taussig, occasionally giving them somewhat lavish credit and praise for their roles in various undertakings... Initially, it was only because of Blalock's custom of giving generous recognition to his associates that Helen Taussig began to receive a share of the acclaim. As time wore on, however some thought that Taussig's somewhat contentious nature and her tendency to assume a greater degree of credit for the success of the procedure than was justified began to undermine this mutually productive relationship; indeed a quite subtle distrust slowly evolved into a thinly suppressed hostility. Blalock, I know, became quite annoyed by some of her statements, reactions, and claims. Fortunately, I believe that there was never any public or open disruption of the Blalock-Taussig team.

Harry Muller, Stephen H. Watts professor of Surgery Emeritus at the University of Virginia, has recounted, in a letter to me, the point to which this controversy degenerated during his tenure as chief resident on the cardiac team (1948-1949):

'At this time [Blalock] was having a great deal of difficulty with Dr. Helen Taussig because she would not recommend patients for operation even though to most of us the patient seemed to merit an operative procedure...' Thomas Turner, dean of the Johns Hopkins School of Medicine during the latter part of the Blalock era, wrote to Longmire recently: 'I knew Al Blalock from his house officer days on; upon his return to Hopkins my admiration for him continued to grow and our friendship deepened. I view with dismay the tendency to underestimate the seminal role he played in developing the so-called Blue Baby operation and related surgery' (24a).

It is certain, however, that Helen Taussig's idea that an increase in pulmonary blood flow would be beneficial was not correct. It was not the diminution in pulmonary blood flow, but the right to left shunt, or the decrease in effective pulmonary blood flow, which was responsible for the cyanosis and clinical symptoms of these patients. Nonetheless, the idea led Blalock to the correct surgical treatment (25; Figure 3). Blalock had already carried out experimental anastomoses between the subclavian and the pulmonary arteries many years prior at Vanderbilt together with Sanford E. Levi to see whether he could produce pulmonary hypertension by increasing pulmonary blood flow (26). But an operation is a surgical and not a medical or pediatric procedure. The best ideas often run afoul in the experimental laboratory, or worse, the operating room. Thus, the early surgical treatment of some types of cya-

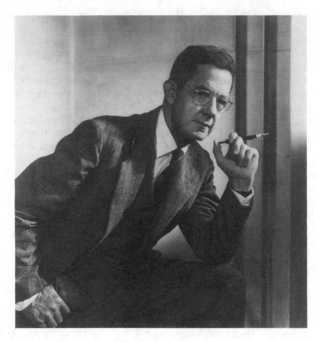

Figure 3.   Alfred Blalock (*Courtesy of The New York Academy of Medicine*)

notic congenital heart disease should be credited to Blalock (27). It was certainly fortunate for the future of cardiac surgery that these divergent and completely different personalities happened to be there at the same time and at the same place.

The world-wide acceptance of the designation of the Blalock-Taussig shunt (B-T shunt as it is colloquially referred to) speaks for itself. Suffice to say that the shunt operation (systemic artery to pulmonary artery) was a landmark achievement. For the first time, miserable, blue, squatting little children became pink, and could run, play, and join the human race. With all the enormous progress in the surgery of congenital heart disease since 1944, one could still argue that more actual suffering was alleviated by this palliative procedure than with any other subsequent corrective operation.

Taussig was born in 1898 (Figure 4). Her father was the Henry Lee Professor of Economics at Harvard. Helen went to Radcliffe for the first two years of her college education; she transferred to the University of California at Berkeley and graduated from that institution. She wanted to study medicine,

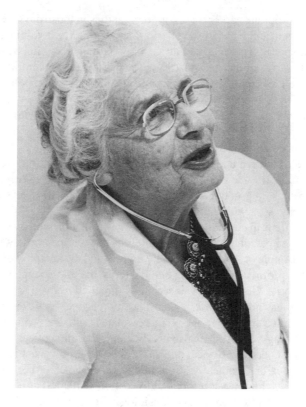

Figure 4. Helen Taussig (*Courtesy of Johns Hopkins University Library*)

but the president of Harvard, a frequent visitor to the house, advised her that as a woman in 1922, she had no chance of being admitted: but she should try the Harvard School of Public Health. The dean of that institution told her that she could audit classes but would not obtain a degree. This was Harvard's first rebuke to Taussig.

Taussig then applied to the Johns Hopkins School of Medicine where she was admitted. (Nearly 50 years before, a wise and wealthy lady had pledged one-half a million dollars to Hopkins under the condition that the school would admit women on the same basis as men). After graduating from medical school, Taussig wanted to be a cardiologist. (In those days, and even 25 years later, this meant a cardiologist for adults). She was steered toward pedi-

atrics, an appropriate career track for young ladies in those days. Edward A.
Park, Chairman and Head of the Harriet Lane Home for Invalid Children, a
major influence in American pediatrics, took Taussig under his wing and encouraged her to establish a cardiac clinic which would concentrate on rheumatic as well as congenital heart conditions. This clinic at Harriet Lane
became her base of operations for the next 50 years. With the virtual disappearance of rheumatic fever in the United States and the growing surgery of
congenital heart disease, the clinic population shifted largely toward congenital malformations. Taussig hovered over her large patient population;
she knew the children and their families intimately and as time went on the
cardiology fellows also became her children. This was her family, a tightly
knit group of young patients and young doctors from all over the United
States and overseas with a marvelous esprit de corps.

Taussig's tools in understanding cardiac malformation were based first on
pathology. She personally dissected hundreds of specimens and was a close
friend and disciple of Abbott. She really understood the anatomy of congenital cardiac malformations. Among clinical tools, the fluoroscope might have
been her favorite. Her hearing was seriously impaired from an early age, thus
auscultation was not her forte. Under the fluoroscope, however, she could
see the anatomy very clearly and could correlate it with her profound knowledge of pathology. Significant also was her understanding of each individual
child as a total person, physical and emotional. Taussig was at first antago-
nistic toward cardiac catheterization. It is not clear whehter her antagonism
was due to aversion to performing additional invasive tests on children, or
due to her lack of understanding of physiological concepts. Seeing many cyanotic children, she gradually defined the clinical, radiologic, and electrocardiographic profile for Tetralogy of Fallot, the most common subgroup of
blue babies. She noticed that among this group, those who had continuous
murmurs were significantly less blue than the others. From this observation
came the original idea of attempting to create an artificial ductus to increase
pulmonary flow of children with tetralogy of Fallot.

Taussig's idea led to her second rebuke from the Harvard Medical School.
One of Taussig's most striking characteristics was her straight, uncluttered,
even unsophisticated thinking. In many ways she was similar to Gross in this
regard. She knew well that Gross, had successfully interrupted a patent ductus arteriosus in 1938 and had done this new operation many times since
then. If a surgeon could ligate and divide the ductus, why couldn't he create
an artificial one? Taussig actually travelled to Boston in the early 1940's to
propose the shunt operation for blue babies to Gross. He listened but was not
interested. He was at the crest of his career and ductus surgery was highly
successful and safe. Coarctation treatment was on the horizon. Taussig re-

turned to Baltimore, where Blalock had been appointed Professor and Head of Surgery. Baltimore became the Mecca for blue babies. When the Harvard Medical School, years later, gave Taussig an honorary degree she recited both earlier Harvard rebuffs (28).

Blalock and Taussig were indeed completely different personalities (29). Probably because of her deafness, Taussig guarded her territory closely. Blalock appeared on the surface as an urbane Southerner, suave and polite. Actually, he was a determined surgeon and the glove hid an iron fist. In contrast to Taussig, he was thoroughly trained in physiology and experimental surgery. Blalock had the ability to cut through nonessentials and arrive at the core of a problem, an important attribute of greatness. This ability demands a singularity of purpose and simplicity of thought. Minds of greater intellectual capacity who lack this quality sometimes cannot find their way through the maze of false leads to arrive at the goal of discovery. Directness of thought, mistaken by some as simplemindedness, is essential to scientific discovery. Directness of thought combined with tenacity, or doggedness, were characteristics of Blalock. For years, he and his assistant Vivien Thomas worked on animals before attempting surgery for the Tetralogy of Fallot (30).

Clearly, fundamental changes have occurred in the care of patients with heart disease in this century. The changes are not only quantitative (establishment of boards and sub-boards with a dramatic increase in the number of certified cardiologists) and qualitative (the technical advances), but also philosophical. Today the cardiologist must be like the surgeon, a technically involved clinician who is familiar with invasive as well as noninvasive techniques.

A man who best represents the new breed of cardiologist was William J. Rashkind. He took the great step forward from diagnostic to therapeutic catheterization in congenital heart disease. Rashkind, born in New Jersey in 1922, had both his undergraduate and graduate education at the University of Louisville, Kentucky, with an MD degree in 1946. After a rotating internship at Michael Reese Hospital in Chicago, he entered the Navy and worked for two years in physiology and hemodynamics at the Naval Medical Institute in Bethesda, Maryland. He pursued his hemodynamic interests for another four years in the Physiology department at the University of Pennsylvania. Rashkind finally decided that he really wanted to be a doctor and began his training in Pediatrics in 1953 at The Children's Hospital of Philadelphia, where he remained for the rest of his life, eventually becoming professor, senior staff member, and head of the catheterization laboratory.

Conceptualization and practical application of balloon atrial septostomy for palliation of transposition of the great arteries was Rashkind's major contribution to the field. The results were presented first at the annual meeting of the American Academy of Pediatrics in Chicago in 1965, and published in the Journal of the American Medical Association (JAMA) in 1966 (31). This relatively simple, ingenious maneuver consists of introducing a deflated balloon into the foramen ovale through a catheter inserted into the inferior vena cava through fluoroscopy control. Once the balloon is lodged in the left atrium, it is blown up with contrast material and pulled back forcefully into the right atrium, causing a large tear in the atrial septum, resulting in an increase in arterial oxygen saturation and venting of the high pressure left atrium. The procedure was simple but needed consummate courage and skill. As Rashkind, with characteristic wit, once said, "The important thing is the big jerk at the end of the catheter." Balloon atrial septostomy significantly improved the clinical course of critically ill babies with transposition of the great arteries. The maneuver was accepted globally and became an eponym. "The Rashkind" was announced with distortion, but clearly recognizable in all languages.

Important as this brilliant maneuver was in the care of children, perhaps more important was establishment of the principle that the cardiac catheter may also be used for treatment purposes in congenital heart disease. This approach had been used for some time in the treatment of coronary heart disease but its application in pediatric cardiology should be credited to Rashkind. Following publication of his paper on balloon septostomy (31), he reported on catheter closure of atrial defect, patent ductus arteriosus, and on animal experiments conducted with closing of ventricular defect (32).

Rashkind was a spectacular human being. Academically, he was brilliant; he was a consummate gadgeteer and physiologist; clinically he was a warm, dedicated, compassionate physician and he enjoyed life. He loved good food and good wine; in search of these devotions he travelled widely in the disguise of medical education. He loved and was very knowledgeable in the fine arts, good books, movies, theater, and opera. He said once that one of the major advantages of living and working in Philadelphia was that you could take the train to New York early Saturday afternoon, go to dinner and the theater in the city, pick up the Sunday New York Times, read it on the train and still be at home in bed at a reasonable hour.

The prototype of the modern cardiac pediatric surgeon is Aldo R. Castaneda. Castaneda was born in Genoa, Italy, where his parents landed, in transit from Guatemala to Germany. He spent his childhood and adolescence in Munich; he was deeply affected, fascinated, and repelled by the horrors of the Nazi regime. Castaneda came from a distinguished medical family in Guatemala; both his father and his uncle were professors at the medical school there. It was, thus, a logical move for him to return home from post-war Germany and enroll in the Medical School of the University of Guatemala, obtaining his M.D. degree in 1957.

While a medical student in Guatemala, Castaneda had his initial contact with the Children's Hospital in Boston, MA. Louis K. Diamond, Senior Physician at Children's and Professor of Pediatrics at the Harvard Medical School, visited Guatemala as the guest of the local Pediatric Society to give a few lectures and, of course, to admire the Inca treasures of Tical and the scenic beauties of Lake Atitlan. Young Castaneda acted as an interpreter to Diamond, a brilliant teacher and an expert talent scout, who was much impressed by Castaneda, and was anxious to help him obtain the best possible training in surgery, his chosen career. He arranged for Castaneda to come to Boston and be interviewed by his good friend Robert E. Gross for a job in his surgical training program. Castaneda indeed came to Boston, saw Gross, but nothing came of it. His internship was at the Guatemala General Hospital.

Castaneda entered the surgical training program at the University of Minnesota, from where he obtained a Ph.D. in Surgery in 1963, and an M.S. in Physiology in 1964. These were heady days in surgery in Minnesota. Owen Wangenstein was Chief and Walt Lillehei was deeply involved in developing circulatory support for open heart surgery first through cross circulation and later through the use of a pump oxygenator, a modification of the Gibbon pump. Castaneda was strongly influenced by these two mentors, as well as by Richard Varco, whose right-hand man he eventually became. Castaneda's surgical brilliance was recognized early, and by 1970 he became full Professor of Surgery at Minnesota.

It is interesting to contemplate the cosmopolitan background of Castaneda. Born in Italy, of Guatemalan parents, raised in Germany, educated to the M.D. level in Guatemala, and trained in surgery in the United States. Castaneda arrived in Boston in September of 1972. Gross retired on June 30th of that year. Gross was very pleased by the selection of the committee; he liked the fact that a practical, no-nonsense operating surgeon was chosen as his successor. He appreciated Castaneda's youth and liked the fact that he was interested in the laboratory (having worked on lung auto-transplants in primates prior to leaving Minnesota). However, there was no doubt that his prime responsibility was meticulous care of patients. He espoused close collaboration and mutual support, among surgeons and cardiologists, intensivists, anesthesiologists, radiologists, nurses, basic scientists, and pathologists. The result is the cardiology department at the Children's Hospital, a highly successful experiment in patient care, medical education and research.

Congenital heart disease is a field of medicine in which the surgeon has shown the way. Without the surgical pioneers, cardiac malformations would have remained interesting abnormalties with no further hope for successful therapy.

REFERENCES

1. Stensen, N. Embryo monstro affinis Parisiis dissectus 1665. Acta Med. Philos. Hafniensis, 1:200–304, 1673.
2. Warburg, E. Niels Stensen's Beskrivelse af det forste publicerede Tilfaede af "Fallots Tetrade". Nord. Med., 16:3550–3551, 1942.
3. Moller-Cristensen, A. G. The Medical Faculty 1479-1842. Copenhagen, Kobenhavns Universitet, 7:39–43, 1979.
4. Miller, W. S. Niels Stensen. Johns Hopkins Hosp. Bull., 25:44–51, 1914.
5. Willius, F. A. An unusually early description of the so-called Tetralogy of Fallot. Cardiac Clinics 124. Proc. Staff Meetings Mayo Clinic, 23:316–320, 1948.
6. Scherz, G. Pioneer der Wissenschaft: Niels Stensen in seinen Schriften. Copenhagen, Munksgaard, 1963.
7. Bennet, L. R. Sandifort's "Observationes," Chapter 1, concerning a very rare disease of the heart. I. Tetralogy of Fallot or Sandifort? Bull. Hist. Med., 20:539–570, 1946.
8. Peacock, T. B. On malformations of the human heart: with original cases and illustrations. 2nd ed. London, Churchill, 1866.
9. The London and Provincial Medical Directory, 1858.
10. Spitzer, A. Ueber den Bauplan des normalen und missbildeten Herzens. Versuch einer phylogenetischen Theorie. Virchows Arch. Pathol. Anat. Physiol. Klin. Med., 243:81–272, 1923.
11. Mann, R. J. and J. T. Lie. The life story of Wilhelm Ebstein (1836–1912) and his almost overlooked description of a congenital heart disease. Mayo Clinic Proc., 54:197–204, 1979.
12. Bartalos, M. Wilhelm Ebstein: a forgotten founder of biochemical genetics. Humangenetik, 1:396, 1965.
13. Ebstein, W. Das chronische Rueckfallfieber, eine neue Infektionskrankheit. Berliner Klin. Wochenschr., 24:565–568, 1887.
14. Ebstein, W. Ueber einen sehr seltenen Fall von Insufficienz der Valvula Tricuspidalis, bedingt durch eine angeborene hochgradige Missbildung derselben. Arch. Anat. Physiol. Wissenshaftl., 33:238–254, 1866.
15. Arnstein, A. Ein seltene Missbildung der Trikuspidalklappe (Ebsteinsche Krankheit). Virchows Arch. Pathol. Anat. Physiol. Klin. Med., 266:247–254, 1927.
16. Dobell, A. Maude Abbott: Portrait of a Pioneer. The Second Clinical Conference on Congenital Heart Disease: B.L. Tucker, G.G. Lindesmith, and M. Takahashi. Gruber and Stratton, Inc., 1982.
17. MacDermot, H. E. Maude Abbott: a memoir. Toronto, Macmillan, 1941.
18. Osler, W. The principles and practice of medicine. New York, Appleton, 1892.
19. Gross, R.E. Hubbard, J.P. Surgical ligation of patent ductus arteriosus. Report of first successful case. JAMA 112:729, 1939.
20. Ladd and Gross. Abdominal Surgery of Infancy and Childhood, W.B. Saunders Co., Philadelphia, PA, 1941.
21. Folkman, M.J. Harvard Medical Alumni Magazine, obituary, 1988.

22. Craafoord, C. Congential coarctation of the aorta and its surgical treatment, J. Thorac. Surg., 14:347, 1945.

23. Ravitch, M. M. Alfred Blalock, 1899–1964. In: The Papers of Alfred Blalock. Baltimore, Johns Hopkins Press, 1966.

24. Ravitch, M. M. Progress in resection of the chest wall for tumor with reminiscences of Dr. Blalock. Johns Hopkins Med. J., 151:43–53, 1982.

24a. Longmire, W.P, Jr. Alfred Blalock: His Life and Times, 1991 William Longmire Jr.

25. Bahnson, H. T. Classics in thoracic surgery: Surgical treatment of pulmonary stenosis: a retrospection. Ann. Thorac. Surg., 33:96–98, 1982.

26. Levy, S. E. and A. Blalock. Experimental Observations on the Effects of Connecting by Suture the Left Main Pulmonary Artery to the Systemic Circulation. J. Thorac. Surg., 8:525–530, 1939.

27. McNamara, D. G. The Blalock-Taussig operation and subsequent progress in surgical treatment of cardiovascular diseases. JAMA, 251:2139–2141, 1984.

28. Nadas, A. Personal communication.

29. Bing, R. J. The John Hopkins: The Blalock-Taussig Era. Persp. Biol. Med., 32:85–90, 1988.

30. Thomas, V. Pioneering Research in Surgical Shock and Cardiovascular Surgery: Vivien Thomas and his work with Alfred Blalock. University of Pennsylvania Press, Philadelphia, PA 1985.

31. Rashkind, W.J., Creation of an atrial septal defect without thoractomy. A pallative approach to complete transposition of the great arteries. JAMA, 196:991, 1966.

32. Rashkind, W.J., Proc. Assoc. of European Ped. Cardiologists, 14:8, 1976.

Chapter 5

Transplantation Of
The Heart

J. BALDWIN AND R.J. BING

Fifty years after Alexis Carrel's pioneering contributions to vascular surgery his work was largely forgotten. Julius Comroe, in his article on Alexis Carrel, reported that when he interviewed 111 cardiovascular scientists, only 7 knew of Carrel's great contribution to vascular surgery, most of them writing after Carrel's name, "Never heard of him" (1). And yet, Carrel (1873 to 1944) pioneered in all fields of vascular surgery, tissue culture, and culture of organs (Figure 1). Among publications which dealt with the transplantation of blood vessels, their preservation in cold storage, with transplantation tolerance and immunity of isografts, allografts and xenografts, Carrell made several references to the transplantation of the heart.

Carrel's surgical innovations were vital to his cardiac transplantation work. His work on the technique of blood vessel sutures, which he perfected as a young physician in Lyon, France, became the cornerstone of his research. His purely technical accomplishment, the anastomosis of blood vessels by triangulation, became the basis of his research. It shows that a simple, rather limited technical advance can lead to extraordinary physiological and technical progress, to specify a few: transplantation of the kidney, of the heart, of an organ from a cadaver to a recipient, of tumors, and the discovery of transplantation immunity. Carrel was quick to recognize that even the most perfect technique with avoidance of infection, was inadequate to guarantee successful transplantation of organs, because of the rejection of the

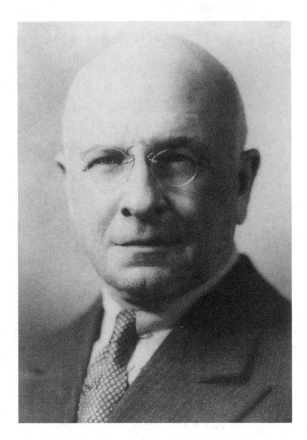

Figure 1.   Alexis Carrel (*Courtesy of The New York Academy of Medicine*)

transplant. Stress on transplantation immunity was one of Carrel's outstanding contributions. As he wrote in his article on "The Transplantation of Organs:"

> As yet these methods (surgical) cannot be applied to human surgery, for the reason that homoplastic transplantations are almost always unsuccessful from the standpoint of the function of the organs. All our efforts must now be directed toward the biological methods, which will prevent the reaction of the organism against foreign tissue and allow the adapting of homoplastic grafts to their hosts (2).

In line with transplantation immunity, Carrel discovered, together with James Murphy of the Rockefeller Institute, that while tumor cells grew very rapidly on chick fetuses to which they had been grafted alone or together with chicken kidney, liver or connective tissue, they grew very little or not at all when pieces of spleen or bone marrow were grafted to the fetus. At the same time, he and Murphy discovered that when they grafted a mouse tumor onto rats, which previously had never taken on rats, splenectomy led to active growth of the tumor for 12 or 13 days, that is longer than in the controls. In the presence of benzol, which diminishes activity of leukocytes and lymphocytes, the duration of life of the mouse tumor was longer and resorption did not occur before 15 days (2). Equally, x-ray exposure to rats led to prolonged survival of mouse tumor. After 35 days, the tumor was still growing. Carrel concluded that the power of the organism to eliminate (reject) foreign tissue was due to organs such as the spleen and bone marrow and that when the activity of these organs was lessened, a foreign tissue can develop rapidly after it had been grafted. This was an early recognition of the role of lymphoid cells in the rejection of transplants (2). Carrel received the Nobel Prize for these studies.

When discussing the surgery of blood vessels in the Johns Hopkins Hospital Bulletin, Carrel noted that the wall of a vein, used as an arterial transplant conduit, reacted very quickly by thickening as a sequence of an increase of blood pressure (3). Using his blood vessel suture technique, Carrel anastomosed the peripheral end of the renal artery to the splenic vein (spleno-renal shunt) and produced a stenosis of the portal vein near the liver. "Venous blood flowed through the renal artery, the kidney, the renal vein and into the vena cava." All kinds of veins were transplanted to all kinds of arteries, end to side, or end to end. An accidental finding was that transplantation of one or two large veins of the thyroid gland into the carotid artery produced a "strong arterial hyperemia, which, in one animal suffering from myxedema, led to improvement of this state; the animal lost excess fat, hair grew rapidly on the bald spots and it became very lively and pugnacious."

In addition, replantation of the kidney was performed several times; for instance the kidney was implanted in the abdominal cavity with anastomosis of the vessels (4,5). Replantation of the leg was also successfully performed.

Experimental bypass operations, in which veins were transplanted to arteries, were repeatedly carried out and led to coronary bypass operations (6,7). Carrel also described that xenografts of blood vessels were possible if the blood vessels had been previously maintained in cold storage for several days prior to implantation (8). He also transplanted skin and, on December 6, 1911 he wrote (8):

The cadaver of an infant who had died during labor was used for the extirpation of cutaneous and other grafts. Several hours after death, the body of the child was washed with soap and water and with ether. Dermoepidermic grafts and flaps of skin were extirpated in large numbers and washed in Ringer's solution. Bones were also extirpated. With the Wassermann reaction negative, the dermoepidermic grafts and the flaps of skin, preserved in petrolatum and in Ringer's solution, were used at the Rockefeller Hospital for the treatment of three large ulcers and one circular ulcer of the leg in two patients.

Reference to transplantation of the heart was made in several publications of Carrel's prior to 1912. In 1905, in a paper in American Medicine, Carrel described the transplantation of the heart of a small dog into the neck of a larger one, by anastomosing the cut ends of the jugular vein and the carotid artery to the aorta, the pulmonary artery, the vena cava and a pulmonary vein (9). Circulation was reestablished through the heart about one hour and 15 minutes after the cessation of the beat; 20 minutes after the reestablishment of the circulation, the blood flowed actively, circulating through the coronary system. Strong fibrillar contractions were seen. Afterward, contractions of the auricles appeared, and, about an hour after the operation, effective contractions of the ventricles began. The transplanted heart beat at the rate of 88 per minute, while the rate of the normal heart was 100/minute. A little later, tracings were taken. Owing to the fact that the operation was made without aseptic technique, the experiment had to be terminated.

Alexis Carrel was cut from a different cloth than other members of the Rockefeller Institute (10,11). He was gregarious, interested in matters other than science such as politics, religion and philosophy. He published articles in popular journals and wrote a popular book dealing with his philosophy concerning primarily man's relationship to his environment and his fellow man. He was a hardworking and dedicated scientist who collaborated in the laboratory every day with his associates, but what distuingished him from his colleagues was primarily his desire to extrapolate his research into the general panorama of the world outside the laboratory. He used his scientific observations as springboards into philosophical, cultural, even parapsychological fields. In this respect he was akin to men of the Renaissance such as Roger Bacon who could not separate the occult from the proven truth and saw no distinction between truth and speculation.

Carrel's work had the most profound effect on the development of cardiovascular surgery, organ transplantation, and tissue culture. His work developed from a relatively simple technique, that of blood vessel suture. He once said that he became interested in "suturing things together" from watching a seamstress who came to the Carrel home. With blood vessel sutures, based on triangulation, and carried out with unusual dexterity (having practiced the suture technique in a match box with one hand), he transplanted organs including the heart, performed the first experimental coronary bypass operation, and the reimplantation of blood vessels preserved in vitro. He realized immediately that the technique of organ transplantation was easy, compared to overcoming the rejection phenomenon. His experiments with Lindbergh to invent methods for cardiopulmonary bypass, originating from Lindbergh's wish to operate on a bloodless heart, were indeed a farsighted idea for the early 1930s. This visionary approach was premature and Carrel and Lindbergh settled for the development of a technique to maintain viability of organs outside the body (12).

What got Carrel into trouble was his tendency to discuss general politics in public and his admiration for strong personalities which offended many of his colleagues. He was a genius of a highly contradictory nature, who had the comforting gift to justify his prejudices to himself with a high degree of naivete and honesty. Simon Flexner, the Director of the Rockefeller Institute, was well aware that Carrel did not fit the pattern of the rest of his flock of scientists at the Institute. Flexner was patient with Carrel considering him an asset to the Institute. When Flexner retired and Herbert Gasser became director of the Institute all of this changed. Gasser, a Nobel Prize winner himself, was the antithesis of Carrel. A punctilious and proper man, administrator and investigator, he considered Carrel a gadfly and a foreign body at the Rockefeller Institute. He soon made Carrel feel unwelcome and this also expressed the feelings of a majority of the faculty.

Carrel returned to his native France, a most ill advised venture, given the Nazi occupation. He must have suffered a great deal during his last years isolated from his friends and his adopted country (13). Carrel was a multifaceted, scintillating but eventually tragic genius, whose charasteristics were bound to conflict with those of his colleagues who saw in him a proponent of scientific and political extravagance.

Carrel's work was the stimulus for subsequent studies on cardiac transplantation. In Carrel's experiment the transplanted heart was in essence an in situ Langendorff preparation, with the heart muscle performing little work. The main purpose was perfusion of the coronary circulation.

His example was followed by Frank C. Mann (1887–1962) from the Mayo Clinic, Director of the Mayo Foundation Institute of Experimental Medicine from 1914 to 1948, who was a world authority on the physiology of the liver, gastrointestinal surgery, and surgery of the kidneys and blood vessels (14). Dr. Mann pioneered in experimental surgery by bringing rigid surgical technique to the experimental laboratory. One of Mann's most remarkable achievements was his work on complete removal of the liver, which made it possible to study the function of this organ. Mann published an article on transplantation of the intact mammalian heart in which he followed the procedure outlined by Carrel (15). He describes that the heart usually began to contract immediately after the coronary circulation had been established. He made the statement, already previously formulated by Carrel that "Failure of the homotransplanted heart to survive is not due to the technique of transplantation but to some biologic factor which is probably identical to that which prevents survival of other homotransplanted tissues and organs."

It is clear from the nature of the preparation that the heart transplanted to the neck can serve primarily one purpose, that of determining its metabolism and speed of rejection. Since the heart does not perform work, the model is dissimilar to the heart transplanted into the chest, serving as a replacement for the recipient heart. However, valuable information has been obtained with the Carrel preparation. For example, Downie using the Carrel method, speculated that rejection was the result of a "humoral agency" which was responsible for the destruction of the transplant (16). The preparation was used by Reemtsma and his associates, to study the metabolism of the transplanted heart (17). They reported on myocardial oxygen consumption and carbohydrate utilization. The former showed distinct variations; no marked difference in myocardial glucose consumption of the transplant as compared to the working heart of the recipient in situ was found. However they observed myocardial lactate production rather than consumption in the majority of their experiments. Similar results were obtained by Lee and Webb (18). Sinitsyn in Soviet Russia, in 1948, maintained the coronary circulation of a homografted heart through the action of its own ventricle (19). Lee and Webb found that in the normothermic homograft the coronary flow in the dog averaged 128 cc/100g of left ventricle per minute and the myocardial oxygen consumption 6.4 cc/minute.

Chiba and Bing and their co-workers described in detail the metabolism of the heart transplanted to the neck of a recipient dog by the method of Carrel and Mann (20,21). They also found that the homografted heart released lactate as well as pyruvate together with malic dehydrogenase and aldolase, while extraction of glucose by the graft usually remained positive. However, when there was accelerated rejection the release of pyruvate and lactate was more pronounced and even glucose appeared in increased concentration in coronary vein blood. The respiratory quotient of the transplanted heart was elevated possibly signifying conversion of carbohydrate to fat (21). An interesting finding was the absence of anoxia of the transplant as indicated by a positive redox potential across the transplanted heart. Rejection of a transplant is not apparently accompanied by myocardial hypoxia. Some histologic findings were similar to those later found in the human cardiac transplant. For example, accumulation of lymphocytes and swelling of vascular endothelium together with polar perivascular cellular infiltration by lymphocytes, plasma cells, macrophages and histiocytes were found. Some other pathological changes appeared in this preparation, such as Aschoff and Anitschkow-like cells. After eight days, necrosis of the myocardium became prominent and endothelial hyperplasia occurred at 14 days. It is possible that this endothelial hyperplasia was an early stage of the severe coronary artery changes later reported in human transplant.

These reports were preliminary to performing transplants in man. Several groups laid the groundwork. Marcus and co-workers, for example, described techniques for the transplantation of a heart in the chest of a dog and speculated on the ultimate use of a transplanted heart as a replacement functioning organ (22). Marcus was not optimistic and wrote, "The latter [transplant heart or heart-lung preparation to be used for replacement of a diseased organ] must be considered at present a fantastic dream and does not fall within the scope of present considerations." Webb and co-workers also described in 1958 a practical method of homologous cardiac transplantation (23). They referred to the work of Neptune and associates who were the first to transplant the combined canine heart and lungs into the mediastinum to replace the recipient's own heart and lungs and reported on a six-hour survival (24). Of 12 technically successful transplants utilizing refrigerated hearts, ten were able to maintain normal blood pressure from 30 minutes to seven and one-half hours (23). Similar to Webb, Hardy carefully explored different operative procedures, using the heart of a lower primate to replace a human heart (25). Unfortunately the primate heart became increasingly unable to handle the large venous return and one hour after the removal of the bypass catheter, the heart was judged incapable of accepting the large venous return without intermittent decompression by manual cardiac massage.

Much credit for human heart transplantation should go to Norman Shumway (26; Figure 2). Shumway's work with Dick Lower in the late 1950s was facilitated by the move of the Stanford Medical School from San Francisco to Palo Alto and the reluctance of many of the senior clinical scientists to join those who were willing to make the risky trek. Shumway and Lower borrowed from a wide range of other experiences and assimilated the accumulating knowledge culminating in the landmark studies which were reported in *Surgical Forum* in 1960 (26). Shumway had a strong interest in myocardial preservation and was a pioneer in the use of cold immersion for induction of hypothermic metabolic inhibition in cardiac tissue. He combined this work with the availability of the early heart-lung machine and the mid-atrial excision and reimplantation technique of Lord Russell Brock to achieve the first successful orthotopic cardiac transplant in the canine model (26,27).

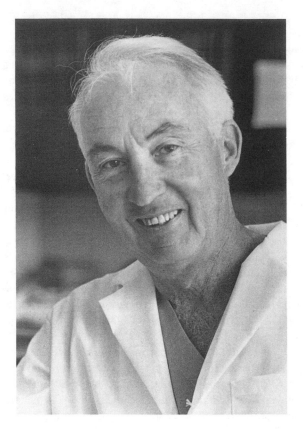

Figure 2.   Norman E. Shumway (*Courtesy of the New York Academy of Medicine*)

Later, Shumway and others in the Stanford transplant laboratory borrowed from those interested in kidney transplantation and in cytotoxic chemotherapy for malignant disease to establish the means for prevention of rejection. R. Lower and others observed the loss of electrocardiographic voltage occurring in transplanted canine hearts, and this made clinical cardiac transplantation truly feasible (28). Prior to that time, without a noninvasive means of diagnosing rejection of the organ, cardiac transplantation was not truly conscionable, because of the fact that survival of the graft was equivalent to the survival of the host. The electrocardiographic finding, which was based upon the development of intramyocardial edema and which was therefore correlated with other clinical findings such as the development of a gallop, remained useful and reliable up until the introduction of cyclosporine. After the introduction of cyclosporine for heart transplantation, intramyocardial edema was found to be a less prominent histological feature, and the electrocardiogram, even with signal averaging, was insufficiently sensitive (29).

The rapid progress made in the late 1950s and early 1960s ushered in the era of clinical cardiac transplantation, which began with the first human transplant in 1964, a xenograft operation performed by Dr. James Hardy in Mississippi (29a). Hardy's patient did not survive, but his report of this experience in the Journal of the American Medical Association accelerated progress toward widespread clinical implementation.

Shumway's 1960 *Surgical Forum* paper is, to this day, the paradigm for cardiac transplantation technique, and it was based upon this technique that Christian Barnard performed the first allograft operation in December of 1967 at the Groote Schuur Hospital in Cape Town (30). The patient survived a mere 18 days, but the widespread publicity associated with this effort served further to accelerate the clinical implementation of cardiac transplantation.

Norman Shumway began his clinical program at Stanford two weeks later in January of 1968 and this proved to be the only uninterrupted program in the world during the period from January of 1968 to the present.

While the operation had been based upon the assimilation of a wide range of laboratory experiences, clinical implementation required even greater collaboration of cardiac surgeons, cardiologists, infectious disease specialists, clinical immunologists, pulmonary medicine specialists, and nephrologists. Even with the tremendous collaborative effort at Stanford, the early experience was difficult. During the first year, approximately 20% one-year survival was obtained (31). This was a spectacular outcome in view of the fact that no candidate survived more than a year without an operation and that the mean survival time for waiting recipients was only three months. One hundred cardiac transplants were attempted at more than 60 centers worldwide during 1968 with abysmal results. The poor results brought about a widespread condemnation of cardiac transplantation as a procedure, and by 1971, the September 17th issue of *Life Magazine* ran a cover story entitled "The Tragic Record of Heart Transplants." The conclusion of the scientific community seemed to be that heart transplantation was a good example of clinical medicine outstripping the associated basic science and resulting in tragically unsuccessful clinical outcomes.

Shumway had to overcome many other types of adversity, including the absence of brain death laws, when he began his program. Newspaper headlines suggested that those removing donor hearts from gunshot wound victims were in fact the real murderers. A tremendous political and legislative effort was required to establish brain death criteria for organ procurement, and this was only a fraction of the overall public and scientific skepticism. Opposition was pervasive in the medical and scientific community, and those who did accept the Stanford program regarded it as an exotic hybrid which could be tolerated but which should not be emulated elsewhere. Nonetheless, the Stanford results steadily improved through refinement of surgical technique, improved immunosuppression with the introduction of anti-thymocyte globulin derived from rabbits in 1977, improving antibiotics, and meticulous attention to detail in recipient selection and postoperative care. The results were difficult to ignore, but many outstanding academic medical institutions rejected introduction of cardiac transplantation, often with great fanfare, attracting the attention of the federal government and others.

Shumway and his Stanford colleagues doggedly persisted and by the end of the decade of the 70s, 80% of the transplant recipients were surviving to one year with 87% rehabilitation—better than any other cardiac surgical operation available.

Cyclosporine was introduced in December of 1980 for cardiac transplantation at Stanford (32). The incidence of rejection was not reduced, nor was the incidence of infection. However, these two major complications of cardiac transplantation were both ameliorated by the introduction of the new agent. Rejection episodes tended to be less catastrophic, and outpatient treatment of rejection was introduced for the first time. While infection was not less frequent, patients tended to respond more reliably to appropriate antimicrobial therapy. While cyclosporine was associated with improvement in results, it also gave an opportunity for many institutions to cite a reason for re-thinking their acceptance of cardiac transplantation, other than the fact that they had been unconvinced before. A multitude of programs sprang up across the nation, and by the mid-1980s, more than 2,000 cardiac transplants were being performed in more than 100 centers in the United States each year. In addition, active programs began in England at the Papworth Hospital in Cambridge and at the Harefield Hospital in London, and in France at LaPitié in Paris and elsewhere. In 1981, the International Society For Heart Transplantation was founded, with Norman Shumway as its Honorary President. Cardiac transplantation is now established worldwide as an effective mode of therapy for patients with endstage heart failure.

Replacement of the entire heart-lung block has also been accomplished. Elevation of pulmonary vascular resistance has made this combined procedure necessary. Early, the Stanford group considered elevation in pulmonary vascular resistance beyond 6–8 Wood units which is unresponsive to vasodilator infusions to be a strict contraindication to orthotopic cardiac transplantation, because of the inability of the normal donor right ventricle to sustain the circulation against the high pressures. Because of the frequent finding of fixed pulmonary hypertension, the Stanford group was keenly interested in pursuing the work of Neptune, Webb, Castaneda, and others in replacement of the entire heart-lung block. The absence of the Herring-Breuer reflex in dogs had made this a difficult problem to study experimentally, but it was found that when the phrenic nerves were carefully preserved, the operation could be successfully performed in monkeys and that they would resume normal ventilation and be able to be weaned from the ventilator. With the introduction of cyclosporine in clinical cardiac transplantation in 1980, successful intermediate term survival in monkeys was demonstrated in the lab by Shumway, Reitz, and others (33), therefore clinical implementation was contemplated.

The first successful combined heart-lung transplant operation was performed in March of 1981 (34). While this operation is technically considerably more demanding than the heart transplant operation and while lung preservation has been a formidable laboratory and clinical problem, heart-lung transplantation has emerged as a highly successful mode of therapy for patients with endstage pulmonary and pulmonary vascular disease. Presently, more than 250 heart-lung transplant operations are performed per year with more than 60% one year survival (35,36).

The future of cardiac transplantation will involve wider application of the operation, particularly in cases of congenital heart disease. Newer immunosuppressive agents will reduce the toxicity associated with immunosuppression and reduce postoperative rejection. The problem of the shortage of available organ donors can be solved through refinement of mechanical heart replacement devices and the introduction of xenograft transplantation. Past experience would indicate that biological placement is likely to be preferable to mechanical devices in terms of quality of life, and xenograft transplantation will be achieved through better understanding of the basic immunology of cardiac transplantation and, quite possibly, through the creation of transgenic lines of animals which have decreased or absent expression of histocompatibility antigens.

Carrel had already clearly demonstrated that the problem in cardiac transplantation was not surgical technique, but rejection of the graft. It is not within the scope of this chapter to describe the development of our knowledge of homograft immunity and tolerance. But reference will be made to the contributions of Peter Medawar. Dr. Peter Brian Medawar was Director of the National Institute for Medical Research in London and received the Nobel Prize in physiology and medicine in 1960. He was born in Rio de Janero, studied at Oxford under Sir Howard W. Florey and became

Professor of Zoology in the University College, University of London (37). One of his greatest accomplishments was to focus on the problem of cellular versus humoral mechanism of rejection, the host versus graft, and graft versus host reactions and the importance of sensitized lymphoid cells. As Medawar wrote,

> In the orthodox homograft reaction a relatively small graft is transplanted into a relatively large animal, whereupon it excites and eventually succumbs to an immunological response. In the graft versus host reaction the cells suspected of being responsible for that reaction are removed from one animal and injected into another, so that they can attack the animal into which they are put, the host now playing the part of the graft in the conventional reaction. The host animal is either rendered incapable of counter-attacking the injected cells by irradiation, or is naturally incapable of doing so by being too young... (38).

The best known example of graft versus host disease is the runt disease, a stunting of newborn animals by the injection into them of allogenic adult lymphocytes" (39).

Graft versus host reaction was discovered by James B. Murphy of the Rockefeller Institute whom we encountered previously in his work with Carrel. To grow neoplastic cells in an embryo, he carefully cut out a rectangular opening in the shell of fowl eggs, inoculated the exposed chorioallantoic membrane with the neoplasm, and reincubated the eggs. He found when the eggs were opened that the chick embryo displayed changes such as nodules in the membranes and enlargement of the spleen. To Murphy's great surprise, similar changes occured also in embryo's injected with normal spleen cells or spleen fragments, indicating that the changes in the heart had nothing to do with any neoplastic nature of the inocculum. In 1956 the graft versus host reaction was rediscovered by Brent and Medawar (40). They wanted to induce tolerance in mice of one strain to tissues from another strain; they injected donor spleen cells into the veins of newborn mice and later grafted the adult mice with the skin from the same donor. They observed that while tolerance could be induced in a high proportion of injected mice in some strain combinations, the injected animal in other combinations stopped growing and runted as if suffering from a mysterious runt disease. This disease was interpreted as being the consequence of an immunological attack by grafted cells on the immunologically immature recipient.

In his Nobel lecture, Medawar pays tribute to the remarkable work of Ray Owen, (Figure 3) now at the California Institute of Technology in Pasadena, who discovered that most twin cattle are born with, and may retain throughout life a stable mixture—not necessarily a 50-50 mixture—of each other's red cells (41); it followed then, that the twin cattle must have exchanged red-

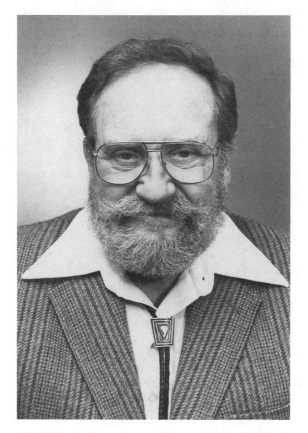

Figure 3.   Ray Owen (*with permission*)

cell precursors, and not merely red cells, in their mutual transfusion before birth. This was the first example of chimerism; the red cells could not have adapted themselves to the strange environment because they were in fact identified as native or foreign by those very antigenic properties which, had an adaptation occurred, must necessarily have been transformed. It was shown that most dizygotic cattle twins would accept skin grafts from each other and that this mutual tolerance was specific for skin transplanted from third parties and was cast off in the expected fashion. Owen's phenomenon was also duplicated in chickens by Hasek making a deliberate synchorial parabiosis between chick embryos in the shell (42). At hatching, the parabions separated and from then on they were incapable of making anti-bodies against each other's red cells and accepted each other's skin grafts. Brent and Medawar also drew attention to the importance of immunosup-pressive agents which he divided into nitrogen mustards, deoxyribo-nucleicacid (DNA) base analogues, folic-acid acid antagonists, and anti-biotics degrading DNA. This was about 20 years before the advent of cyclosporin (40).

The discovery of cyclosporin is an example of serendipity (43,44). In 1970 antimycotic activity in products of two fungi were discovered at Sandoz Laboratory in Basel, Switzerland. This was the outcome of a fundamental search from soil samples from Norway and Wisconsin. Fermentation of Trichoderma Polysporum and Cylindrocarpon Lucidum produced a com-pound with disappointing antibody potential, but some evidence of im-munosuppressive properties. In January 1972 Borel observed important immunosuppresive reactions which were not related to general toxicity. The drug certainly was a "bust" as far as antimicrobial activity was concerned but it was an unsuspected success in a completely different field. If the workers at Sandoz had used a different cell strain, cyclosporin A would not have been discovered. Stähelin writes,

> The results obtained in December and January 1971 and 1972 in the screening program already disclosed the three most important features of the biological effects of this preparation which was later found to consist mainly of cyclosporin A: effective immunosuppression with a well tolerated dose, no general inhibition of cell proliferation and impairment of kidney function at high doses. Elucidation of the chemical structure soon followed and a purer preparation of cyclosporin A was found to reduce the immune response in a number of tests: hemaglutinin production, formation of antibody-producing cells, rejection of skin grafts and grafts versus host disease. The drug exerts its main effect on T lymphocytes by interfering with the activity of Interleukin-2. The first public report on the biological effects of cyclosporin A was an oral presentation at the meeting of the Union of Swiss Societies Experimental Biol-ogy in 1976. Later, Borel reported his findings before the British Society for Immunology. In 1978, Calne of Cambridge, England undertook the first clini-cal trials in renal transplantation (44).

The pathways of cyclosporin discovery, so writes Stähelin, is a good ex-ample to show that,

> pharmaceutical research quite often proceeds in a path with many windings; and they illustrate how many people, groups of people, strokes of luck, seren-dipity, preceding events, etc. contribute to research endeavors of this kind and that they are those factors which make the difference between the usual, fre-quent failures and the rare success (44).

REFERENCES

1. Comroe, J. "Who was Alexis, Who?", Cardiovascular Diseases: Bulletin of the Texas Heart Journal, 6:251–270 (1979).
2. Carrel, A. The Transplantations of Organs, 1915
3. Carrel, Alexis "The Surgery of Blood Vessels, etc.", The Johns Hopkins Hosp. Bull., 190:18–26,1907.
4. Carrel, A., and C.C. Guthrie. Successful transplantation of both kidneys from a dog into a bitch with removal of both normal kidneys from the latter, Science, 23:394–395, 1906.
5. Carrel, A., and C.C. Guthrie. Complete amputation of the thigh with replantation, Am. J. Med. Sci., 131:297–301, 1906.
6. Carrel, A. and C.C. Guthrie. Results of the biterminal transplantation of veins, Am. J. Med. Sci., 132:415–422, 1906.
7. Carrel, A: Results of the transplantation of blood vessels, organs and limbs, J. Am. Med. Assoc., 51:1662–1667, 1906
8. Carrel, A.. The preservation of tissues and its applications in surgery, J. Am. Med. Assoc. 59:523–527, 1912.
9. Carrel, A. and C.C. Guthrie. The transplantation of veins and organs, J. Am. Med. Assoc., 10:1100–1102, 1905.
10. Edwards, W.S. and P.D. Edwards. Alexis Carrel, Visionary Surgeon, Charles C. Thomas publisher, Springfield, Illinois 1974.
11. Malinin, T.I. Surgery and Life: the Extraordinary Career of Alexis Carrel, Harcourt, Brace, Jovanovich, New York and London, 1979.
12. Bing, R.J. Lindbergh and the biological sciences: a personal reminiscence. Texas Heart Inst. J., 14:231–237, 1987.
13. Chambers, R.W. and J.T. Durkin. Papers of Alexis Carrel centennial conference, Georgetown University, 1973, Georgetown University, Washington.
14. Institute's Dr. Mann dies at 75. Mayovox, 13:2, 1962.
15. Mann, Frank C., Priestley, James T., Markowitz, J. and Yater, W.M. Transplantation of the intact mammalian heart, A.M.A. Arch. of Surg. 26:219–224, 1933.
16. Downie, H.G. Homotransplantation of the dog heart, A.M.A. Arch. Surg., 66:624–636, 1953.
17. Reemtsma K., J.P. Delgado, O. Creech. Transplantation of the homologous canine heart: serial studies of myocardial blood flow, oxygen consumption, and carbohydrate metabolism. Surgery, 47:292–300, 1960.
18. Lee, S.S., and W.R. Webb. Metabolism of the isolated normothermic and rewarmed heart, Surg. Forum 9:284–291, 1958.
19. Sinitsyn H. Transplantation as a new method In: Experimental Biology and Medicine, Moscow 1948. as quoted by S.F. Sayegh and O. Creech. Transplantation of the homologous canine heart. J. Thor. Surg., 34:692–703, 1957.
20. Bing R.J., C. Chiba, A. Chrysohou, P.L. Wolf, and S. Gudbjarnason: Transplantation of the heart. Circ. 25:273–275 1962.
21. Chiba C., P.L. Wolf, S. Gudbjarnason, A. Chrysohou, H. Ramos, B. Pearson, and R.J. Bing. Studies on the transplanted heart: Its metabolism and histology. J. Exp. Med. 115:853–866, 1962.
22. Marcus E., S.N. Wong, and A.A. Luisada. Homologous heart grafts, A.M.A. Arch. Surg., 66:179–191, 1953.

23. Webb, W.R., H.S. Howard, and W.M. Neely: Practical methods of homologous cardiac transplantation. J. Thor. Surg. 37:361–366, 1959.
24. Neptune, W.B., B.A. Cookson, C.P. Bailey, R. Appler and F. Rajkowski: Complete homologous heart transplantation. A.M.A. Arch. Surg. 66:174–178, 1953.
25. Hardy J.D., C.M. Chavez, F.D. Kurrus, W.A. Neely, S. Eraslan, M.D. Turner, L.W. Fabian, and T.D. Labecki. Heart transplantation in man. J. Am. Med. Assoc., 188:1132–1140, 1964.
26. Lower, R.R. and N.E. Shumway. Studies on orthotopic homotransplantation of the canine heart. Surg. Forum, 11:18–19, 1960.
27. Cass, M.H. and R. Brock. Heart excision and replacement. Guys Hosp. Rep. 108:285, 1959.
28. Lower, R.R., E. Dong, Jr., and F.S. Glazener. Electrocardiograms of dogs with heart homografts. Circ. 33:455–460, 1966.
29. Keren, A., A.M. Gillis, R.A. Freedman, J.C. Baldwin, M.W. Billingham, E.B. Stinson, M.B. Simson, and J.W. Mason. Heart transplant rejection monitored by signal-averaged electrocardiography in patients receiving cyclosporine. Circ. 70:I124–I129, 1984.
29a. Hardy, J.D., C.M. Chavez, F.D. Kurrus, W.A. Neely, S. Eraslan, M.D. Turner, L.W. Fabian, T.D. Labecki: Heart transplantation in man. JAMA, 188:1132, 1140, 1964.
30. Barnard, C.N.: The Operation. A human cardiac transplant: an interim report of a successful operation performed at Groote Schuur Hospital, Cape Town. S. Afr. Med. J., 41:1271–1274, 1967.
31. Baldwin, J.C., E.B. Stinson, P.E. Oyer, V. Starnes and N. Shumway. Cardiac Transplantation and Followup Care. In: The Heart, 7th Edition, ed. by J. W. Hurst, New York, McGraw Hill, 1990, pp. 2248–2254.
32. Oyer, P.E., E.B. Stinson, S.W. Jamieson, S.A. Hunt, B.A. Reitz, C.P. Bieber, J.S. Schroeder, M.B. Billingham, and N.E. Shumway. One year experience with cyclosporin A in clinical heart transplantation. Heart Trans. 1:4, 285–289, 1982.
33. Reitz, B.A., N.A. Burton, S.W. Jamieson, J.L. Pennock, E.B. Stinson and N.E. Shumway. Heart and lung transplantation. J. Thorac and Cardiovasc. Surg. 80:360–372, 1980.
34. Reitz, B.A., J.L. Wallwork, S.A. Hunt, J.L. Pennock, M.E. Billingham, P.E. Oyer, E.B. Stinson and N.E. Shumway, N.E. Heart-Lung Transplantation. N. Engl. J. Med. 306:557–564, 1982.
35. Franco, K.L., and J.C. Baldwin. Heart-lung transplantation for cystic fibrosis: an overview. J. Appl. Cardiol. 4:571-580, 1989
36. Baldwin, J.C., W.H. Frist, T.D. Starkey, A. Harjula, V.A. Starnes, E.B. Stinson, P.E. Oyer and N.E. Shumway. Distant graft procurement for combined heart and lung transplantation using pulmonary artery flush and simple topical hypothermia for graft preservation. Ann. Thorac. Surg., 43:670–673, 1987.
37. Medawar, P.B.: Do advances in medicine lead to genetic deterioration. Mayo Clinic Proceed. 40:23–33, 1965.
38. Gibson, T., and P.B. Medawar. Homografts, Chapter 1–15, in Modern Trends in Plastic Surgery, Volume 2, 1966.
39. In: Immunology the Science of Self–Nonself Discriminatino by Jan Klein,

A.Wiley—Interscience Publication, John Wiley & Sons, New York, Westchester, Brisbaine, Toronto, Singapore, page 192.

40. Brent, L., and P.B. Medawar. Cellular immunity and the homograft reaction. Brit. Med. Bull. 23:55–60, 1967.

41. Medawar, P.B. Immunological tolerance, the phenomenon of tolerance provides a testing ground for theories of the immune response, Science 133:303–306, 1961.

42. Hasek, M. Vegetative hybridization of animals by joining their blood circulations during embryonic development. Cs. Biol. 2:265–277. 1953.

43. Heimbecker, R.O. Transplantation: the cyclosporine revolution by Can. J. Cardiol. 1:354–357, 1985.

44. Stähelin, H. (Cyclosporin) Historical background. Prog. Allergy, 38:19–27, 1985.

Chapter 6

Atherosclerosis

R.J. BING

Atherosclerosis manifests itself in a variety of cardiovascular abnormalities, such as cerebral vascular accidents, myocardial infarction, and peripheral vascular disease. We know that the disease has been present since ancient times, as it has been discovered in Egyptian mummies dating from 1580 B.C. to 525 A.D. During embalming, the whole of the viscera and most of the muscles of the body were removed, while the body cavity and the holes, left in the limbs after removal of the muscles, were filled with mud, sand, or rags. The sole of the foot was packed with sawdust mixed with some resinous material. The aorta fortunately owing to its deep location, often escaped the embalmer's knife. In 1911, M.A. Ruffer isolated the mummy's aorta by placing the parts to be examined in a solution containing carbonate of soda and formalin, and soaking it for 24–48 hours when the skin could be taken off. The arteries could then be dissected out (1). Atheromas were found in almost all of the arteries examined. As Ruffer stated, "The lesions were of the same nature as we see at the present day, namely calcification following an atheroma." He said, he "could not exclude the theory that a high meat diet was the cause of the severe atherosclerosis in the mummies, as the mummies examined were mostly those of priests and priestesses who, owing to their high position, undoubtedly lived well (1)."

Arteriosclerosis was first described by the anatomists; the early reports were concerned with "bone in the heart," a condition which already had been described by Aristotle in certain animals (2). It is likely that this calcification of the heart was synonymous with calcified aortic valves, a fact already recognized by Morgagni (2). While Antonio Benevieni did not define atherosclerosis, he reported that on 15 necropsies "wounds of the arterial system" were among them (possibly atheromata) (2). It is, however, known that Vesalius was familiar with aortic aneurysms (2). At that time, no distinction was made between aneurysm due to syphilis or arteriosclerosis. The Dutch anatomist Volcher Coiter, while in Bologna, heard from "men worthy of credit" that they had seen the great artery (aorta) universally bony in a body dissected by Fallopius at Padua. By the year 1600, it was likely that all educated physicians had become aware of the condition of ossification of arteries, particularly the aorta. William Harvey, forever the physiologist, had emphasized the difficulty of transmission of the pulse in these arteries (2).

A fascinating description of early atherosclerosis was by Johann Conrad Brunner, who witnessed the necropsy of his father-in-law, Johann Jacob Wepfer (1620–1695). Wepfer was the discoverer of the relationship of cerebral hemorrhage and stroke. Brunner described the aorta which contained bone-like plaques throughout, especially in the upper abdominal aorta, "touching this structure hurt the fingers from the roughness of the bones (2)." In 1740, Johann Frederich Crell published his findings in which hardening of the coronary arteries was described (2). He took a great step forward by writing that the ossifications were in fact not bony, but of tophaceous nature and were derived from atheromatous matter. In 1755, Haller, of Bern, discussed the indurations of the aorta, placing particular emphasis on the atheromatous element existing in senile changes of this artery (2). Morgagni, in 1761, noticed the increased size of the heart in some cases with extensive hardening of the arteries; he was the first who took notice of the changes in the smaller arteries. Antonio Scarpa, who was Morgagni's pupil, while teaching in Modena and Pavia, Italy, was particularly interested in the relationship of the atheromatous ulcer to the aneurysm and rupture of the vessel. He referred to the report of Nichols on the necropsy of George III of England, in whom at postmortem, a fissure in the internal coat of the artery was discovered into which blood had diffused to form an ecchymosis. In 1801, Bichat stated that the initial lesions of arteriosclerosis were in the intima; he reached this conclusion by careful dissection (2).

We owe the term arteriosclerosis to Jean Frederick Martin Lobstein, the incumbent of the chair of pathological anatomy at the University in Strasbourg (3) (Figure 1). In his textbook we find the term "arteriosclerosis" ("nom composé d'artere et de sclerose"). He published a chemical analysis of the calcified arterial plaques. In 1839, the Viennese pathologist C. Rokitanski spoke of "excessive deposition in the inner membrane of the vessel," and believed that abnormalities in blood lay at the bottom of these conditions (4). But the idea of imbibition of the aortic wall by material in blood

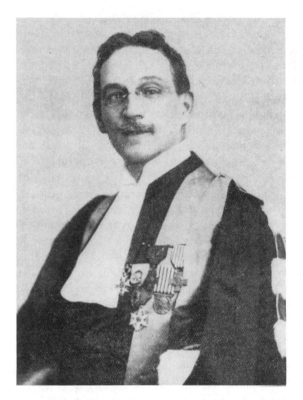

Figure 1.   Jean Frederick Lobstein (*Courtesy of The New York Academy of Medicine*)

was proposed in a more complete form by the great German pathologist R. Virchow, who postulated a deposition (imbibition) of material from the blood stream into the arterial intima (5). The alterations following blood imbibition were not purely passively degenerative, because he noticed proliferation of the connective tissue together with an increase in the associated ground substance. An amazing look into the future! The participation of blood pressure in imbibition was later suggested by Virchow's pupils.

The second phase in atherosclerosis research was concerned with the etiology of this condition. This quest continues unabated to the present and undoubtedly will continue into the future.

At the onset, it was necessary to develop an animal model to study the mechanism and etiology of atherosclerosis. This development is credited to

A. Ignatowski, N.W. Stuckey, Sergius Saltykow, and N. N. Anitschkow. Ignatowski, from Odessa, who worked in the laboratory of Diagnostic Clinical Science in St. Petersburg, had the good sense, favored by serendipity, to use the rabbit in his experiments (6). In 1907, he presented a lecture before the Military Medical Academy in St. Petersburg, titled, "To the Question of the Influence of Animal Nutrition on the Organism of the Rabbit." An article on the influence of animal nutrition on the organism of young rabbits appeared in the transaction of the Clinical Military Hospital in St. Petersburg in May, 1907 (7). In these lectures and articles, Ignatowski demonstrated that a high "protein" diet produces atherosclerosis in the aorta of rabbits. However, the "protein" was in reality a mixture of milk and egg yolk. Among other pathological findings, he discovered atheromata of the aorta. Thus, he should be given credit for developing the rabbit model which is still used in the study of atherosclerosis. At the time, laboratory-bred rats were unavailable, fortunately, because rats fed cholesterol do not show these changes. Stuckey, also in St. Petersburg, was quick to follow and in 1910 discovered similar changes resulting from administration of egg yolk and "brain extracts (8)." In the paper, "On the Changes of Rabbit Aorta after Feeding Different Fatty Material," he reported that the administration of egg yolk was responsible for the aortic changes (9). Stuckey reported identical results with the feeding of brain substances. After four months, he noticed atherosclerotic changes in the aorta.

In 1908, Saltykow, prosector at the Kanton Hospital in San Gallen, Switzerland, experimented with the effect of staphylococcal injection on experimentally produced atherosclerosis in rabbits, reporting that he had observed typical yellow spotted thickening of the mitral valve (10,11; Figure 2). Saltykow also administered cholesterol-rich food to these animals and the changes observed probably were the result of the diet rather than the staphylococcal injection, although the presence of bacterial endocarditis was a remote possiblity. In several articles, Saltykow summarized his findings which consisted of meticulous descriptions of the histological changes in the aorta (10-12). Of interest here is that he mentioned the work of Alexis Carrel and Guthrie, then in Chicago, who transplanted the terminal aorta to the venous network of an organ with diminished vascular capacity. After a few months they discovered medial hypertrophy followed by sclerosis and calcification of the intima and adventitia. This is an example of the application of Carrel's surgical technique which he used so successfully in the investigation of physiological phenomena.

The central figure in these early Russian studies was Anitschkow (Figure 3). Anitschkow's life straddled both Imperial Russia and the early revolutionary period. His papers from 1913 are listed as from the Pathologic Ana-

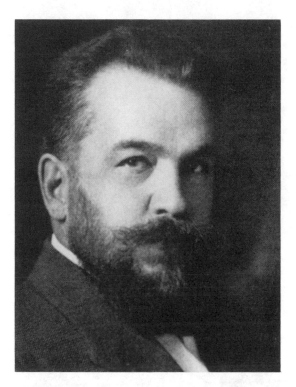

Figure 2. Sergius Saltykow (*Courtesy of The New York Academy of Medicine*)

tomical Institute of the Imperial Medical Military Academy at St. Petersburg, while his later publications are from Leningrad, USSR, (now again St. Petersburg). Some of his articles originated from Ludwig Aschoff's Institute in Freiburg, Germany. He mentions the role of cholesterol in the production of experimental atherosclerosis in the rabbit (13, 15–22). Anitschkow concluded that the deposit was cholesterol, since the double refringence of the crystals, according to Aschoff, "consists in the living organism primarily of fatty acid esters or cholesterol." He mentions further the work of A. Windaus, the chemist, who found lipids in the aortic wall in human atherosclerosis (14). He concluded that "previous and present authors can come to a complete agreement because it is now completely clear why such nutritional elements, as for example, egg yolk or brain substance produce changes in the organism." Cholesterol has since then, achieved a central

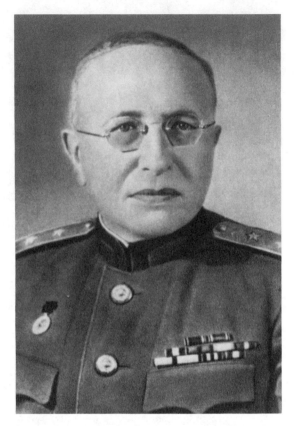

Figure 3. Portrait of N.N. Anitschkow as a General in the Red Army.
(*Courtesy of The New York Academy of Medicine*)

position in experimental, clinical, and pharmacological studies on atherosclerosis.

Anitschkow was a prolific writer; most of his publications are more than
30 pages long (13, 15–20). The role of cholesterol in atherosclerosis remains
however, the most important of his discoveries. Anitschkow proposed another farsighted concept: participation of smooth muscle fibers in the formation of atherosclerotic processes. "Sometimes one sees layer upon layer of
smooth muscle fibers close to the most superficial layers of the intima." The
role of smooth muscle proliferation in atherosclerosis has become an important field of research (20). Anitschkow also produced atherosclerotic

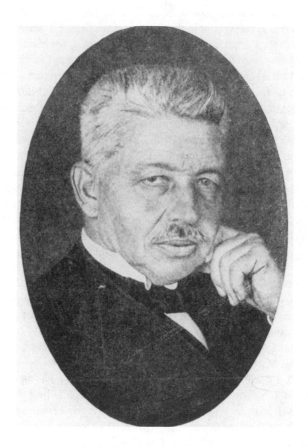

Figure 4.   Ludwig Aschoff (*Courtesy of The New York Academy of Medicine*)

changes in mitral and aortic valves. This breakthrough could not have been made without the work of the pathologist Aschoff, whose studies in pathologic anatomy pointed to the role of cholesterol, and of Windaus, who demonstrated the presence of cholesterol in human tissue (14) (Figure 4). Windaus, in a paper written at the suggestion of Aschoff, concluded that in atheromatous aortas the content of cholesterol is significantly increased. This increase is partially due to the presence of free cholesterol (14). In 1907, Aschoff discussed his finding that cholesterol had been taken up "by the fatty globules, which then became anisotropic (23)." One of Anitchkow's students, W. D. Zinserling, showed in 1932 that spontaneous atherosclerotic changes could also be present in the aorta of dogs (24). He admits that in the rabbit, spontaneous arterial lesions resembling human atherosclerosis are not observed, just as these animals do not exhibit pronounced thickening of the intima in advanced age. In 1924, Zinserling published an extensive article on the presence of fatty changes occuring in the arteries of children (24). He considered fat deposits (fatty streaks) as precursors of atherosclerosis in the adult. He described the typical distribution in children and their increase with age; he found that they originate in the hypertrophic intima, and that they consist of cholesterol. Zinserling mentions that three factors are, in general, important for their origin: cholesterolemia; mechanical influences; and the condition of the arterial wall. Thus, Zinserling clearly foresaw the most important problems of atherosclerotic research during the next 60 years. He believed that, with time, the lipid mixture which had infiltrated the intima decomposes but that together with the decomposition and resorption of lipid material, reactive tissue originates which is formed in close proximity to the initial infiltration process.

In this historial review, one must recall the work of Rudolph Schoenheimer (25), whose research stands at the beginning of the modern era of cholesterol metabolism. His work led to the exploration and definition of the pathways leading to cholesterol formation by Konrad Bloch (26), F. Lynen (27), and the discovery of the low density lipoprotein receptors by J.L. Goldstein and M.S. Brown (28).

Schoenheimer was born in 1898, in Berlin (Figure 5). His first studies on cholesterol metabolism were published when he was a young physician at a Berlin hospital. In order to obtain additional training in his chosen field, biochemistry, he worked for three years with Karl Thomas in Leipzig where he developed a new method for peptide analysis. In 1926, Schoenheimer moved to Freiburg where he began his studies with Aschoff which were to be of fundamental importance in the area of cholesterol metabolism. In 1930, he joined the University of Chicago, strangely enough in the department of surgery, where he became a Douglas Smith Fellow. In 1931, he returned to Germany and became the director of the division for physiological chemistry. In 1933, he left Germany and joined the Department of Biochemistry of the College of Physicians and Surgeons at Columbia University, New York, which was under the direction of Hans Clarke (29).

Schoenheimer published his paper on the synthesis and destruction of cholesterol in 1933. The work was done in Aschoff's department in Freiburg, Germany. By the time the paper appeared, Schoenheimer had joined Columbia University. Schoenheimer described studies on the influence of food stuffs on the synthesis and decomposition of cholesterol in mice. The paper

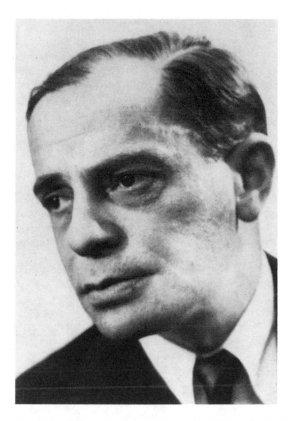

Figure 5.   Rudolph Schoenheimer at Columbia University College of Physicians and Surgeons, (New York). (*Courtesy of the New York Academy of Medicine*)

preceded Schoenheimer's studies on the use of isotopes and elucidation of biochemical pathways.

Schoenheimer was able to follow quantitatively the synthesis and destruction of cholesterol. He confirmed previous work indicating cholesterol can be synthesized in the body. He also showed that in the field of total metabolism, synthesis can play an exceptionally important part. On a diet of bread or bread and fat, mice synthesize as much cholesterol in one month as they had in their bodies at the beginning of the experiment. The administration of large amounts of fat was without significant effect. He furthermore con-

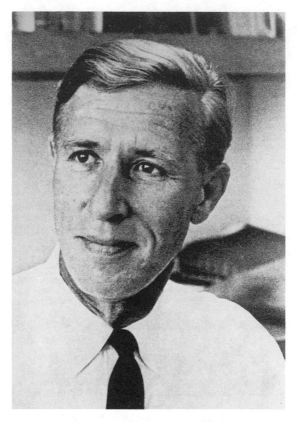

Figure 6.   Konrad Bloch (*with permission*)

firmed the data of others according to which cholesterol could also be de-
composed.

One of the advances in atherosclerotic research, which was to become the
basis of clinical treatment, was the elucidation of cholesterol synthesis by
Bloch (26) and Lynen (27). Bloch, who played a major role, was born in
Silesia, Germany (Figure 6). He trained with Wieland and Hans Fischer in
Munich. After the advent of the National Socialists, he worked in Davos,
Switzerland, where he studied the cholesterol content of tubercle bacilli.
Like Schoenheimer, he later joined Clarke's department at the College of
Physicians and Surgeons, Columbia University. After some period at the

University of Chicago, he joined the Department of Chemistry at Harvard. This work, for which he was awarded the Nobel Prize together with Lynen, culminated in the elucidation of cholesterol synthesis. Bloch fed acetate, isotopically labeled in its carbon atoms, to rats and found that the cholesterol which synthesized contained the isotopic label (26). All 20-7 carbon atoms of cholesterol were derived from acetyl CoA. Of particular importance was the finding that 3-hydroxyl-3-methylglutaryl CoA, an intermediate compound in cholesterol synthesis, can be reduced to mevalonate and that the enzyme catalyzing this step, 3-hydroxyl-3-methylglutaryl CoA reductase is the control site in cholesterol synthesis which progresses via squalene and lanosterol to cholesterol. This fundamental discovery, made by Folkers et. al. in the Merck Laboratories, together with the finding of Brown and Goldstein (28) on receptor mediated uptake of low density lipoproteins, is the basis for the astonishing progress made in treatment of atherosclerosis by means of HMG-CoA reductase inhibitors.

The discovery demonstrates again the value of fundamental research in the treatment of disease. Bloch, at the end of his article "Summing Up," expresses the feelings of scientists in a manner that might well reflect that of scientists who have enjoyed a lifelong dedication to research:

> Whatever the motives, whether curiosity or ambition—usually a combination of both—only near the end does one fully appreciate the rewards and privileges that go with a career in science. So much the better if the results should prove to have some degree of permanence. Science is indeed a glorious enterprise and it has been for me, I admit, glorious entertainment (26).

Why did Konrad Bloch like so many others such as Rittenberg, Schoenheimer, and Chargaff flock to Columbia University in New York to the Department of Biochemistry of Hans Clark? The reason was a nurturing environment, particularly because of a departmental chairman whose interest was the promotion of excellent science and scientists. Hans Clark was a cultured individual who tolerated divergent personalities and understood different cultural backgrounds.

An important discovery in the field of atherosclerosis which shifted the emphasis from cholesterol to lipoproteins was made by John W. Gofman and his co-workers in 1955, working at the Donner Laboratories at the University of California at Berkeley (30; Figure 7). Gofman proceeded to undertake a physiochemical investigation of the giant molecules of serum composed of cholesterol, phospholipids, fatty acids, and protein as building blocks. The basic premise was that it is entirely possible that a defect might exist in certain of these giant molecules, which could be responsible for the development of atherosclerosis, whereas the mere analytical levels of any of these

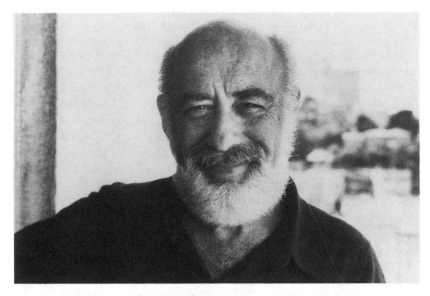

Figure 7.   John William Gofman (*with permission*)

building blocks in serum might be of little or no significance. This work was made possible by the development of the analytical ultracentrifuge. Their studies revealed a considerable diversity of components existing in the low density group which they termed B_1-lipoproteins (now beta lipoproteins). By analyzing the ultracentrifugal flotation diagrams of lipids and lipoproteins of humans and rabbits, they concluded that the mechanism of cholesterol transport in the serum of rabbits and humans was in giant lipid and lipoprotein molecules of low density. Defining them as "low or lower density molecules," they showed that these molecules were present in increased amounts in the cholesterol-induced atherosclerosis in the rabbit, as well as in patients with proved myocardial infarction. They furthermore illustrated that cholesterol intake by the human, as well as by the rabbit, influences the blood level of low density lipoproteins. This discovery opened the way for the classification of hyperlipoproteinemia of individuals with dominant and recessive types and eventually led to the discovery of abnormal receptors for low density lipoproteins.

The latest chapter in the study of atherosclerosis deals with the fusion of genetics, biochemistry, and molecular genetics. The central themes are concerned with cholesterol synthesis and transport in blood, cholesterol ho-

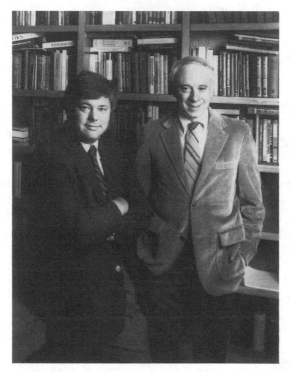

Figure 8. M.S. Brown *(left side)* and J.L. Goldstein *(right side)*

meostasis within the cell, and analysis of the origin and progression of vascular lesions of atherosclerosis with special reference to proliferation of smooth muscle cells.

A large number of publications on the low density lipoprotein, (LDL) receptor have appeared from the laboratories of Brown and Goldstein (Figure 8).. Their most fundamental contribution concerns the origin of LDL receptors in cell membranes and the mechanism of cellular uptake and transportation of LDL in the cell. Goldstein trained in biochemistry and medical genetics at the National Institute of Health and at the University of Washington in Seattle, and Brown trained at the National Institutes of Health, before joining the University of Texas in Dallas.

In 1972, because of their interest in genetics, Goldstein and Brown developed an interest in familial hypercholesterolemia (28). In the two forms of the disease, the heterozygous and homozygous type, the blood cholesterol is markedly elevated. Patients with the heterozygous form carry a single copy of a mutant LDL receptor gene and they may suffer from coronary artery disease at thirty to forty years of age. The homozygotes inherit two mutant genes of the LDL receptor location. These latter individuals may develop heart attacks as children. LDL is internalized into cells after binding to the LDL receptor. Following endocytosis the LDL is delivered to lyosomes, where cholesteryl esters of the LDL are hydrolized to cholesterol and fatty acids. The cholesterol may be used in the biosynthesis of plasma membranes, bile acids and hormones. The most interesting finding concerns receptor-mediated endocytosis of LDL and the rapidity of internalization in coated pits of the cell membrane. The astonishing fact about these receptors is that they shuttle back and forth: LDL is dissociated from the receptors within intracellular endosomes and receptors shuttle back to the cell surface, to bind another lipoprotein. Each LDL receptor makes a round trip every ten minutes in a continuous fashion whether or not it is associated with LDL.

The impact and ramifications are broad for the therapy of atherosclerosis, for the structure of LDL, for genetics and molecular biology in general. The action of cholesterol lowering drugs represents an example of feedback mechanisms, involving cholesterol synthesis and LDL receptor activity. HMG-CoA reductase inhibitors inhibit cholesterol synthesis in the liver; this inhibition *triggers* regulatory mechanisms that result in reduction of the plasma LDL-cholesterol level. Inhibition of cholesterol synthesis in the liver by inhibitors of HMG-CoA reductase elicits a dual compensatory response: hepatocytes synthesize increased amounts of both HMG-CoA reductase and LDL receptors. The increase in HMG-CoA reductase is probably sufficient to neutralize the inhibitors effects of compactin or mevinolin. As a result of the increase in hepatic LDL receptors there is increased clearance of LDL out of the plasma and into the liver and a subsequent decline in plasma LDL levels. Goldstein's earliest papers in this field were published in 1972. His first joint article with Brown appeared in 1973. A new chapter was opened in atherosclerotic research. It represents another victory of basic research, which began with the structure of cholesterol, progressed to its synthesis, and finally to its metabolic fate at the cellular level.

Receptor related and low density lipoprotein uptake and disposition are but only one facet of present research work on the pathogenesis of atherosclerosis. Research also continues on the morpholoy of the disease. Confirmation of studies of Anitschkow on the morphology of atherosclerosis are being pursued using electron microscopy. Research studies have led to clarification of the fatty streak, the earliest lesion of atherosclerosis, and to the advanced fibromuscular lesions. The role of macrophages and of smooth muscle cells in plaque formation has been studied by means of monoclonal antibodies. The sequence of changes occurring in the development of atherosclerotic lesions has been followed by Russell Ross and his co-worker in monkeys during diet-induced atherosclerosis (31). The role of leukocytes and monocytes, which become macrophages, has been elucidated. Endothelial cells play a major role in the development of atherosclerotic lesions. After exposure to elevated plasma low density lipoproteins, endothelial cells may become altered (in some as yet undefined way) and thus affect their normal function. In addition LDL may enter the subendothelial space and become oxidized and stimulate endothelial cells to release various cytokines. The net result is the entry of blood monocytes and LDL into the subendothelial space. Mitogens, derived from adhered platelets may subsequently result in smooth muscle cell proliferation. There is therefore a close connection between monocytes, macrophage accumulation, endothelial damage, platelet adherence and smooth muscle proliferation. Endothelial cells also produce vasoactive agents, growth factors, and growth inhibitors. Platelet-derived growth factor (PDGF) was first described by Ross (32). PDGF is not only a mitogen but also a chemoattractant, thus promoting movement of smooth muscle cells from the media to the intima.

Few subjects in medical research are more challenging than atherosclerosis, which involves biochemistry, genetics, morphology, and molecular genetics. It is therefore not surprising that so many different approaches have been used which have been fruitful and rewarding. We now see the spin off of these fundamental studies in the therapy and prevention of atherosclerosis. From Aristotle's description of "Bone in the Heart," to the experimental production of atherosclerosis in animals by the Russians, and to the discovery of cholesterol synthesis and lipoprotein receptors, the progress has been crescendo, because the basic sciences such as chemistry, physics, and molecular genetics have presented us with the tools. But, we should by all means avoid the spirit conveyed by Galen when he wrote "It is certainly no small advantage that we enjoy living at the present day with the medical arts already brought to such perfection." This concept, expressed by some even now, would surely lead to complacency, scientific stagnation, and the end of progress.

REFERENCES

1. Ruffer, M. A. On arterial lesions found in Egyptian mummies (1580 B.C. - 525 A.D.). J. Path. Bact., 15:453–462, 1911.
2. Long, E. R. Development of our knowledge of arteriosclerosis. In: Arteriosclerosis, edited by E. V. Cowdry. New York, Macmillan, 1933, pp. 19–25.
3. Lobstein, J. F. Traité d'Anatomie Pathologique. Paris, Levrault, 1829–1833.

4. Rokitanski, C. Handbuch der Pathologischen Anatomie. Wien, Braumueller und Seidel, 1842–46.

5. Virchow, R. Die Cellularpathologie in ihrer Begruendung auf Physiologische und Pathologische Gewebelehre. Berlin, A. Hirschwald, 1st ed. 1858, 2nd ed. 1859, 3rd ed. 1862, 4th ed. 1871.

6. Ignatowski, A. Influence of animal feeding on the rabbit organism. Trans. Military-Med. Acad. Petersburg, 16:174, 1908.

7. Ignatowski, A. Ueber die Wirkung des tierischen Eiweisses auf die Aorta and die parenchymatoesen Organe der Kaninchen. Virchows Arch. Path. Anat., 198:248–270, 1909.

8. Stuckey, N. W. Ueber die Veraenderungen der Kaninchenaorta unter der Wirkung reichlicher Tierischer Nahrung. Centralbl. Allg. Path. u. Path. Anat., 22:379, 1911.

9. Stuckey, N. W. Ueber die Veraenderungen der Kaninchenaorta bei der Fuetterung mit verschiedenen Fettsorten. Centralbl. Allg. Path. u. Path. Anat., 23:910, 1912.

10. Saltykow, S. Atherosklerose bei Kaninchen nach wiederholten Staphylokokkeninjektionen. Beitr. Path. Anat., 43:147–171, 1908.

11. Saltykow, S. Zur Kenntnis der alimentaeren Krankheiten der Versuchstiere. Virchows Arch. Path. Anat., 213:8–22, 1913.

12. Saltykow, S. Die experimentell erzeugten Arterienveraenderungen in ihrer Beziehung zu Atherosklerose und verwandten Krankheiten des Menschen. Centralbl. Allg. Pathol., 19:321–369, 1908.

13. Anitschkow, N., and S. Chalatow. Ueber experimentelle Cholesterinsteatose und ihre Bedeutung fuer die Entstehung einiger pathologischer Prozesse. Centralbl. Allg. Pathol., 24:1–9, 1913.

14. Windaus, A. Ueber den Gehalt normaler und atheromatoeser Aorten an Cholesterin und Cholesterinestern. Hoppe-Seyler's Zeitschr. Physiol. Chem., 67:174–176, 1910.

15. Anitschkow, N. Ueber die Veraenderungen der Kaninchenaorta bei experimenteller Cholesterinsteatose. Beitr. Path. Anat., 56:379–404, 1913.

16. Anitschkow, N. Ueber die experimentelle Arteriosklerose der Aorta beim Meerschweinchen. Beitr. Path. Anat., 70:265–281, 1922.

17. Anitschkow, N. Ueber die experimentelle Atherosklerose der Herzklappen. Virchows Arch. Path. Anat., 220:233–256, 1915.

18. Anitschkow, N. Ueber die Rueckbildungsvorgaenge bei der experimentellen Arteriosklerose. Verhandl. Deutsch. Path. Gesellsch., 23:473, 1925.

19. Anitschkow, N. Ueber die Atherosklerose der Aorta beim Kaninchen und ueber deren Entstehungsbedingungen. Beitr. Path. Anat., 59:306–348, 1914.

20. Anitschkow, N. Development of our knowledge of arteriosclerosis. Experimental arteriosclerosis in animals. In: Arteriosclerosis, edited by E. V. Cowdry. New York, Macmillan, 1933. .

21. Anitschkow, N. Das Wesen und die Entstehung der Atherosklerose. Ergebn. Inn. Med. u. Kinderh., 28:1–46, 1925.

22. Anitschkow, N. Zur Histophysiologie der Arterienwand. Klin. Wochschr., 4:2233–2235, 1925.

23. Aschoff, L. Ein Beitrag zur Myelinfrage. Verhandl. Deutsch. Path. Gesellsch., 166–170, 1906.

24. Zinserling, W. D. Untersuchungen ueber Atherosklerose. Virchows Arch. Path. Anat., 255:677–705, 1925.

25. Schoenheimer, R., and R. Breusch. Synthesis and destruction of cholesterol in the organism. J. Biol. Chem., 103:439–448, 1933.

26. Bloch, K. The Biological synthesis of cholesterol. Les Prix Nobel, 179–203, 1964.

27. Lynen, F. The Pathway from "activated acetic acid" to the terpenes and fatty acids. Les Prix Nobel, 205–246, 1964.

28. Goldstein, J. L. and M. S. Brown. The low-density lipoprotein pathway and its relation to atherosclerosis. Ann. Rev. Biochem., 46:89–930, 1977.

29. Schoenheimer, R. (1898-1942) Ueber den Beginn deu Tracer-Technik bei Stoffwechseluntersuchungen. Inaugural-Dissertation zur Erlangung der Doktorwuerde der Medizinischen Fakultaet der Universitat Zuerich. Juris Druck & Verlag Zurich, 2–6, 1972.

30. Gofman, J. W., F. Lindgren, H. Elliott, W. Mantz, J. Hewitt, B. Strisower, and V. Herring. The role of lipids and lipoproteins in atherosclerosis. Science, 111:166–171,186, 1950.

31. Ross, R., The pathogenesis of atherosclerosis - an update. New Engl. J. Med. 314:488, 1986.

32. Ross, R., J. Glomset, B. Kariya and L. Harker. A platelet-dependent serum factor that stimulates the proliferation of arterial smooth muscle cells in vitro. Proc. Natl. Acad. Sci., 71:1207–1210, 1974.

Chapter 7

Coronary Artery Disease

O. PAUL AND R.J. BING

Credit for the early work on coronary artery disease should go to clinical observations and judgement. More recently increased speed of scientific advance has led to a decline in emphasis on purely clinical observations, while at the same time extolling the diagnostic and therapeutic benefits of scientific technology. For a medical student in the late 1920s and early 1930s, training was primarily based on observations and personal experience—the art of medicine—with little hope for successful therapy. Then we paid a price for our ignorance by inability to cure many diseases; today, we pay a price for the emphasis on science and technology, because we are less aware of the patient as a distinct personality, his social and economic concerns, and his personal response to disease. Reading the early 18th and 19th century descriptions of coronary artery disease, we see how much can be accomplished by one's eyes, ears, and mind.

Vesalius and Vieussens (1), contributed greatly to the anatomy of the coronary circulation. William Harvey clearly described the second or coronary circulation, "For what should the coronary arteries pulsate in the heart; save to drive blood on by the impulse? And why should there be coronary veins except to acquire blood from the heart?" (2).

The pathologic state of the heart in angina pectoris was recognized by Morgagni (1,2). In 1761, he published his famous "De Sedibus et Causis Morborum." Written in the form of letters, De Sedibus contains the clinical

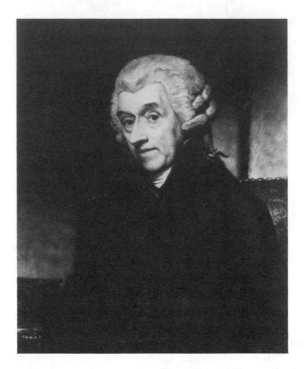

Figure 1.   William Heberden (*Courtesy of the Wellcome Institute for the History of Medicine, London, United Kingdom*)

and pathological description of approximately 700 cases. Regarding one of the patients who died of an incarcerated hernia, he wrote; "the left coronary artery appeared to have been changed into a bony canal from its very origin to the extent of several fingers (2)." Morgagni himself died of a ruptured ventricle, presumably infarcted in his 90th year, just seven years before William Heberden's famous lecture on angina pectoris (2).

Heberden was one of the great British physicians who described angina pectoris, without relating it to diseases of the coronary artery (Fig. 1). Other clinicians were John Hunter (Fig. 2), Edward Jenner (Fig. 3), C.H. Parry, J. Fothergill, Marshall Hall, and Allan Burns (1,2,3;Fig.4). A vivid description of these great clinicians is contained in James B. Herrick's book, "A Short History of Cardiology" published in 1942 and in the chapter on the coronary circulation and cardiac metabolism in *Circulation of the Blood: Men and Ideas* (1). These men, except for Burns, were primarily clinical observers,

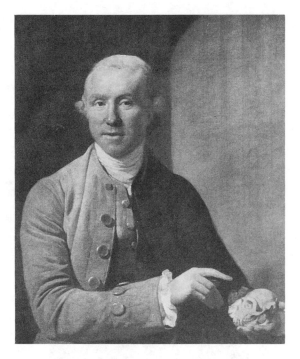

Figure 2.   John Hunter (*Courtesy of Special Collections, Health Sciences Library, Columbia University, NY*)

rather than experimentalists. The story of Hunter is well known and remains a landmark in medical history (Fig. 2). At the age of 40, he began to suffer from recurring attacks of angina pectoris with severe pain in the stomach. He died during an attack which was provoked by a hospital board meeting on October 16, 1793, when "in his usual state of health, he went to St. George's Hospital meeting with some things which irritated his mind and not being perfectly master of his circumstances, he withheld his sentiments in which state of restraint he went into the next room and turned around to Dr. Robertson, one of the physicians of the hospital, gave a deep groan and dropped down dead." On autopsy, performed by Jenner, the discoverer of small pox vaccination, there was intense "ossification of the coronary arteries (1)."

Parry wrote a book entitled "Syncope Anginosa" which was based on cases similar to those of Hunter (1,2,3). He too correlated the clinical symptoms with autopsy findings. Parry paid more attention to the suddenness of

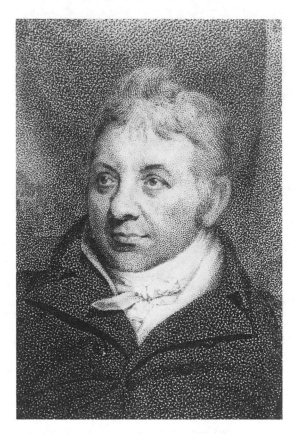

Figure 3.   Edward Jenner (*Courtesy of The New York Academy of Medicine*)

the attack of weakness "due to the loss of strength of the heart muscle" than to the pain.

It remained for Heberden, who studied many patients with angina pectoris, to draw a clear picture of what he called angina pectoris. Heberden was not concerned with the relationship between chest pain and coronary artery disease (1). Yet, his description of angina pectoris became a classic and the disease has sometimes been referred to as Heberden's angina. He described clearly the symptoms: "They who are afflicted with this disease, are seized while they are walking (more especially if it be uphill, and soon after eating), with a painful and most disagreeable sensation in the breast which seems as it would extinguish life if it were to increase or to continue; but the moment

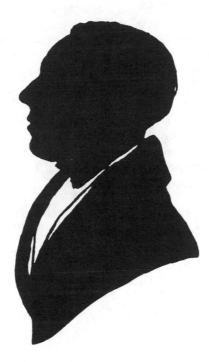

Figure 4.   Allan Burns (*in silhoutte*) (*University of Glasgow Medical Library*)

they stand still, all this uneasiness vanishes." He mentions many times that the pain may be localized in several places, that males are more likely to be afflicted than females, and that the pain will appear not only when the person is walking, but when they are lying down. He ended his chapter by stating, "I know one who set himself a task sawing wood for half an hour every day, and was nearly cured. In one also, the disorder ceased of itself. Bleeding, vomiting, and purging, appear to me improper (1,4)."

Of all these men, Burns deserves a special place, not only because he related clinical symptoms to pathophysiology, but because he was a most unusual personality in the field of cardiology (1). At 14, he began to study medicine and at 16 he took over the sole direction of the dissecting room from his elder brother (Figure 4). He never obtained a university degree, (today he would be without licensure and board certification in internal medicine and cardiology and therefore would be unable to practice!), but he gained experience as a physician and surgeon chiefly by attending and studying the patients of his brother and his friends. Burns accumulated drawings which were subsequently used to prepare his books on the diseases of the heart, on the blood vessels and on surgical anatomy. He wrote two books during his brief career. The second book, entitled "Observations on the Surgical Anatomy of the Head and Neck," is illustrated by cases and engravings. Published in 1811, this book had two printings of the second edition, as well as a German and American edition. Burn's first book entitled, "Observations on Some of the Most Frequent and Important Diseases of the Heart," was published in 1809 (5). Chapter 7 is of special interest, because here he connects angina pectoris to coronary blood flow.

> The heart like every other part has particular vessels set apart for its nourishment. In health, when we excite the muscular system to more energetic action than usual, we increase the circulation in every part, so that to support this increased action, the heart and every part has its power augmented. If, however, we call into vigorous action a limb, around which we have with a moderate degree of tightness, applied a ligature, we find then that the member can only support its action for a very short time; for now its supply of energy and its expenditure do not balance each other; consequently, it soon, from a deficiency of nervous influence in arterial blood, fails and sinks into a state of quiescence. A heart, the coronary vessels of which are cartilaginous or ossified, is in nearly a similar condition; it can, like the limb, begin with a moderately tight ligature, discharge its function so long as its action is moderate and equal. Increase, however, the action of the whole body and along with the rest that of the heart, and you will soon see exemplified the truth of what has been said; with this difference, that as there is no interruption to the action of the cardiac nerves, the heart will be able to hold out a little longer than the limb.

He continued, "If however, a person with the nutrient arteries of the heart diseased in such a way as to impede the progress of the blood among them, attempts to do the same, he finds that the heart is sooner fatigued than the other parts are, which remain healthy (1,5)." Thus, Burns clearly saw the connection between a decrease in coronary blood flow and angina pectoris.

When Burns was 23, he accepted an invitation of the Empress Catherine of Russia to go to St. Petersburg as director and surgeon of a hospital. But he soon returned home to again take up lectures on anatomy and surgery. Burns died in 1813, at the age of 31, probably of a ruptured appendix.

The correlation between coronary artery disease and fatty changes of the cardiac muscle was recognized by Sir Richard Quain, who published a book on fatty diseases of the heart in 1850 (1,6). To quote him, "I have seen the coronary arteries extremely ossified going directly to the only part of the heart affected ... this connection between fatty softened heart and obstructed arteries suggests an analogy with softening of the brain, in which a like condition of the vessel is known to exist."

M. Hall, who became senior president of the Royal Medical Society of Edinburgh two years after registering as a medical student, expressed the belief that sudden death was often due to arrest of the coronary circulation (1,7). This suggestion was taken up by another English clinician, J.E. Erichsen, who posed the problem in the following way, "The question, then, is to determine what effect the arrest of the coronary circulation would have on the action of the heart." He therefore ligated coronary vessels of dogs and observed that ventricular action continued for about 20 minutes (1,8).

Julius Friederich Cohnheim was the initiator of the concept that coronary arteries are end-arteries, in other words, occlusion of one artery would lead to immediate cessation of blood flow to the area of the heart muscle supplied by this artery. Occlusion of a coronary artery would be fatal because blood supply to that part of the heart muscle cannot be furnished from collateral sources (9). Cohnheim, a pupil of R. Virchow, was one of the early experimentalists: he cannulated the carotid, femoral and pulmonary arteries of dogs. He fitted cannulae to manometers for the recording of pressures. He and his colleague A. von Schultheiss-Rechberg examined the possibility that the consequences of ligating a coronary artery arose from lack of oxygen (9). They did not think this likely however, since oxygen deprivation of the whole animal had quite different results. Cohnheim even believed in the release of a poison by the heart muscle after occlusion. In the new Sydenham Society lectures on General Pathology, an extensive memoir of Cohnheim was published which gives credit to this unusual and interesting personality (10). Cohnheim (1839-1884) commenced the study of medicine in 1856, in Berlin (Fig. 5). As a boy of 15, his father was compelled by his affairs to leave home for Australia, where misfortune crowded upon him and whence he returned only to die. In Berlin, Cohnheim worked under Virchow's guidance in the Pathological Institute. It was there that he resolved to devote his life to science. Following this, he assumed the pathology chair at Kiel. In 1872, Cohnheim removed to Breslau and hence to Leipzig where he made his mark as one of the early experimental pathologists and commenced his experiments on the effect of ligation of a coronary artery in dogs.

By the end of the 19th century, the clinical consequences of coronary occlusion had been clearly defined by two German pathologists, C. Weigert and E. Ziegler. Weigert wrote, "If the occlusion occurs gradually in the absence of collateral circulation producing chronic changes, a slow atrophy and destruction of the muscle fibers without damage to the connecting tissue can be observed—the disappearing muscle fibers are then replaced by connective tissue (1,2,11,12)." Weigert was an extremely productive worker in the

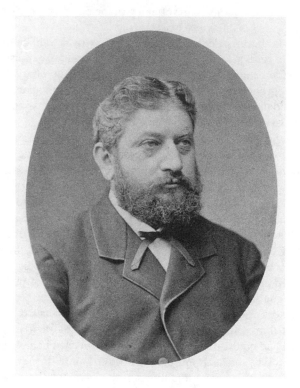

Figure 5.   Julius F. Cohnheim (*Courtesy of Special Collections, Health Sciences Library, Columbia University, NY*)

field of medicine as well. In 1901, he proposed that myasthenia gravis was related to an abnormality of the thymus (2,12). He was concise and clear in his description of the pathologic anatomy of myocardial infarction and coronary artery disease. To quote him,

> Atheromatous changes of the coronary arteries are frequently associated with thrombotic or embolic occlusion of their branches. If the occlusion occurs slowly or in such a way that collateral pathways, even though they are insufficient, exist, we will find a slow atrophy degeneration of the muscle fibers without damage to the connective tissue. These injured muscle fibers are then replaced by fibrous connective tissue. The so-called chronic myocarditis is nothing else but such a process certain parts of the heart, we will find yellowish, dry masses resembling coagulated fibrin. In the surrounding areas there is a reactive infiltration of round and spindle cells (2,12).

Ziegler also published a concise description of the "gross and histologic" features of myocardial infarction from onset to healing (1,2,13). He wrote, "The appearance of the shortened areas varies according to their age and blood content. Shortly after beginning of the anemia they are firm and manifest themselves only by a dull yellow coloration of the heart muscle." He then describes the changes that occur with time and he also described necrosis of muscle cells and what he called "homogenous degeneration." The great step forward was that he anticipated the work of Herrick when he wrote, "When a certain stage is reached, the reparatory process starts." Thus, he realized that occlusion of the coronary artery may not be fatal, as Cohnheim had proposed, but may lead to chronic changes in the heart muscle which are compatible with life (13).

In a field where great clinicians and personalities abound, Adam Hammer certainly was unique (14;Fig. 6)). He had a checkered career. Born in Germany, he graduated from the University of Heidelberg in 1842, but after participating in the revolution of 1848, Hammer had to flee Germany and sought refuge in America. In St. Louis, Missouri, he first established a practice and later a medical school which survived for only one year. Nine years later, he established another medical school in St. Louis, the Humboldt Institute, where instruction was given in German; this school existed for ten years. In 1877, Hammer returned to Europe and, in 1878 he started a medical practice in Vienna. He died the year after he had presented his detailed report of a patient with coronary thrombosis. Hammer's case report deals with a 34 year old patient who apparently had rheumatic fever and collapsed. His heart rate was 23 beats per minute. Later, the pulse rate dropped to 8 beats per minute. Hammer reasoned, "In this desperate situation, I wondered if a disturbance of the nourishment of the heart could explain such a condition, and whether this could have been caused by a thrombotic occlusion of at least one coronary artery." At autopsy there was a thrombus in the sinus of Valsalva, which extended all the way into the take off of the right coronary artery. Incidentally, for some time Hammer was also Felix Mendelssohn's physician (15).

It remained for Herrick to state, in 1912, that a sudden occlusion of the coronary artery might be comparable with life (1,16). Herrick was a great clinician and innovator and shared with William Osler the ability to present his thoughts and observations in an original and poignant style (1,17; Figure 7). He knew medical history and presented it with humor and a personal perspective, acquired during his 70 years as a physician (18). Aside from his clear presentation of the clinical symptoms of coronary occlusion, he recognized for the first time the clinical entity, sickle cell anemia. Richard S. Ross has written a delightful essay on Herrick (17). He quotes from Herrick's Billings lecture of 1934, "he would be rash indeed, who would venture to predict

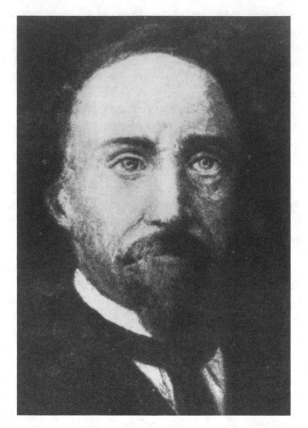

Figure 6.   Adam Hammer (*Courtesy of The New York Academy of Medicine*)

what will be the exact stages of medicine or the relation between physician and patient a century from now, yes, even a decade ahead. Toppling thrones, scrapped constitutions, unsettled economic conditions, hostile industrial and social groups, angry nations brandishing loaded weapons, all these things not alone upset the world at present but threaten the stability and tranquility of the future." A truly prophetic statement! Herrick himself made a dramatic attempt to keep abreast of emerging medical science, and Ross reports that, in 1904, when Herrick was 43 years old and busy with consultation practice, he matriculated at the University of Chicago to take courses in biology and physical and organic chemistry. He subsequently left his practice, went to Germany and studied with Emil Fischer.

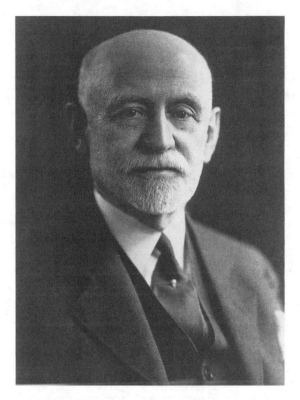

Figure 7.   James B. Herrick (*Courtesy of Special Collections, Health Sciences Library, Columbia University, NY*)

As is the case with many new concepts, it is not surprising that no critical discussion followed Herrick's classical paper on coronary thrombosis presented in 1912 before the Association of American Physicians. Herrick wrote later,

> You know I never understood it. In 1912 when I arose to read my paper at the Association, I was elated, for I knew I had a substantial contribution to present. I read it, and it fell flat as a pancake. No one discussed it except Emanuel Libman, and he discussed every paper read that day. I was sunk in disappointment (17).

In 1918, Herrick again spoke to the Association of American Physicians on coronary thrombosis and this time he included some experimental work done by his colleague, Fred Smith, on occlusion of the coronary artery in dogs (19). He presented electrocardiograms taken on these animals after experimental occlusion and showed the similarity to those obtained from patients. Herrick observed that work done in the laboratory on a dog attracted more attention than that done in the ward on patients. Herrick's broad interest in matters other than medicine is shown by the fact that at the age of 70 he presented a talk on Chaucer at the evening program of the Association of the American Physicians (17). One of the young men in the audience was heard to remark, "Well, I know who Dr. Herrick is, but who in hell is Chaucer?" Herrick took this to indicate that there was a serious lack of cultural background in the physicians of the day and made a strong case for a liberal arts education as a background for medicine (17).

After Herrick, the flood gates opened and today we have seen a substantial reduction in mortality from myocardial infarction. Two factors are responsible for this fortunate development. First, an extension of surgical techniques together with the introduction of special catheterization procedures, such as selective coronary angiography and coronary angioplasty. Secondly, advances in the basic sciences have lent a helping hand through biochemical-pharmacological, electro-physiological, and molecular-biological research. Yet, without the clinical and experimental observations of these pioneers, advanced developments would not have been possible. In medicine, as in science, there is no peak of final accomplishment. If society continues to respect and promote scientific projects, our present advances will seem but the forerunners of greater accomplishments.

Following the work of Herrick, numerous clinical cardiologists made important contributions to the study and treatment of coronary heart disease. In several instances, their contributions were not totally new; others had done somewhat similar preliminary work but had failed to be as persuasive and effective in their reasoning and presentations.

Paul Dudley White is an example (20;Fig. 8). He was raised in the Boston area, attended the Harvard Medical School, and received additional training at the Massachusetts General Hospital. In 1913, he went to London to study under Thomas Lewis (later Sir Thomas Lewis), and then saw service as a medical officer in World War I. White became the head of cardiology at the Massachusetts General Hospital, where he soon developed a busy clinical service with a heavy load of teaching, research, and patient care. Gifted with boundless energy, a large measure of common sense, broad experience, and a warm and attractive personality, he soon became an international leader. His successful textbook entitled "Heart Disease" was first published in 1931, and went into four editions including translations into Spanish and Italian. White's many research publications included reports about neurocirculatory

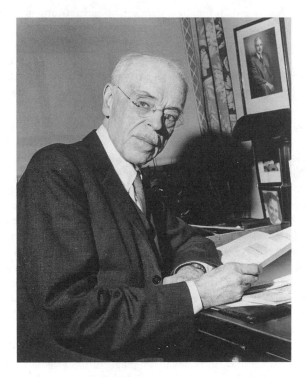

Figure 8.   Paul D. White (*Courtesy of The New York Academy of Medicine*)

asthenia in civilians, descriptions with Ed Churchill of the first resection of the pericardium for chronic constrictive pericarditis to be performed in the English-speaking world (1930), the first report on what came to be called the Wolff-Parkinson-White syndrome (also in 1930), and clinical and electrocardiographic findings in acute cor pulmonale. He served as President of the American Heart Association and of the International Society of Cardiology.

White's role in coronary heart disease was highly influential, not only through the clinical reports published by him and his associates, but especially through his exposition of a prescription for living which he applied with great effectiveness not only to healthy individuals, but also to patients with angina pectoris or who had a history of myocardial infarction. His philosophy had three components: an attitude of optimism, regular physical activity, and avoidance of premature invalidism and retirement from useful living.

As the diagnosis of clinical coronary heart disease became relatively common following upon the work of Herrick and others, there was a tendency for physicians and members of the lay public to regard persons with such a label as delicate, liable to sudden catastrophe including sudden death, and in need of inordinate protection from the nervous and physical strains of everyday life. Individuals with such diagnoses were often counseled to give up or greatly alter their employment for a routine of rest and quiet living. Surrounding all this was an atmosphere of resignation and pessimism. It was here that White, using his own large experience, but not reflecting any specific physiologic investigations or controlled clinical studies, intervened with great effect.

Beginning as early as 1927, White began to speak and write about the benefits of a routine of regular moderate physical exercise, such as walking and bicycling, for most patients with coronary heart disease; and beginning in 1932, he initiated a campaign to replace pessimism with optimism for such individuals, emphasizing that many persons with coronary heart disease could look forward to years of useful and satisfying living. This more cheerful view was coupled with an admonition to avoid unnecessary invalidism.

White's philosophy was not only presented widely to the medical professions; it was also extensively discussed before lay audiences, as White was a master in lay education. He reached the peak of his influence in this area when he was called in as consultant to President Dwight D. Eisenhower, when the President had a myocardial infarction while in Denver, Colorado, in September 1955. Fascinated by the daily bulletins regarding this very visible illness, the media concentrated on the often quotable pronouncements of White at periodic press conferences. He became the center of attention on the medical aspects of the heart attack, particularly when he stated that despite the history of an undoubted recent myocardial infarction, the President might resume playing golf and campaign for a second term. This decision was of course influenced by the uncomplicated course of Eisenhower's illness, his good recovery, and the absence of unfavorable factors such as hypertension, diabetes, or hyperlipidemia. White's optimistic prognosis was borne out, and Eisenhower not only lived through his second term, but survived eight more years after he left the White House. This Boston physician's realistic message regarding coronary heart disease was widely disseminated, and without question permitted many patients with angina pectoris or a history of myocardial infarction to look to the future without the grim foreboding so common earlier in the century.

A major correlation of the pathology of coronary artery disease, and its complications, with its clinical manifestations appeared in 1940. This undertaking began with the work of Monroe J. Schlesinger, pathologist at the Beth Israel Hospital in Boston, who described in 1938 an ingenious technique for injecting coronary arteries postmortem with a colored radiopaque lead phosphate in agar mass, followed by cutting open the heart and completely dissecting the coronary tree (21). In this fashion, he was able to accurately locate areas of narrowing and obstruction, as well as to visualize anastomoses. Two years later, making good use of this new approach, Schlesinger and Herrman L. Blumgart, who would soon become Physician-in-Chief at Beth Israel, completed the classic paper "Studies on the Relation of the Clinical Manifestations of Angina Pectoris, Coronary Thrombosis, and Myocardial Infarction to the Pathologic Findings (22;Fig.9)." Blumgart had received his training at the Harvard Medical School and the Peter Bent Brigham Hospital, followed by a year in London, and then four years at the Thorndike Memorial Laboratory of the Boston City Hospital, a famous incubator of research talent. He was a gracious and charming teacher and physician, in many ways resem-

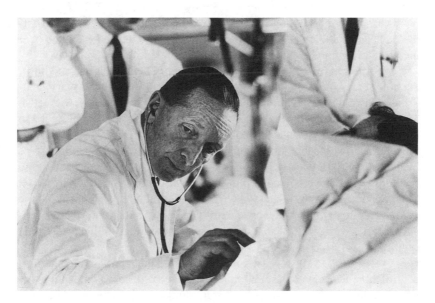

Figure 9.   Herrman L. Blumgart (*Courtesy of The New York Academy of Medicine*)

bling his mentor, Francis W. Peabody. Blumgart and Schlesinger had taken a series of 125 autopsy cases, in which "all subjects were studied who, during life, had had angina pectoris, coronary thrombosis, or congestive failure, or, on postmortem examination, showed coronary occlusion or myocardial infarction or fibrosis." This was a large and detailed undertaking, and the report of the findings occupied 91 pages of the American Heart Journal.

Blumgart and Schlesinger's conclusions were important and have stood the test of time. The cardiologist and the pathologist together found that normal hearts did not show intercoronary anastomoses of any size, and that larger anastomoses clearly developed in response to the presence of stenotic or occlusive disease. Cases with a history of angina pectoris were usually associated with one or more coronary occlusions; on the contrary, coronary occlusions existed in several cases with no history of angina. Congestive heart failure most often was seen when hearts showed a diffuse fibrosis. Blumgart and Schlesinger also found that the presence of coronary thrombosis and occlusion did not "necessarily produce any characteristic clinical manifestations," and the clinical syndrome called at that time "coronary occlusion" in reality signified the presence of myocardial infarction. Finally, they emphasized "the extraordinary significance of the collateral circulation in bridging the discrepancy between supply and demand." This significant publication was indeed a high point in the collaboration between clinical cardiologist and pathologist. Its conclusions were supported and extended over the years as technological advances permitted other new approaches.

Very different from the work of Blumgart and Schlesinger was the introduction of an exercise test for patients suspected of having coronary heart disease; such a test was promoted chiefly in its early phase by Arthur M. Master, of Mt. Sinai Hospital, New York. Others had also been involved in its development. Master and Oppenheimer had published, in 1929, tables setting out criteria for a test employing repeated ascent and descent of two steps by the patient (23). Each step was nine inches high, and the pulse and blood pressure were to be recorded two minutes after completion of the exercise. This was first described in general terms as "helpful in the diagnosis and the grading of circulatory efficiency and insufficiency," but with further experience, Master wrote in 1935 that the test "is particularly useful in the anginal syndrome (24)."

Six years later, in 1941, Master modified his original protocol by taking a control three-lead electrocardiogram prior to the exercise, and repeating this immediately after completion of the step-climbing. He referred in his first brief report on the revised technique to a 58-year-old man with a history of chest and arm discomfort, both with and without effort, who had a normal control electrocardiogram, but "immediately after the climb of the required number of steps, the RS-T segment became depressed in the three standard leads, the depression reaching 3 mm. in lead 2 (25)." The findings were thus helpful in confirming a diagnosis of underlying coronary artery disease. Actually, others had made similar observations a few years before this. Katz and Landt in 1935 reported on the use of arm exercise with the patient reclining in bed, and produced typical ischemic changes in the electrocardiogram (which included a single chest lead) (26). Also, Missal (27), and independently Puddu (28), in 1938, had comparable experiences, the former employing Master's own two-step test, and the latter a slightly different stair-climbing technique. Because the Master protocol was a standard one, required no large expensive equipment, could provide valuable information, and was associated with minimal risk, it was widely used during the 1940's and 1950's. It was gradually supplanted by the treadmill and the stationary bicycle with improved monitoring capability. Thus, the application of exercise testing to the study of coronary heart disease, first introduced in 1929, became a much-used and sometimes over-used, feature of office and hospital cardiologic practice and research.

A controversial aspect of the therapy of coronary heart disease and its complications was the use of oral anticoagulants to retard thrombin formation, introduced in the years immediately after the Second World War and widely prescribed for some years thereafter. Spotty use of these anticoagulants, with and without heparin, had been undertaken for a decade beginning in the late 1930's. Irving S. Wright, Professor of Clinical Medicine at Cornell, became a forceful proponent of their use in 1945. Wright a large genial bald-headed physician led a multi-hospital cooperative controlled study, with a distinguished group of clinical investigators, which was sponsored by the American Heart Association. This short-term study, employing the drug dicumarol, included 1,031 patients with acute myocardial infarction (29). It was found that after six weeks of drug treatment, the mortality in the treated group was seven percent lower than in the controls and that thromboembolic events were almost twice as frequent among the controls as among those receiving dicumarol.

The report of this study, published in 1954, was praised and criticized. Certain other investigators obtained quite similar results; others did not. Expectations of great benefit from the short-term use of such an agent in the management of acute myocardial infarction were not realized. In addition, a small number of patients experienced serious and even fatal hemorrhage. Further, the design and execution of the project were, in retrospect, far from ideal. Despite its shortcomings and the findings of only modest benefit, the 1954 report by Wright and his collaborators was a useful stepping-stone to further investigations.

Wright's study ushered in an era of multi-institutional controlled tests for coronary heart disease, studies which steadily became more sophisticated in design, quality control, and statistical expertise. They focused attention on the role of clotting, not just in the coronary circulation but also in the complications of venous thrombosis and pulmonary and peripheral embolism. General conclusions of these studies were supported in 1977 by Chalmers et al after they had reviewed thirty years of experience in the treatment of acute myocardial infarction with oral anticoagulants; this was at a time when the enthusiasm for the routine use of these agents had waned (30).

In the decades after 1954, a vast number of other investigations approached the issue of clotting complications in coronary disease, including the use of aspirin and other drugs to alter platelet aggregation, and of several potent thrombolytic substances to attack the clot directly (the observations of DeWood and his collaborators in 1980 pointed once again to the importance of the freshly formed occlusive thrombus in a major coronary artery in the first few minutes and hours of the acute process) (31). In the 1990s as in the 1950s, the complex subject of clotting and its modification was at the forefront of scientific interest.

It was a clinician Samuel A. Levine who revolutionized the medical treatment of myocardial infarct by drastically shortening the period of bed rest. He was a feisty, astute, experienced cardiologist, short in stature, and widely respected for his diagnostic ability and good sense. Born in Poland and trained at the Harvard Medical School, his professional career was spent in Boston at the Peter Bent Brigham Hospital, where he was deservedly popular as a teacher and practitioner. In 1936, he published a short, readable, and wise text titled "Clinical Heart Disease," which went into five editions. He and his associates contributed numerous clinical articles to the medical literature, with one on the "'Armchair' Treatment of Acute Coronary Occlusion," written with Bernard Lown and published in 1952, becoming a classic (32). This was in a time in which strict and prolonged bed rest for several weeks had become enshrined as a prerequisite for recovery from acute infarction.

Levine and Lown stated that "It has been our view that recumbency in bed affords less rest to the heart than the sedentary position in a chair with the feet down." In this brief but influential study, patients with acute myocardial infarction were allowed to be lifted from the bed to the chair for increasing periods, beginning not later than seven days after the onset of the attack, with apparent benefit and without deleterious consequences. The authors wrote: "The prompt improvement shown by some of those desperately ill with congestive heart failure after being placed in a chair was particularly impressive," and "This method of treatment also appeared to have beneficial effects on the psychological state of the patient, and facilitated the rehabilitation process." This was not an impressive publication in terms of later standards. The number of patients in the series was not large, there were no true controls, and the modification of the treatment routine was minor (32). But, the senior position of Levine and the influence of his writings (this was a lead article in the Journal of the American Medical Association) were such that this recommendation served to encourage others to open the door to successive steps to liberalize the care of acute myocardial infarction. In a few years, earlier use of the bedside chair and of ambulation became widely accepted. These changes brought great economic and psychological advantages, facilitating and not compromising the optimal recovery of the patient.

Cardiac arrest had long been known to occur in a variety of situations including in the presence of underlying heart disease. With the introduction of routine electrocardiograms, documentation of terminal ventricular arrhythmias and of asystole was frequenty made. This "act of God" was usually viewed as irreversible, although several methods of resuscitation had been proposed since 1880, including mouth-to-mouth artificial respiration, and attempts to maintain the circulation. In 1947, Beck et al reported the first successful open chest defibrillation of a human heart by a technique developed by Hooker, W. B. Kouwenhoven and Langworthy (33). This was followed by the important work of Zoll (34), and of Lown (35), making closed chest defibrillation feasible.

No satisfactory method of restoring both ventilation and circulation of patients experiencing cardiac arrest, especially as a consequence of coronary heart disease, was available until the 1961 landmark work of James R. Jude from the Department of Surgery at Johns Hopkins, assisted by the same Kouwenhoven and by G.G. Knickerbocker (36). These investigators introduced a remarkably simple combination of closed chest cardiac "massage" by compression of the lower sternum toward the thoracic spine sixty to eighty times a minute, coupled with intermittent mouth-to-mouth or mouth-to-nose ventilation. Their original report included 138 cardiac arrests in 118 patients, 24 of whom had acute myocardial infarction, and in many of whom external electrical defibrillation was also attempted. Five of the 24 with infarction were successfully resuscitated, but only three survived to leave the hospital. This technique was soon widely adopted and became the established one for treating the earliest phase of cardiac arrest. Hospital personnel including physicians and nurses were trained in the method, as were policemen, firemen, and emergency staff. Many lay individuals attended classes in the technique.

The combination of the ability to sustain life for a precious few minutes using the Jude-Kouwenhoven-Knickerbocker approach, better trained emergency staff and improved equipment in emergency rooms and ambulances, and the capacity for closed-chest external cardiac defibrillation as described by Zoll and by Lown, permitted the rescue of a significant number of lives which would otherwise have been lost. (*See also chapter on Electrophysiology and Electrocardiography.*)

Dovetailing nicely with the growing popularity of this active program for treating cardiac arrest was the appearance of the coronary care unit. For many decades, patients hospitalized with signs of acute myocardial infarction or unstable angina had been placed on the regular hospital medical wards, or in single or two-bed units. The advantage of doing otherwise were not obvious. With the availability of a more effective approach to the management of cardiac arrest, should it occur, and the ability to monitor the electrocardiogram constantly, there was a reason for change. In June 1962, Wilburne and Fields, from the Cedars of Lebanon and Mt. Sinai Hospitals in Los Angeles, described before a meeting of the American Medical Association "a central coronary care unit together with 1) a program of physiologic and closed circuit television monitoring, and 2) an organized step-by-step plan of resuscitation in cardiac arrest due to coronary artery disease (37)." Simultaneous with this innovative report day at the Bethany Hospital, Kansas City, and Meltzer at the Presbyterian University of Pennsylvania Medical Center in Philadelphia published similiar studies (38). Such a sequestration of acute coronary cases, together with provision for a specially trained nursing staff and monitoring equipment, was rapidly adopted by most hospitals in the belief that patient lives might thus be saved.

The existence of an acute coronary care unit became overnight not only a useful facility, but also a hospital status symbol, as well as providing business for manufacturers of electronic equipment. Equally important was the delegation of new duties to nurses. Of necessity, nurses became well trained in recognizing cardiac arrest, and often they were the ones to initiate and carry out resuscitative measures. Their level of competence, and their role in applying techniques previously applied only by physicians, increased their professional image and, enhanced their importance especially in the area of coronary heart disease,. A true cardiac team was usually the result, a happy and unexpected dividend.

The history of coronary heart disease in the twentieth century would be incomplete without reference to the recognition of risk factors in coronary heart disease formulated by scientists and epidemiologists. Now accepted without question as important in the genesis of coronary atherosclerotic disease, it was not always so. Earlier in the century, investigators working in the areas of nutrition, blood lipids, cigarette smoking, and other factors, were often regarded as harmless and of no significance. Recognition therefore should be given to a few whose often lonely work has proved fundamental in the risk factor concept. A recent review of the background of cardiovascular disease has pointed to individuals or groups who have been particularly significant in the area of coronary heart disease (39). "Information on this subject is also available from the comprehensive textbooks on cardiology by Braunwald (40) and Hurst (41)." In the field of diet, the lineage of contributing investigators goes back one hundred years. Ancel Keys of the University of Minnesota was one individual who in the twentieth century has provided especially significant additions to our knowledge, particularly as to blood lipids.

In the area of hypertension, Fisher in 1914 was the first to associate an elevated arterial pressure with an excess mortality among life insurance policy holders. Allan in 1934 correctly concluded, from uncontrolled observations, that hypertension was a major factor in the occurrence of angina pectoris and coronary occlusion. Later, several long-term population studies amply confirmed this. The cigarette smoking habit was first linked to coronary heart disease by English, Willius, and Berkson of the Mayo Clinic, in 1940, but was paricularly well documented by the classic investigation of Hammond and Horn of the American Cancer Society in 1954. These few examples—and many other pertinent reports—have served to provide the basis for the current expanding field of the prevention of coronary heart disease. (*See also chapter on Atherosclerosis*) .

REFERENCES

1. Bing, R. J. Coronary circulation and cardiac metabolism. In: Circulation of the Blood. Men and Ideas, edited by A. P. Fishman, and D. W. Richards. Oxford University Press, 1964, pp. 199–264.
2. Lie, J. T., Recognizing coronary heart disease. Selected historical vignettes from the period of William Harvey (1578–1657) to Adam Hammer, (1818–1878). Mayo Clin. Proc., 53:811–817, 1978.
3. Herrick, J. B. A Short History of Cardiology. Springfield, IL, Thomas, 1942.
4. Heberden, W. Commentaries on the History and Cure of Diseases. London, Payne, 1802.
5. Burns, A. Observations on some of the most frequent and important diseases of the heart; on aneurysm of the thoracic aorta; on preternatural pulsation in the epigastric region; and on the unusual origin and distribution of some of the large arteries of the human body. Edinburgh, Bryce, 1809.
6. Quain, R. On fatty acid diseases of the heart. Med. Chir. Trans., 33:121, 1850.
7. Hall, M. On the mutual relations between anatomy, physiology, pathology and therapeutics, and the practice of medicine. The Golstonian Lectures for 1842. London, Bailliere's, 1842.
8. Erichsen, J. E. On the influence of the coronary circulation on the action of the heart. London Med. Gaz., 2:561–564, 1842.

9. Cohnheim, J. F. and A. von Schultheiss-Rechberg. Ueber die Folgen der Kranz-arterienverschliessung fuer das Herz. Virchows Arch. Path. Anat., 85:503–37, 1881.

10. McKee, A. B. Lectures on General Pathology. Trans. of Julius Cohnheim, Vorlesungen ueber allgemeine Pathologie. London, New Sydenham Society, 1889–90.

11. Talbott, J. H. A biographical history of medicine; Excerpts and essays on the men and their work. New York, Grune and Stratton, 1970, pp. 837–840.

12. Weigert, C. Ueber die pathologischen Gerinnungsvorgaenge. Virchows Arch. Path. Anat., 79:87–123, 1880.

13. Ziegler, E. Lehrbuch der allgemeinen Pathologie und der pathologischen Anatomie fuer Aertze und Studierende. Jena, Fischer, 1881–1906.

14. Lie, J. T. Centenary of the first correct antemortem diagnosis of coronary thrombosis by Adam Hammer (1818–1878): English translation of the original report. Am. J. Cardiol., 42:849–852, 1978.

15. Neumayr, A. "Musik und Medizin: am Beispiel der deutschen Romantik" Edition Wien, p. 118, 1989.

16. Herrick, J. B. Clinical features of sudden obstruction of the coronary arteries. J. Am. Med. Assoc., 59:2015–2020, 1912.

17. Ross, R. S. A parlous state of storm and stress. The life and times of James B. Herrick. Circulation, 67:955–959, 1983.

18. Herrick, J. B. The coronary artery in health and disease. Harvey Lectures, 26:129–151, 1931.

19. Herrick, J. B. Concerning thrombosis of the coronary arteries. Trans. Assoc. Am. Physicians, 33:408–418, 1918.

20. Paul, O. Take Heart: The life and prescription for living of Paul Dudley White. Boston, MA. Harvard University Press for the Francis A. Countway Library of Medicine, 1986.

21. Schlesinger, M.J. An injection plus dissection study of coronary artery occlu-sions and anastomoses. Am. Heart J., 15:528–568, 1938.

22. Blumgart, H.L., M.J. Schlesinger and D. Davis. Studies on the relation of the clinical manifestations of angina pectoris, coronary thrombosis, and myocardial infarction to the pathologic findings. Am. Heart J., 19:1–91, 1940.

23. Master, A.M. and E.J. Oppenheimer. A simple exercise tolerance test for circu-latory efficiency with standard tables for normal individuals. Am. J. Med. Sci., 177:223–243, 1929.

24. Master, A.M. The two-step test of myocardial function. Am. Heart J., 10:495–510, 1935.

25. Master, A.M. and H.L. Jaffe. The electrocardiographic changes after exercise in angina pectoris. J. Mt. Sinai Hospital, 7:629–632, 1941.

26. Katz, L.N. and H. Landt. The effect of standardized exercises on the four-lead electrocardiogram. Am. J. Med. Sci., 189:346–351, 1935.

27. Missal, M.E. Exercise tests and the electrocardiograph in the study of angina pectoris. Ann. Int. Med., 11:2018–2036, 1938.

28. Puddu, V. Alterazioni elettrocardiografiche da sforzo, in sogetti normali e anginosi, con particolare riguardo alla derivazione foracica. Cardiologia, 2:183–192, 1938.

29. Wright, I.S., C.D. Marple, and D.F. Beck. Myocardial Infarction: Its clinical

manifestations and treatment with anticoagulants; a study of 1031 cases. New York. Grune and Stratton, 1954.
30. Chalmers, T.C., R.J. Matta, H. Smith, Jr., and A-M. Kunzler. Evidence favoring the use of anticoagulants in the hospital phase of acute myocardial infarction. N. Engl. J. Med., 297:1091–1096, 1977.
31. DeWood, M.A., J. Spores, R. Notske, L.T. Mouser, R. Burroughs, M.S. Golden, and H.T. Lang. Prevalence of total coronary occlusion during the early hours of transmural myocardial infarction. N. Eng. J. Med, 303:897–902, 1980.
32. Levine, S.A. and B. Lown. Armchair treatment of acute coronary thrombosis. J. Am. Med. Assoc., 148:1365–1369, 1952.
33. Beck, C.F., W.H. Pritchard, and H.S. Feil. Ventricular fibrillation of long duration abolished by electric shock. J. Am. Med. Assoc., 136:985–986, 1947.
34. Zoll, P.M., A.J. Linenthal, W. Bibson, M.H. Paul, and L.R. Norman. Termination of ventricular fibrillation in man by externally applied electric countershock. N. Engl. J. Med, 254:727–732, 1956.
35. Lown, B., J. Neuman, R. Amarasingham, and B.V. Berkovits. Comparison of alternating current with direct current electroshock across the closed chest. Am. J. Cardiol., 10:223–233, 1962.
36. Jude, J.R., W.B. Kouwenhoven, and G.G. Knickerbocker. Cardiac arrest. Report of application of external cardiac message on 118 patients. JAMA, 178:1063–1069, 1961.
37. Wilburne, M. and J. Fields. Cardiac resuscitation in coronary heart disease. JAMA, 184:453–457, 1963.
38. Meltzer, L.E. and A.J. Dunning, editors. Textbook of coronary care. Philadelphia, Charles Press 1972, pages 5–7.
39. Paul O. Background of the prevention of cardiovascular disease. Circulation, 79:1361–68; 80:206–214, 1989.
40. Braunwald, Eugene. Heart disease: a textbook of cardiac medicine. Edited by Eugene Braunwald, Saunders, Philadelphia, 4th ed. 1992.
41. Hurst, John W. The Heart, Arteries and Veins. Seventh edition, McGraw-Hill, New York, NY, 1990.

Chapter 8

Coronary Artery Surgery

J. BALDWIN, J. SANCHEZ AND R.J. BING

Coronary artery disease, the greatest killer in the Western world, has compelled the attention of cardiologists and surgeons more than any other single affliction. The earliest attempt at the surgical relief of angina pectoris in man is believed to have been undertaken in 1916 by Jonnesco (1). He treated angina by ablation of the upper thoracic sympathetic ganglia. Non-operative approaches to sympathetic ablation, which included paravertebral alcohol injection, were ultimately abondoned due to the high incidence of complications and the frequency of inducing increased angina (2).

With the knowledge that diminished coronary blood flow was the cause of angina, attempts to increase collateral blood flow or introduce extracardiac sources of blood to affected areas of the heart were undertaken. In 1931, Moritz made the observation that pericardial adhesions appeared to confer a beneficial effect on the course of coronary artery disease. This notion had first been suggested by Thorel in 1903 in a patient with complete obliteration of both coronary arteries and extensive pericardial adhesion. (3).

Claude S. Beck (Figure 1) joined the faculty at the Western Reserve University in Cleveland following training in surgery at the Peter Bent Brigham Hospital in Boston. Beck was interested in the problem of cardiac blood flow and made the astute observation that adhesions between the pericardium and the heart bled profusely from both ends when severed (4). This led to discussions with Moritz regarding his study of naturally occurring collaterals to the

169

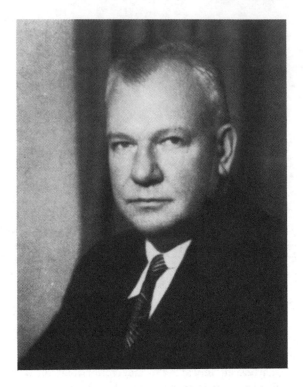

Figure 1.   Claude S. Beck (*Courtesy of Dr. Mary Ellen Wohl*)

heart and the early studies of treatment of suppurative pericarditis by instilla-
tion of Dakin solution into the pericardium. Beck began a series of brilliant
experiments in dogs in 1932, which demonstrated the efficacy of recruiting
collateral blood flow between coronary arteries and from the adjacent pericardium by mechanical and chemical irritation (4,5). His paper, published in
1935, began "It is perversity of nature that the most important muscular
structure in the body is the most defenseless" (5).

By 1943, Beck had published his experience with the procedure on 30
patients reporting partial or complete relief of pain in survivors (6). The
technique initially involved the installation of mechanical irritants such as
ground beef bone dust. Later, Beck found chemical irritants more efficacious
and suggested the use of asbestos. The use of talc and magnesium silicate,
was popularized by Thompson who reported favorable results in 70% of 30

patients (7). Later, mechanical abrasion of the epicardium was performed using specially designed burrs and even sandpaper (6). Vineberg proposed placement of the Ivalon sponge in the pericardial space to achieve adhesion and improved blood flow (8). Others reported an increase in the vascular supply of the pericardium following ligation of the internal mammary arteries (9).

Although the pericardium became a convenient vehicle for the enhancement of blood supply, through development of adhesions it soon became clear that more direct means were required to increase supply of blood to the myocardium. Beck and O'Shaughnessy, independently tried various vascular conduits including the pectoral muscles and the omentum in "cardiopexy" procedures (10,11). Lezius, working in Germany in 1939, established that lung adhesions to the heart after pericardiectomy allowed ligation of a coronary artery without adverse effects in animals in 1939 (12). These "pneumopexy" techniques were later popularized by Carter and by Vidone (13,14). Other ideas included the use of pediculted grafts of jejunum by Key and of skin by Moran, as sources of augmented blood supply to the heart. (15,16). Deaths occurred often with these techniques and were thought to be a result from coronary thrombosis brought about by release of thromboplastic materials from the abraded tissues, as well as by direct injury to already diseased coronary intima (17).

Beck's subsequent experimental efforts revolved around the feasibility of increasing myocardial tissue perfusion by "arterialization" of the coronary venous system (18). This concept was an expansion of work done by Gross who reported his results with coronary sinus occlusion to the Society of Experimental Biology and Medicine in 1935 (19). Fauteux later studied the effect of coronary vein ligation, which was believed to result in an increase in oxygen uptake by an ischemic myocardium (20). Beck, however, focused on the establishment of retrograde perfusion through the coronary sinus via arterial or venous conduits such as the internal mammary artery or venous grafts to the descending aorta (18). This technique was subsequently incorporated clinically by Beck and by others as part of revascularization operations and the bold concept of retrograde perfusion has now been resurrected, with the use of retrograde infusion of cardioplegia solutions through the coronary sinus for intra-operative myocardial protection (21).

Methods for perfusion of the myocardium directly from the cardiac chambers were investigated by several groups. These efforts were based on studies of Wearn on the capillary bed of the heart and those of Beck on venous stasis in the coronary circulation (22,23). Goldman placed explanted carotid grafts into the myocardium which communicated with the left ventricle (24). The grafts contained a number of small openings which directed theoretically ventricular blood into the sinusoidal network within the myocardium. This procedure reportedly protected against ligation of the anterior descending coronary artery in dogs. Similarly, Massimo and Boffie inserted T-shaped polyethylene tubes of 4 mm. in diameter which were imbedded in the myocardium of dogs (25).

The direct implantation of the internal mammary artery into ischemic myocardium by Dr. Arthur Vineberg of Montreal in 1945 was a continuation of the search for optimal sources of extracardiac blood (26,27). Although the clinical results were difficult to assess, experimental and clinical data suggested significant increases in myocardial blood flow with this approach (28). Furthermore, recognition that many of these patients had persistently patent mammary arteries and established collateral blood flow when studied many years later sustained interest in the internal mammary artery as a conduit. By 1965, Vineberg had reported on 115 patients with an operative mortality of only 2.9% and a graft patency rate of approximately 75%. Based on these encouraging findings, 76 Vineberg procedures were performed at the Cleveland Clinic by Effler between April of 1962 and December of 1963 (29). However, the long time period required to achieve maximal revascularization, at least nine months, significantly diminished the appeal of this approach to the urgent problem of myocardial ischemia.

Confidence derived from surgical successes in the treatment of congenital lesions of the heart and in "closed" techniques for relief of mitral stenosis suggested bolder methods in the treatment of coronary disease. Coronary endarterectomy was pursued by *Szilagyi* and others in animals and in postmortem specimens (30). As a result, a series of endarterectomy procedures were performed on patients and reported by Bailey and by Longmire the following year, 1958 (31,32). As experience accumulated, improvements in survival followed. Modifications, such as the use of the vein patch in 1959 by Senning, were incorporated (33). A high operative mortality, however resulted in restrained enthusiasm and remained as a impetus for the search of safer methods of myocardial revascularization.

The introduction of selective coronary arteriography by Sones in 1959 offered precise localization of lesions preoperatively as well as an assessment of surgical results postoperatively (34). The Cleveland Clinic group studied various techniques in the surgical treatment of coronary artery disease including Vineberg's operation, endarterectomy, and techniques involving direct coronary artery anastomoses (34,35).

In 1910, Carrel bypassed coronary arteries in the laboratory, using a segment of explanted carotid artery which was interposed between the aorta and the left coronary artery (36). Sustained experimentation with direct coronary artery anastomoses, however, was not undertaken until the early 1950's when Murray reported interposition arterial grafts following resection of proximal segments of coronary arteries in dogs (37). Experimental work at the University of Minnesota in the late 1950's investigated the feasibility of direct anastomosis to coronary arteries with the internal mammary artery (38,39). These experiments with internal mammary graft pedicles were expanded by Ormond Julian in Chicago (40). Julian used free arterial grafts interposed between the aorta and the left circumflex coronary artery in dogs on cardiopulmonary bypass. Several other studies were conducted with refinements in the technique (41,42,43,44).

The use of aorto-coronary bypass in man was first reported in 1962 by David C. Sabiston at Duke University in a patient following an unsuccessful right coronary endarterectomy (45; Fig. 2). Sabiston described a patient in whom a complete occulsion of the right coronary artery was demonstrated by

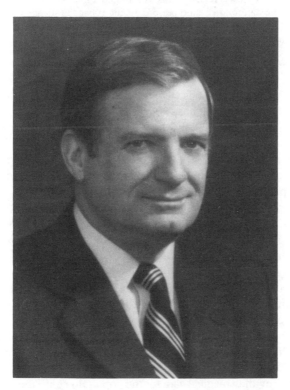

Figure 2. David C. Sabiston (*with permission*)

coronary arteriography. Endarterectomy was unsuccessful and a reversed saphenous vein graft was placed. The patient died of a cerebral vascular accident three days later, and, at autopsy, a thrombus was present at the aortic end of the coronary anasotmosis. Two years later, again as a result of difficulties following endarterectomy, Garret performed aorto-coronary bypass to the left anterior descending artery (46). This case, however was not reported until seven years later.

In the popular medical mind, the origin of the current era of coronary surgery was the Cleveland Clinic, and the prodigious efforts of Effler, Favaloro, and Grove which were truly historic in gaining wide acceptance for this procedure in a relatively short period of time. Their experience began in May of 1967 when surgery on an occluded right coronary artery required its excision and replacement with an interposed segment of saphenous vein. The patient recuperated fully and was discharged.

> With timidity, we slowly repeated this experience. First to the right and later to the left coronary artery. In a short period, the interposed grafts gave way to the bypassed grafts from aorta to coronary artery. As results improved and enthusiasm escalated, all combinations of single and multiple grafts were tried and efforts were made to find the simplest and best procedures and then to standardize them. *Letter from Dr. Effler to Dr. Bing.*

In 1967, 37 bypass operations were performed at the Cleveland Clinic. By 1968, the number rose to almost 200. In 1969, 1,500 patients underwent coronary artery bypass procedures at the Clinic and, in 1976, the number was 3,000. The surgical results by Effler and his colleagues were singular for their low operative mortality and the Clinic became a magnet for surgeons around the world interested in learning these techniques. The success of the operation depended upon careful selection of low-risk patients and standardized teamwork, as emphasized by the Cleveland group. This approach involved coordination of surgeons, anesthesiologists, cardiologists, as well as nursing and other health care personnel committed to caring for these patients in a reliable and consistent fashion.

Although no one individual can be credited for the ultimate success of the bypass procedure, Rene Favaloro stands out as one of the most innovative surgeons of this era. The career of Favaloro, like many of the pioneers, was a circuitous one (Figure 3). After graduation from La Plata University School of Medicine in 1948, and obtaining an MD degree in 1949, Favaloro moved to a small village in a farming area of Argentina with approximately 1,100 inhabitants. There he worked as a country doctor with the help of his physician brother, providing medical care for the population until the end of 1961. As Favaloro wrote, "I could no longer watch the revolution in cardiac sur-

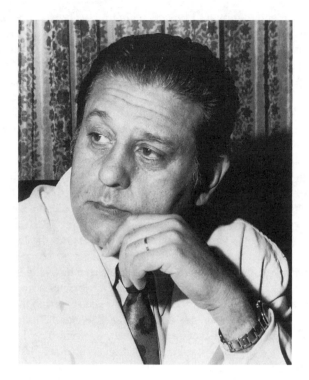

Figure 3.   Ray G. Favaloro (*Courtesy of the New York Academy of Medicine*)

gery any longer. I wanted to be part of it (47)." In early 1962, he moved to the United States and started work in the Department of Thoracic and Cardiovascular Surgery at the Cleveland Clinic, under the guidance of Effler. Favaloro also credited Sones saying "there is no question that without his introduction of coronary arteriography the operation would have not been feasible. Initially there was considerable concern about the prolonged patency of the saphenous vein graft." Favaloro quotes Sones who would often shake his head, saying to him, "Oh Rene, I wonder what will happen to all of us if those grafts occlude two or three months after the operation." Favaloro mentions that the first operation was performed on one of the relatives of an executive at the Cleveland Clinic who had suffered a myocardial infarct. A single by-pass was performed to the anterior descending coronary artery and the patient made an uneventful recovery.

The medical community was slow in accepting the bypass operation as a legitimate surgical procedure. Favaloro remembered a discussion during a meeting of the World Congress of Cardiology in London in 1979, when he and Charles Friedberg, a prominent clinical cardiologist, had serious arguments about this type of surgery (47). Finally, in the discussion, when Friedberg said that it was difficult to accept the very low mortality rate, Favaloro wrote, "My Latin blood flared up and I said emphatically that the work of our team was an honest effort under the leadership of Effler and Sones and that our records at the Cleveland Clinic were at the disposal of anyone who wanted to study them."

Although the mammary arteries were identified early as suitable arterial conduits for coronary bypass, they were employed sparingly in the United States during this time (48). In Leningrad, Professor Vasilii Kolessov, as Chairman of the Surgical Department of the First Medical Institute performed a series of internal mammary anastomoses to the left coronary circulation. His accomplishments and contributions to coronary surgery were virtually unkonwn in the western medical literature at the time, 1967 (49,50). He used direct internal mammary artery to coronary artery anastomoses, describing his procedure in detail and reporting the results on five patients. The main difference between the Cleveland Clinic group and Kolessov was that the latter eschewed coronary angiography "lest it should result in fibrillation of heart ventricle." Kolessov graduated in 1931, from the Second Leningrad Institute. After serving in the war, he returned to Leningrad where he was awarded the title of Professor, in 1949. In 1952, he became the Chief of the Department of Military Surgery in the Military Medical Department in Leningrad. At the time of his publication, he was the Chairman of the Surgical Department of the First Leningrad Medical Institute.

As cardiopulmonary bypass technology improved and familiarity and safety were achieved, longer pump runs and more complete revascularizations were undertaken. Important in this regard was the refinement of the techniques of myocardial protection. Although the concept of cardioplegia was initially advanced by Melrose, it received intensive and widespread attention with the advent of the "bypass revolution." More recently, the work of Buckberg and many others has made possible extended periods of arrest, thereby allowing surgeons of widely varying skills and speed to operate with relative safety (51).

Given the lack of long-term follow-up data, bypass operations were not initially embraced by the general medical community. Acceptance came slowly as the efficacy of the procedure at relieving angina was recognized. Large multicenter trials were instituted to investigate the efficacy of coronary bypass in comparison to standard medical therapy. The first of these studies was the Veterans Administration Cooperative Study which began its pilot phase in 1970 (52). Although this study was undertaken during the early days of the coronary artery bypass operation, it clearly demonstrated the benefit of surgery for patients with significant (>50%) left main coronary artery stenosis. This was followed by the European Cooperative Surgery Study which demonstrated the superiority of surgery over medical management for symptomatic patients with three-vessel coronary disease or two-vessel disease in which the left anterior descending coronary artery is involved (53). This study also corroborated the findings of the VA study for patients with left main coronary artery disease. The Coronary Artery Surgery Study, which was sponsored by the National Institutes of Health, studied patients who were randomized to medical or surgical therapy between 1975 and 1979 (54). This study attempted to define the role of surgery as initial therapy for patients with significant coronary disease and limited symptoms. It demonstrated a benefit for surgery in those patients with coronary artery disease in three vessels and depressed ventricular function (ejection fraction between 0.35 and 0.5). Although these studies have been instrumental in defining the benefits of surgery, differences in study design and data collection have resulted in continued controversy. Nonetheless, proponents of the need for national statistical and longitudinal analysis of the efficacy of new medical interventions can find gratification in the area of coronary surgery. It is perhaps the best studied of the newer technological innovations in medicine.

Newer developments in the surgical treatment of coronary disease, include the use of other arterial conduits as bypass grafts such as intra-abdominal vessels (55,56). The use of laser technology in artherectomy devices, while largely experimental, may ultimately be useful as an adjunct to bypass procedures. In addition, transmyocardial laser channels are being used to revascularize the ischemic myocardium (57). This approach is a modification of methods described by Goldman and by Massino and based on the myocardial sinusoidal network concept developed by Wearn and Beck nearly 40 years ago.

The dramatic success with cardiac transplantation for "ischemic cardiomyopathy" has resulted in a trend toward increasing prevalence of ischemic disease as an indication for transplant. At present, the majority of patients awaiting heart transplant have ischemic disease. Ultimately, replacement of the heart with a biological (allograft or xenograft) or mechanical substitute will establish itself as a fundamentally new approach to ischemic heart disease, one which conceptually transcends this century's remarkable efforts at repair and palliation.

REFERENCES

1. Jonnesco, T. Traitement chirurgical de l'angine de poitrine par la résection du sympathique cervico-thoracique. Presse. med., Par., 29:193, 1921.
2. White, J.C. Cardiac pain: anatomic pathways and physiologic mechanisms. Circulation. 16:644, 1957.
3. Thorel, C.H. Pathologie der Kreislauforgane. Ergebn. Allg. u Path. Anat. 9:559–1116, 1903.
4. Beck, C.S. The effect of surgical solution of chlorinated soda (Dakin's Solution) in the pericardial cavity. Arch. Surg 18:1659–1671, 1929.
5. Beck, C.S. and V. L. Tichy. The production of a collateral circulation to the heart. [I. An Experimental study.] Am. Heart J., 10:849–873, 1935.
6. Beck, C.S. Principles underlying the operative approach to the treatment of myocardial ischemia. Ann. Surg., 118:788–806, 1943.
7. Thompson, S.A. and M.J. Raisbeck. Cardio-pericardiopexy: the surgical treatment of coronary arterial disease by the establishment of adhesive pericarditis. Ann. Int. Med. 16:495–520, 1942.
8. Vineberg, A.M., T. Deliyannis and G. Pablo. The Ivalon sponge procedure for myocardial revascularization. Surgery 47:268–289, 1960.
9. Battezzati, M., A. Tagliaferro, and G. DeMarchi. La legatura delle due arterie mammarie interne nei disturbi di vascolarizzazione del miocardio. Minerva Med. 11:1178–1188, 1955.
10. O'Shaughnessy, L. An experimental method of providing a collateral circulation to the heart. Brit. J. Surg. 23:665–670, 1936.
11. O'Shaughnessy, L. Surgical treatment of cardiac ischaemia. Lancet 1:185–194, 1937.
12. Lezius, A. Die anatomischen und funktionellen Grundlagen der kuenstlichen Blutversorgung des Herzmukels durch die Lunge bei Coronarterienverschluss. Arch. Klin. Chir. 191:101, 1938.
13. Carter, B.N. Discussion of Beck, C.S. Revascularization of the heart. Ann. Surg. 128:861–864, 1948.
14. Vidone, R.A., J.L. Kline, M. Pitel and A.A. Liebow. The application of an induced bronchial collateral circulation to the coronary arteries by cardio-pneumopexy. Am. J. Path. 32:897–925, 1956.
15. Key, J.A., F.G. Kergin, Y. Martineau and R.G. Leckey. A method of supplementing the coronary circulation by a jejunal pedical graft. J. Thorac. Surg. 28:320–330, 1954.
16. Moran, R.E., C.G. Neumann, G. von Wendel, J.W. Lord, P.W. Stone, and J.W. Hinton. Revascularization of the heart by tubed pedicle graft of skin and subcutaneous tissue. Plastic and Reconstruct. Surg. 10:295–302, 1952.
17. King, E.S.J. Surgery of the Heart. William and Wilkins, 1941, p. 437.
18. Beck, C.S. Revascularization of the heart. Ann. Surg., 128:854–864, 1948.
19. Gross, L. and L. Blum. Effect of coronary artery occlusion on the dog's heart with total coronary sinus ligation. Proc. Soc., Exp. Biol. Med. 32:1578–1580, 1935.
20. Fauteux, M. Experimental study of the surgical treatment of coronary disease. Surg. Gynecol. Obst., 71:151–155, 1940.
21. Beck, C.S., E. Stanton, W. Batiuchok, and E. Leiter. Revascularization of the

heart by graft of a systemic artery into coronary sinus. J. Am. Med. Assoc. 137:436–442, 1948.

22. Wearn, J.R. The extent of the capillary bed of the heart. J. Exper. Med. 47:273–291, 1928.

23. Beck, C.S. and A.E. Mako. Venous stasis in the coronary circulation. Am Heart J. 21:767–779, 1941.

24. Goldman, A., S.M. Greenstone, F.S. Preuss, S.H. Strauss, and E.S. Chang Experimental methods for producing a collateral circulation to the heart directly from the left ventricle. J. Thorac, Surg., 31:364–374, 1956.

25. Massimo, C. and L. Boffi. Myocardial revascularization by a new method of carrying blood directly from the left ventricular cavity into the coronary circulation. J. Thorac. Surg. 34:257–264, 1957.

26. Vineberg, A. and G. Miller. Internal mammary coronary anastomosis in the surgical treatment of coronary artery insufficiencey. Can Med. Assoc. J. 64: 204–210, 1951.

27. Vineberg, A.M. Development of an anastomosis between the coronary vessels and a transplanted internal mammary artery. Canad. Med. Assoc. J. 55:117–119, 1946.

28. Effler, D.B., L.K. Groves, F.M. Sones, Jr., and E.K. Shirey. Increased myocardial perfusion by internal mammary implant: Vineberg's operation. Ann. Surg. 158:526–536, 1963.

29. Effler, D.B., F.M. Sones, Jr., L.K. Groves, and E. Suarez. Myocardial revascularization by Vineberg's internal mammary artery implant. Evaluation of postoperative results. J. Thor. Cardiovasc. Surg., 50:527–533, 1965.

30. Szilagyi, D.E., R.T. McDonald and L.C. France. The applicability of angioplastic procedures in coronary atherosclerosis: an estimate through postmortem injection studies. Ann. Surg. 148:447–461, 1958.

31. Bailey, C.P., A. May, and W. M. Lemmon. Survival after coronary endarterectomy in man. J. Am. Med. Assoc. 164:641–646, 1957.

32. Longmire, W.P., Jr., J.A. Cannon, A.A. Kattus. Direct-vision coronary endarterectomy for angina pectoris, N. Engl. J. Med. 259:993–999, 1958.

33. Senning, A. Strip gratfing in coronary arteries: report of a case. J. Thorac. Cardiovasc. Surg. 41:542–549, 1961.

34. Effler, D.B., L.K. Groves, and F.M. Sones, et al. Endarterectomy in the treatment of coronary artery disease. J. Thorac. Cardiovasc. Surg. 47:98–108, 1964.

35. Effler, D.R., F.M. Sones, Jr., R. Favaloro and L.K. Groves. Coronary endarterotomy with patch-graft reconstruction: clinical experience with 34 cases. Ann. Surg. 162:590–601, 1965.

36. Carrel, A. On the experimental surgery of the thoracic aorta and the heart. Ann. Surg., 52:83–95, 1910.

37. Murray, G., R. Porcheron, J. Hilario, and W. Roschlau. Anastomosis of a systemic artery to the coronary. Can. Med. Assoc. J. 71:594–597, 1954.

38. Absolon, K.B., J.B. Aust, R.L. Varco, and C.W. Lillehei. Surgical treatment of occlusive coronary artery disease by endarterectomy or anastomotic replacement. Surg. Gyn. Obst., 103:180–185, 1956.

39. Thal, A., J.F. Perry, F.A. Miller and O.H. Wangensteen. Direct suture anastomosis of the coronary arteries in the dog. Surgery 40:1023–1029, 1956.

40. Julian, O.C., M. Lopez-Belio, D. Moorehead and A. Lima. Direct surgical

procedures on the coronary arteries: experimental studies. J. Thorac. Surg. 34:654–660, 1957.

41. Botham, R.J. and W.P. Young. An experimental study of experimental systemic coronary anastomosis. Surg. Gyn. Obst. 108:361–365, 1959.
42. Baker, N.H. and J.H. Grindlay. Technique of experimental systemic coronary anastomosis. Proc. Staff Meet. Mayo Clinic. 34:397–501, 1959.
43. Miller, E.W., W.F. Kolff and L.K. Groves. Experimental coronary artery surgery in dogs employing a pump-oxygenator. Surgery 45:1005–1012, 1959.
44. Moore, T.C. and A. Riberi. Maintenance of coronary ciruclation during systemic-to-coronary artery anastomosis. Surgery 43:245–253, 1958.
45. Sabiston, D.C., Jr. and A. Blalock. Physiologic and anatomic determinants of coronary blood flow and their relationship to myocardial revascularization. Surgery 44:406–423, 1958.
46. Garrett, M. E., E. W. Dennis, and M. E. DeBakey. Aortocoronary bypass with saphenous vein graft. Seven-year follow-up. JAMA, 223:792–794, 1973.
47. Favaloro, R. G. Coronary bypass surgery: the first decade. Med. Trib., R4-R12, 1976.
48. Green, G.E., S.H. Stertzer, and E.H. Reppert. Coronary arterial bypass grafts. Ann. Thorac. Surg., 5:443–450, 1968.
49. Kolessov, V. Mammary artery-coronary artery anastomosis as method of treatment for angina pectoris. J. Thor. Cardiovasc. Surg., 54:535–544, 1967.
50. Olearchyk, A.S. Vasilii I. Kolessov: a pioneer of coronary revascularizaton by internal mammary-coronary artery grafting. J. Thorac. Cardiovasc. Surg. 96:13–18, 1988.
51. Buckberg, G.D., G.N. Olinger, D.G. Mulder and J.V. Maloney, Jr. Depressed postoperative cardiac performance. Prevention by adequate myocardial protection during cardiopulmonary bypass. J. Thorac. Cardiovasc. Surg. 70:974–988, 1975.
52. Murphy, M.L., H.N. Hultgren, K. Detre et al. Treatment of chronic stable angina. A preliminary report of survival data of the randomized Veterans Administration Cooperative Study. N. Engl. J. Med. 297:621–627, 1977.
53. European Coronary Surgery Study Group: Long-term results of prospective randomized study of coronary artery bypass in stable angina pectoris. Lancet 2:1173–1180, 1982.
54. CASS Principal Investigators and their Associates; Coronary Artery Surgery Study (CASS) a randomized trial of coronary artery bypass surgery. Survival data. Circulation 68:939–950, 1983.
55. Mirhoseini, M., S. Shelgikar and M.M. Cayton, New concepts in revascularization of the myocardium. Ann. Thorac. Surg. 45:415–420, 1988.
56. Mills, N.L. and C.T. Everson. Technique for use of the inferior epigastric artery as a coronary bypass graft. Ann. Thorac. Surg. 51:208–214, 1991.
57. Hardy, R.I., K.E. Bove, F.W. James, S. Kaplan and L. Goldman. A histologic study of laser-induced transmyocardial channels. Lasers Surg. Med. 6:563–573, 1987.

Chapter 9

Isotopes In Cardiology

H. SCHELBERT AND R.J. BING

The use of isotopes is one of several important technical contributions of fundamental science to medicine. This contribution has been made by inspired and colorful scientists and physicians whose ideas are projecting cardiology into the next century. One of the early pioneers in this field was George Hevesy (Figure 1). His publications give a rare insight into the development of the use of isotopes in biology and medicine. We owe him description of the first use of isotopes in biology and medicine. A native of Hungary, he worked in 1911 with Lord Ernest Rutherford; Hevesy foresaw the possibility of using radioactive radium D as a tracer to study chemical reactions. One of his most important contributions was the discovery of the dynamic state of the body components. Hevesy obtained his Ph.D. in 1908 from the University of Freiburg, Germany, then studied with Rutherford until 1913. He worked at the Vienna Institute of Radium Research and, in 1920, went to the University of Copenhagen on the invitation of Niels Bohr. He then returned to the University of Freiburg as Professor of Physical Chemistry. In 1943, he fled from Copenhagen before the invading Nazis and took refuge in Sweden.

Hevesy's historical papers are informative and entertaining (1–5). He mentioned his cooperation with Rutherford, who asked Hevesy to separate radium D from lead. Rutherford said, "My boy, if you are worth your salt, you try to separate radium D from all that lead." The efforts of Hevesy were unsuccessful. In 1913, Hevesy worked with Paneth at the Vienna Institute of Radium Research; they published the use of labeled lead to determine the solubility of lead chromate and sulphide. Applications of radio sodium in cir-

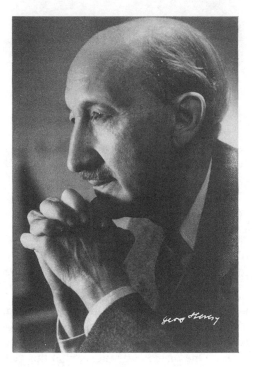

Figure 1.   George Hevesy (*Courtesy of The New York Academy of Medicine*)

culatory studies were to follow. The first use of radioactive indicators in plant physiology was carried out by Hevesy in 1923, using labeled lead in bean seedlings and its release by the plant upon placing it in a culture solution containing non-radioactive lead. Until 1933, only the isotopes of lead, bismuth, thallium, radium, thorium, and actinium had been applied as tracers, none of which played a role in the living organism.

Further advances in this field were not possible until the discovery of heavy water (deuterium) in 1932, by Harold C. Urey, and of artificial radioactivity by Irène and Frederik Joliot-Curie in 1933 (6–14). Use of radioisotopes in medicine and cardiology was entirely dependent on the discovery of artificial radioactivity. The Joliot-Curies were pioneers in this field (Figure 2). They discovered artificial radioactivity which made possible preparation of a large number of radioactive isotopes which became of considerable importance in biology and medicine. Irène Curie became her mother's (Marie

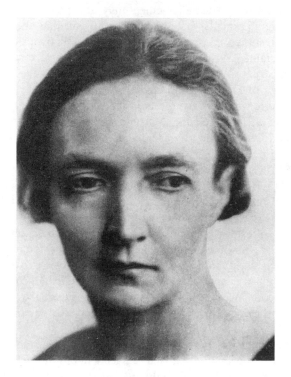

Figure 2. Irène Joliot-Curie (*Courtesy of The New York Academy of Medicine*)

Curie) assistant at the Radium Institute in Paris. In 1925 she received her doctorate on her graduate thesis, "Recherches sur les rayons alpha du polonium." In 1934, the Joliot-Curies succeeded in artificially producing radioactive elements, thereby furnishing proof of the possibility of transforming elements (6–14). On Monday, the 15th of January, 1934, Jean Perrin introduced to the session of the French Academy of Science a communication titled, "A New Type of Radioactivity," with the authors Irene and Frederik Joliot-Curie. The text of the announcement read, ". . . it has been possible, for the first time, to create by means of external causes, radioactivity of certain substances which remain stable for a measurable time (6–14)." The authors demonstrated that when an aluminum foil was irradiated on a polonium preparation, the emission of positive charged electrons did not cease immediately when the active preparation was removed. A new isotope had been produced. They wrote, "the radioelement may be regarded as a known nucleus formed in a particular state of excitation." But they thought it more probable that these new radioactive elements were unknown isotopes which are always unstable (6–14). In 1935, the Joliot-Curies received the Nobel prize in chemistry.

The marriage of Frederik Joliot and Irène Curie was one of opposites. While Irene Curie was quiet and serene, Joliot was impulsive. By nature reserved, she had difficulty relating to people. She cared little for external appearance and dresses, while he was a handsome well-groomed man. Irène loved French, English, and German poetry. As Michel Rouze wrote, "Joliot and Irène had different characters, but they were complimentary, for work as well as life. Often valuable associations are not those of individual characters, but of personality features which compliment each other (13)."

Joliot and Irène Curie's fundamental discovery was followed by that of Fermi and his colleagues, who produced radioisotopes by neutrons emitted from uranium by a mixture of radon and beryllium in an atomic pile. Identical methods were used for the production of ^{32}P by Hevesy in Copenhagen, an isotope which was soon used for biological studies (1–5). As Hevesy wrote, "It was soon made clear that isotopic methods were the only possibility of studying the organism as a whole under practically equilibrium conditions."

Fermi's method to use uranium-produced radioactive isotopes made possible extended application of radioactive tracers in biology. The first radio-iodine was produced by Fermi in Italy, in 1934. Study of the activity of the thyroid gland and the synthesis of thyroid hormones began soon afterwards. In 1940, John Lawrence and Joseph Hamilton utilized ^{131}I in the treatment of hyperthyroidism and treatment of cancer of the thyroid.

The construction of the cyclotron by Lawrence in Berkeley, was an outstanding event in the history of biological application of radioactive tracer (16,17). The cyclotron found immediate use in medicine. The use of ^{131}I commenced soon and the discovery of radio-sodium followed. In 1935, ^{32}P was introduced on both sides of the Atlantic. Lawrence, in 1936, conceived the idea to *selectively* irradiate leukemic cells. This idea was the beginning of what was called metabolic radiotherapy. In 1939, cyclotron produced radiophosphorus was used in clinical studies of leukemia; extensive use of these isotopes in other biological fields followed. Lawrence's paper on the production of high speed light ions without the use of high voltages, appeared in April of 1932 (17). He described the apparatus for generation of 1,220,000 volt protons. It is noteworthy that this work was partially supported by the industry, such as the Federal Telegraph Company and the Chemical Foundation. Soon afterwards cyclotron produced iodine was used in the study of radioiodine uptake by the thyroid. Other isotopes of sodium, potassium, calcium, and strontium soon became available.

The early part of this century was a great period for physics; it was the time of Otto Hahn and Lise Meitner who discovered nuclear fission and of Hess who discovered cosmic rays. The early 20th century was also the time of the introduction of quantum theory of the atomic structure by Niels Bohr (1913), Rutherford's fundamental observation on the structure of the atom, introduction of the first counter for radioactivity by Hans W. Geiger at Kiel, and Einstein's theory of relativity.

The pioneering work of Hevesy was soon followed by the studies of Rudolph Schoenheimer and David Rittenberg at the College of Physicians and Surgeons, Columbia University (18; *See Fig. 5 Chapter 6*). After his work on cholesterol metabolism in the Department of Pathology in Freiburg, Germany under Ludwig Aschoff, Schoenheimer carried out his studies in the United States on the use of isotopes in investigating metabolism with Rittenberg. It was Urey who gave them the isotope needed: heavy hydrogen (deuterium). The epochal discovery of Urey appeared in a letter to Physical Reviews (15,19). An argument immediately ensued regarding what to call this new isotope. Names such as bar-hydrogen and diplogen were proposed by Rutherford, but the name deuterium was maintained. Using deuterium as an isotopic tracer, Schoenheimer and Rittenberg (the latter had worked in Urey's laboratory), developed methods of synthesizing isotopically labeled compounds, for example, linseed oil hydrogenated with deuterium was used to study the isotopte's fate in experimental animals. They showed that labeled fatty acids were deposited in fat depots even during starvation (18).

Later, when ^{15}N was concentrated in Urey's laboratory in the form of heavy ammonia, Schoenheimer and Rittenberg turned to the problem of protein metabolism (18). Administering compounds labeled with ^{15}N or double labeled with deuterium and ^{15}N, they confirmed Hevesy's observation that body constituents are in a highly dynamic state. This led to the concept of a "metabolic pool," with body tissues continually entering and leaving this pool.

Rudolf Schoenheimer, who introduced the application of radioisotopes in the study of metabolic functions was born in May 1898, and died by suicide in September 1941. (*See Figure 5, Chapter 6, Atherosclerosis.*) Son of a physician who practiced in Berlin, he studied medicine at the University of Berlin, receiving his M.D. degree in 1922. After a year in the Department of Pathology, he recognized his deficiency in biochemistry and studied biochemistry at the University of Leipzig under a Rockefeller Foundation Fellowship for three years. Schoenheimer's productive career commenced at the University of Freiburg with the great pathologist Aschoff, with a short interlude at the University of Chicago; he soon became head of the Department of Pathological Chemistry at the University of Freiburg. In 1933, he moved to New York to the College of Physicians, Columbia University. Schoenheimer was an ingenious and scintillating personality. In a moving obituary, Hans T. Clarke, his friend and chief, wrote:

> Schoenheimer died by suicide at the height of his productive career, September 11, 1941 (20). Few men had more reason for desiring to live; his work gave him intense satisfaction, and its increasing importance was widely recognized ... one of Schoenheimer's most striking characteristics was his ability to correlate pertinent facts from highly diversified branches of knowledge and bring them to bear upon problems under immediate considerations.

The application of radioisotopes to cardiology began with G. Liljestrand from Stockholm who, in 1939, determined the normal blood volume in the ventricles of the human heart (21). In 1940 Hevesy used radioactive phosphorus to determine circulation time (2). The method was relatively simple; blood was withdrawn from the patient and mixed with radioactive phosphorus. The mixture was reinjected intravenously, while an intraarterial needle permitted the collection of fractionated specimens of arterial blood for measurement of radioactivity. Nylin, who worked in Stockholm in close proximity to Hevesy, used isotopes for the determination of residual blood in the cardiac ventricles and also measured circulation time (22,23). In a paper published in 1945, he referred to the advantage of radioisotopes over the prevalent measurement of circulation time with decholin, a test which had to rely on the patients subjective judgment (23).

In 1947, H. Blumgart, at the Harvard Medical School, accomplished accurate measurements of the "velocity of blood flow" (circulation time), using intravenous radium and detection time of arrival at another point of the circulation (24; *See Fig. 9 chapter 7*). He cited work at the Memorial Hospital in New York, dealing with the possible therapeutic effect of radium C in patients with advanced generalized carcinomatosis. In this study, repeated intravenous injections of up to 75 millicuries of radium were administered without any consequent ill effects. Blumgart's detection device was complicated, but he was able to measure normal circulation time (approximately 18 seconds) from arm to contralateral arm. Much higher values were obtained in myocardial failure. Blumgart was an outstanding physician and investigator, one of a great group of Harvard cardiologists which included Paul D. White. (*See Chapter on Coronary Artery Disease*)

Similar to Blumgart, M. Prinzmetal used a Geiger counter positioned over the heart to record "radiocardiograms" (25). He summarized his efforts by stating that radiocardiography offers a simple and safe method for the determination of the "pumping qualities of the heart." He also studied patients with congenital heart disease (patent ductus arteriosus) before and after surgical correction. Discussing Prinzmetal's paper presented at the Section on Experimental Medicine and Therapeutics at the 97th Annual Session of the American Medical Association, Chicago, in 1948, Nylin voiced astonishment that "it was feasible to study the filling and emptying of both cavities separately." Prinzmetal affirmed that he consulted several experts in the field of atomic energy in California and elsewhere on the danger of radioactive material, ". . . their opinion was unanimous that the amount of radioactivity used is completely safe by all methods of estimation" (25).

Tracing of isotopes through coronary arteries was described in 1952 by P. von Waser and W. Hunzinger, from Basel, who observed that the descendant slope of the left ventricular component of the radiocardiogram contained a significant amount of radioactivity due to the passage of radioisotopes through coronary vessels (26). In 1955, G. Sevelius attempted to estimate myocardial blood flow with iodinated human serum albumin ^{131}I following the example of Huff and co-workers (27). He employed a "heart channel and a carotid channel." Each channel consisted of a scintillation detector, a rate meter, and a recorder. In this procedure, it was difficult to recognize the coronary flow contribution in the precordial radiogram.

A great step forward for cardiology was achieved by Hal Oscar Anger who developed the Gamma-Ray camera for in vivo studies in 1952, (28,29; Figure 3). Anger was born May 24, 1920, in Denver, Colorado, and received his elementary and high school education in Southern California. During the war (1942), he devised a special unit for use in radar. This was later referred to as the "Anger Circuit." After graduation, he served on the staff of the Radio Research Laboratory at Harvard University. His cooperation with the Donner Laboratory at the University of California at Berkeley, began in 1946, when he became associated with John Lawrence.

"No single person has been as successful as Hal Anger in interrelating physics with nuclear medicine through sound engineering principles and practice" according to William G. Myers (28). Anger first used ^{131}I to visualize thyroid metastases in bone of living patients. In his first device, a 3-mm pinhole in a lead shield was located 20 cm from a photographic plate, placed in contact with a sodium iodine intensifying screen. A useful image was obtained from a 1R exposure to the plate when the ^{131}I density was about 1 mCi per cc thyroid tissue. This instrument pointed the way for development of his more sensitive scintillation camera five years later. In 1958, Anger constructed his scintillation camera, equipped with a sodium iodide crystal only 4 inches in diameter which was viewed by 7 phototubes. In 1963, he completed construction of a larger scintillation camera employing an 11 1/2 inch

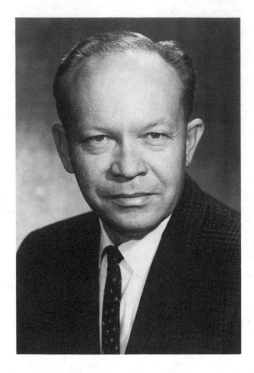

Figure 3.   Hal Oscar Anger (*with permission*)

crystal. This camera and its subsequent models are essential for use in scanning of the heart to the present day. The Anger camera was later used to
measure regional myocardial blood flow (28,29).

Early work on myocardial scanning was performed by H.N. Wagner (30),
by W.D. Love and G.E. Burch (31), by E.A. Carr (32), and by R.J. Bing (33).
Carr, in 1962, used [84]Rb to scan the precordium prior to and after the death of
the animal (32). Accidental counts resulting from the use of single emission
interfered with the accuracy of these determinations.

After these beginnings, the use of isotopes in cardiology increased expo-
nentially. The determination of cardiac wall motions and of cardiac ejection
fraction at rest and during exercise have become important clinical tests in
patient evaluation.

THE USE OF POSITRON EMITTERS

In 1937, Carl D. Anderson published his Nobel lecture entitled "The new particles in physics" (34; Fig.4). These new particles in physics were positive charged electrons (positrons). Anderson had received the Nobel Prize for his work in 1936. It is interesting that, when his Nobel lecture was published in the Bulletin of the California Institute of Technology, Anderson was still an Assistant Professor of Physics (Figure 4). Anderson reported that information of fundamental importance to the general problem of atomic structure had resulted from systematic studies of the cosmic radiation carried out in the Wilson cloud chamber. Energies of atomic particles of 5 billion electron-

VOLUME 46   NUMBER 2

Bulletin of the
CALIFORNIA INSTITUTE
of TECHNOLOGY

THE PRODUCTION *and* PROPERTIES
of POSITRONS

Nobel Lecture presented before the Swedish Royal Academy
of Science at Stockholm, December 12, 1936.

by CARL D. ANDERSON, Ph.D.
Assistant Professor of Physics,
California Institute of Technology

PASADENA, CALIFORNIA
JUNE, 1937

Figure 4.   Title page of the Nobel Prize winning article by Carl D. Anderson, California Institute of Technology (*with permission*)

volts were discovered. It was shown that particles of positive charge occurred about as abundantly as did those of negative charge, and in many cases
several positive and negative particles were found to be projected simultaneously from a single center (34). Anderson had interpreted the particles of
negative charge as electrons, but those of positive charge were first tenta-
tively identified as protons—at that time the only known particle of unit was
a positive charge. It soon became evident, however, that the positive particles
differed in specific ionization only inappreciably from the negative ones. At
first, to avoid this assumption which appeared at the time very radical, Anderson wrote that the positive particles did have electronic mass and appeared to be positively charged, but were in reality negatively charged
electrons which, through scattering, had suffered a reversal of direction and
were projected upwards away from the earth (34). But this explanation soon
appeared to be inadequate.

It became clear that the results could be interpreted only in terms of particles of a positive charge and a mass of the same order of magnitude as that
normally possessed by the free negative electron. The only possible conclusion seemed to be that these were positively charged electrons. These results
were published in September 1932, announcing the existence of free positive
electrons (35). The mass and charge of the positive electrons did not differ by
more than 20% and 10% respectively from the mass and charge of the negative electron. Soon, production of positrons by agents other than cosmic rays
was shown, when it was observed that positrons were produced by the radiation generated in the impact of alpha particles upon beryllium. The Joliot-
Curies measured the yield of positrons as a function of the thickness and
material of the absorber by a lead block and paraphine and concluded that the
positrons arose more likely as a result of gamma rays than of neutrons. Positrons also were soon observed among the disintegration products of certain
radioactive substances.

In 1964, [84]rubidium which emits positrons 19% of the time was used for
determination of coronary blood flow in man (36,37). Positrons (free positive electrons) travel 1.5 mm in the tissue and disintegrate by striking an electron, ejecting two gamma-photons at an energy level of 0.51 mev, 180° apart
or back to back. The coincidence method has the following advantages over
the single proton emission method: since the counting system registers only
coincidence events background counting rates arising from natural radioactivity, cosmic radioactivity, and the presence of background counting rates
are essentially zero. The coincidence counting method gives approximately
five times the counting rates of single photon emission for a given field of
view. Although, coincidence counting is like simple proton counting subject

to tissue absorption of gamma rays (a phenomenon termed attenuation), the relative time of light of the two gamma protons indicates the relative position of the atom emitting the positron particle. Because of the elimination of single gamma photons, the coincidence method provides a means for distinguishing radioactivity of the heart muscle from that of the surrounding tissue, thereby simplifying collimation, and together with the coincidence counting systems, eliminating interference with accidental counts. This principle offers a higher resolution than simple proton techniques in positron emission tomography (PET).

During early attempts, a continuous infusion of ^{84}Rb for determination of coronary blood flow was used (38). A coefficient had to be obtained which made possible definitions of clearances in ml/min. Furthermore, the first derivative of the myocardial clearance of ^{84}Rb had to be obtained in order to calculate uptake of ^{84}Rb at zero time. This was accomplished by extrapolation of the myocardial clearance to zero. At that time, the activity in coronary venous blood was assumed to be zero and the extraction ratio is unity. Later, coronary blood flow was measured after a bolus injection of ^{84}Rb, as performed by L. Donato (39) and by S.B. Knoebel (40). According to L.A. Sapirstein, the uptake of rubidium by the heart muscle can be calculated since cardiac uptake equals the fraction of cardiac output supplying the myocardium (41). This method has the advantage that the coronary sinus need not be intubated. Other methods rely on the use of clearances of radioactive materials such as krypton or xenon (42,43). Superiority of the coincidence method over the use of single gamma photons determination was demonstrated on models (44).

These pioneering experiments with the positron emitter ^{84}Rb sparked future developments in techniques of imaging and in physiological studies. The work became a precursor for the determination of myocardial imaging with thallium-201 and technitium 99 sestamibi using single-photon emission computed tomography (SPECT). Using these isotopes, perfusion defects in the myocardium can be outlined and the amount of myocardium at risk can be estimated. The most important advance originating from the early work on Rb^{84} was the development of positron emission tomography (PET), discussed later in this chapter.

As a positron emitting nuclide, ^{84}rubidium found itself in good company. Cyclotron bombardment of stable atoms with deuterons or protons produced positron emitting isotopes of elements like ^{15}O, ^{11}C and ^{13}N. These elements were major constituents of living matter. Incorporated into biological molecules, their positron emitting nuclides carried considerable promise for tracing biological processes in vivo. For example, Kamen and co-workers (45) recognized the importance of the ^{11}C label for studies of the carbon dioxide utilization by plants and in 1941, Cramer and Kistiakowsky (46) conducted metabolic studies with lactate labeled with ^{11}C in the 1 and 2, 3 positions. Several years later, Buchanan and Hastings (47) applied the same radionuclide to studies of intermediary metabolism; in 1946, Tobias and co-workers (48) studied the metabolism of carbon monoxide in humans with [11]C. The positron emitting ^{13}N also found uses for biological studies of nitrogen metabolism in plants (49,50).

In the mid-1940s interest in these radioisotopes began to fade. Possible reasons were their short physical half-life and associated logistical complexities. Another reason, according to Ter-Pogossian (51), was the availability of more stable isotopes like ^{14}C or ^{3}H which offered more flexibility in the research laboratory. Both isotopes played important roles in delineating aspects of human substrate metabolism. They also proved useful for mapping the spatial distribution of functional processes in organs as autoradiography could quantify their regional tissue activity concentrations. It was at that time that Louis Sokoloff, trained in psychiatry and working at the University of Pennsylvania, devised a novel approach for the exploration of regional cerebral metabolism (52,53). Employing ^{14}C labeled deoxyglucose, he mapped the spatial distribution of regional rates of cerebral glucose utilization and their changes in response to physiologic stimuli in awake rats and cats. Sokoloff's approach took advantage of the specific properties of deoxyglucose. The agent traces the initial uptake and the hexokinase mediated phosphorylation of glucose to glucose-6-phosphate as a key metabolic step in the glycolytic flux of the brain. Unlike its parent substrate, the labeled glucose analog was a poor substrate for glycolysis, the fructose-pentose shunt and for dephosphorylation. Because the phosphorylated analog is rather impermeable to the cell membrane, it becomes virtually trapped in brain in proportion to rates of regional cerebral glucose metabolism. The tissue kinetics of this tracer compound were described by a three-compartmental model which formed the basis for estimating regional metabolic rates. From the arterial tracer input function, the arterial plasma glucose concentrations and the cerebral ^{14}C activity concentrations determined postmortem by quantitative autoradiography, it yielded metabolic rates of glucose in μmol per minute per gram tissue. In fact, Sokoloff's method possessed the ingredients of the later evolving Positron Emission Tomography except of course that measurements of regional tracer activity concentrations relied on quantitative autoradiography. Obviously, the approach was unsuitable for studies in humans. Given the impact more stable radioisotopes had made on biomedical research, Siri in 1949 painted a rather bleak picture of the future of the short-lived positron emitting radionuclides (54). He noted that "the unstable species of the longest half-life is oxygen-15 (126 sec); this has not been employed for tracer work and does not offer much promise."

Ter-Pogossian was the man who revived interest in short-lived positron emitting radionuclides for biomedical research in the mid-1950s. Ter-Pogossian (51) saw the earlier perceived weakness of these short-lived radioisotopes as a major advantage. They permitted serial measurements of biological processes. He recognized the fact that they constituted a major part of living matter. Their insertion into biomolecules caused no adverse effects on their very properties. They could be synthesized in high specific activities. Therefore, they exerted no mass effect and did not perturb the very process to be studied. Early work in Ter-Pogossian's laboratory at Washington University in St. Louis included autoradiographic approaches to the study of tumor oxygenation with ^{15}O. Later work expanded into other areas such as studies of cerebral oxygen metabolism. These pioneering studies gave new impetus to investigations with other positron emitting nuclides at several institutions which commissioned cyclotrons dedicated to biomedical research. Foremost among these institutions were Hammersmith Hospital in London, The Sloan-Kettering Institute in New York City, The University of Chicago, The University of California at Berkeley and later at Los Angeles with Schelbert and Phelps.

It must be remembered that this early pioneering work relied on external radiation detectors for monitoring the uptake and clearance of positron emitting nuclides in whole organs or large organ parts. What these studies lacked were imaging devices for localizing or even mapping the distribution of functional processes evaluated by these radiotracers. Early attempts in Ter-Pogossian's laboratory for determining the spatial distribution of these functional processes prompted the development of the "lead chicken."

The device resembled a lead helmet spiked with 26 detector probes for collecting activity from different regions of the brain. Yet, it proved to be less than satisfactory. The lead collimators lowered the count efficiency and required injection of the tracer directly into the carotid artery. At the same time, Hal Anger demonstrated that two-dimensional images of the distribution of tracers in organs could in fact be obtained. Taking advantage of the simultaneous emission of two 511 keV photons in diametrically opposite directions as a property unique to positron decay, he designed a coincidence circuitry for a double headed gamma scintillation camera. In 1968, Yano and Anger at the University of California at Berkeley presented the first images of the heart and kidney in animals, recorded with the ultra short-lived ^{82}Rb (55). Long-standing interests in Gordon Brownell's laboratory at the Massachusetts General Hospital at that time resulted in the first dedicated positron camera (56). It consisted of two large detector banks of sodium-iodide detectors coupled to 72 photomultiplier tubes. Coincidence circuits connected each detector in one bank with 25 detectors in the opposite bank and provided a total of 2549 lines of coincidence response. Both Brownell's and Anger's devices yielded planar images of the distribution of positron emitting nuclides in organs. They fell short of providing information on their spatial or three-dimensional distribution.

David E. Kuhl, at that time at the University of Pennsylvania, had been keenly interested in the development of techniques that would depict the distribution of radionuclide in the form of transverse images. He demonstrated the utility of back projection techniques which produced transverse section images of the distribution of single photon emitting radionuclides (57,58). Properties specific to positron decay offered distinct advantages for producing truly tomographic images. As early as 1962, Rankowitz built a device for coincidence collimation (59). It consisted of a ring of *discreet* radiation detectors. Ironically, Rankowitz' system preceded its time as mathematical algorithms for image reconstruction had not been developed.

Hounsfield described in 1973 the x-ray computed tomography (60). This event proved pivotal for subsequent advances in the field of tomo-graphic imaging of positron emitting nuclides. The general principles for reconstructing tomographic images from angular projections of an object were formulated. Michael E. Phelps, an Assistant Professor with a doctoral degree in nuclear chemistry, together with his Fellow, Edward J. Hoffman, dissembled in Ter-Pogossian's laboratory the "lead chicken" in order to salvage the 26 detector probes. They positioned sets of four detector probes in a hexagonal array. Phelps and Hoffman rotated by hand the source of positron emitting nuclides placed in the center of this array for proper linear and angular sampling while different computers at different locations, at the Medical School, in a biomedical laboratory several blocks away and a large IBM computer at the University campus, collected and mathematically reconstructed the data. Jerome Cox, Donald Snyder and Sung-Cheng Huang designed the reconstruction algorithms. The first true tomographic image was obtained in 1973. They dubbed the new imaging device as PETT II for positron emission transaxial tomography. The system contained only 12 coincidence lines and offered an intrinsic spatial resolution of only 25 mm in only one single image slice. The initial success led to the development of the first tomograph for human studies, called PETT III, and produced the first images on ^{13}N ammonia uptake in the human brain (61,62) and formed the basis for the first commercially built Positron Emission Tomography (63). The initial, single slice imaging approach formed the basis for the soon following multi-slice positron emission tomographs which today acquire simultaneously as many as 15 to 30 slices with over a million response lines and an intrinsic in-plane resolution of three to five mm. Ironically, Phelps and Hoffman in 1975 moved to the University of Pennsylvania where Sokoloff had conceived the deoxyglucose method for mapping the spatial distribution of metabolic rates of glucose in rat brain and where in David E. Kuhl's laboratory transverse images of the spatial distribution of deoxyglucose in brain labeled with ^{18}F had been acquired (64,65). The following years demonstrated the possibility to measure accurately rather than only to depict the regional F-18 deoxyglucose concentrations with Positron Emission Tomography. This imaging device thus could substitute for quantitative autoradiography. This ability permitted in vivo measurements of regional tracer tissue concentrations and resulted in the application of Sokoloff's approach to the measurements of regional metabolic rates of glucose in human brain (66).

With these accomplishments, Positron Emission Tomography began to evolve as an analytical tool for probing biochemical processes in humans. This development would not have been possible without an increasing number of positron emitting isotopes. Investigators in centers of major activities under Al Wolf at Brookhaven National Laboratory and under Michael Welch at the Mallinckrodt Institute at Washington University, have designed and developed synthesis methods for more than 200 such compounds labeled with positron emitting radionuclides. Processes that can now be evaluated and measured in the human heart include blood flow, biochemical reaction rates, fluxes of glucose, fatty acid, and oxygen, as well as studies of receptors in the human heart.

As Claude Bernard had stated, "No category of sciences exists to which one could give the name of applied sciences. There are science and application of science, linked together as fruit of the tree that bore it (67)."

REFERENCES

1. Hevesy, G. A scientific career. In: Adventures in Radioisotope Research. New York, Pergamon, 1962.
2. Hevesy, G. Some applications of isotopic indicators. In: Adventures in radioisotope research. New York, Pergamon, 1962. (Originally published in Les Prix Nobel 1940–1944, p. 95.)
3. Hevesy, G. Historical progress of the isotopic methodology and its influences on the biological sciences. In: Adventures in radioisotope research. New York, Pergamon, pp. 997-1038. (Originally published in Minerva Nucleare, 1:182, 1957. Lecture delivered in 1956 at the International Meeting of Nuclear Medicine in Turin.)

4. Hevesy, G. The application of radioactive indicators in biochemistry. In: Adventures in radioisotope research. New York, Pergamon, 1962, pp. 961–996. (Originally published in Chem. Soc. J., p. 1618, 1951. Faraday Lecture, delivered before the Chemical Society in Edinburgh on March 29th, 1950.)
5. Hevesy, G. McGraw-Hill Modern Men of Science, edited by J. E. Greene. New York, McGraw-Hill, 1966, pp. 222–224.
6. Joliot-Curie, F. and I. Joliot-Curie. Oeuvres scientifiques complètes. Paris, Presses Universitaires de France, 1961.
7. Amaldi, E., P. Briquard, L. Goldstein, et al. La radioactivité artificielle à 50 ans, 1934–1984. Paris, Centre Nationale de la Recherche Scientifique, 1984.
8. Joliot, F., and I. Curie. Artificial production of a new kind of radio-element. Nature, 133:201–202, 1934.
9. Nobel Prize Winners: Charts, Indexes, Sketches, compiled by Flora Kaplan. Chicago, Nobel Publishing, 1941, pp. 37,38,58.
10. Cotton, E. Les Curies et la radioactivité. From the series: Savants du Monde Entier. Paris, Editions Seghers, 1963, pp. 74–79.
11. Biquard, P. Frederic Joliot Curie; Choix de Textes, Bibliographie, Portraits, Facsimiles. From the series: Savants du Monde Entier. Paris, Editions Seghers, 1961, pp. 26–31.
12. Chaskolskata, M. Frédéric Joliot-Curie. Essais et Documents (Editions de Moscou), 26–31.
13. Rouze, M. Frédéric Joliot-Curie. Editeurs Francais, Reunis, 1950.
14. La radioactivité artificielle et les sciences de la vie. Synelog L'Edition Artistique, Paris (1), 228:26, 40.
15. Urey, H. C. Names for the hydrogen isotopes. Science, 78:602–603, 1933.
16. Lawrence, E. O. and M. S. Livingston. The production of high speed protons without the use of high voltages. Phys. Rev., 38:834, 1931.
17. Lawrence, E. O. and M. S. Livingston. The production of high speed light ions without the use of high voltages. Phys. Rev., 40:19–35, 1932.
18. Schoenheimer, R. and D. Rittenberg. The study of intermediary metabolism of animals with the aid of isotopes. Phys. Rev., 20:218–248, 1940.
19. Urey, H. C. Relative abundance of H1 and H2 in natural hydrogen. Phys. Rev., 40:464–465, 1932.
20. Clarke, H. T. Rudolf Schoenheimer, 1898-1941. Science, 94:553–554, 1941.
21. Liljestrand, G., E. Lysholm, G. Nylin, and C. G. Zachrisson. The normal heart volume in man. Am. Heart J., 17:406–415, 1939.
22. Nylin G. and M. Malm. Ueber die Konzentration von mit radioactivem Phosphor markierten Erythrocyten im Arterienblut nach der intravenoesen Injektion solcher Blutkoerperchen. Cardiologia, 7:153–162, 1943.
23. Nylin, G. The dilution curve of activity in arterial blood after intravenous injection of labeled corpuscles. Am. Heart J., 30:1–11, 1945.
24. Blumgart, H. and O. C. Yens. Studies on the velocity of blood flow. J. Clin. Invest., 4:1–13, 1927.
25. Prinzmetal, M., E. Corday, R.J. Spritzler, and W. Flieg. Radiocardiography and its clinical applications. J.A.M.A., 139:617–622, 1949.
26. Waser, von P., and W. Hunzinger. Radiocirculographische Untersuchung des Coronarkreislaufes mit Na24Cl. Cardiologia, 22:65–100, 1953.

27. Sevelius, G. and P. C. Johnson. Myocardial blood flow determined by surface counting and ratio formula. J. Lab. Clin. Med., 54:669–679, 1959.
28. Myers, W. G. Nuclear Medicine Pioneer Citation—1974, Hal Oscar Anger, D.Sc.(Hon.). J. Nucl. Med., 15:471–473, 1974.
29. Anger, H. O. Scintillation camera. Rev. Sci. Instr., 29:27–33, 1958.
30. Wagner, H. N., J. G. McAfee, and J. M. Mozley. Medical radioisotope scanning. JAMA, 174:162–165, 1960.
31. Love, W. D., and G. E. Burch. A study in dogs of methods suitable for estimating the rate of myocardial uptake of RB86 in man, and the effect of L-norepinephrine and pitressin on RB86 uptake. J. Clin. Invest., 36:468–478, 1957.
32. Carr, E. A., W. H. Beierwaltes, A. V. Wegst, and J. D. Bartlett. Myocardial scanning with rubidium-86. J. Nucl. Med., 3:76–82, 1962.
33. Bing, R. J. Scanning of heart. N.Y. State J. Med., 67:1406–1410, 1967.
34. Anderson, C. D. The production and properties of positrons. Nobel lecture, Bull. Calif. Inst. Tech., 46:3, 1937.
35. Anderson, C. D. The apparent existence of easily deflectable positives. Science, 76:238–239, 1932.
36. Bing, R. J., C. Cowan, D. Bottcher, G. Corsini, and C. G. Daniels. A new method of measuring coronary blood flow in man. JAMA, 205:277–280, 1968.
37. Cohen, A., E. J. Zaleski, H. Baleiron, T. B. Stock, C. Chiba, and R. J. Bing. Measurement of coronary blood flow using rubidium84 and the coincidence counting method: a critical analysis. Am. J. Cardiol., 19:556–562, 1967.
38. Bing, R. J., A. Bennish, G. Blumchen, A. Cohen, J. P. Gallagher, and E. J. Zaleski. The determination of coronary flow equivalent with coincidence counting technique. Circulation, 29:833–846, 1964.
39. Donato, L., G. Bartolomei, and R. Giordani. Evaluation of myocardial blood perfusion in man with radioactive potassium or rubidium and precordial count ing. Circulation, 29:195–203, 1964.
40. Knoebel, S. B., P. L. McHenry, L. Stein, and A. Sonel. Myocardial blood flow in man as measured by a coincidence counting system and a single bolus of 84RbCl. Circulation, 36:187–196, 1967.
41. Sapirstein, L. A. Fractionation of the cardiac output of rats with isotopic potassium. Circ. Res., 4:689–692, 1956.
42. Ross, R. S., K. Ueda, P. L. Lichtlen, and J. R. Rees. Measurement of myocardial blood flow in animals and man by selective injection of radioactive inert gas into the coronary arteries. Circ. Res., 15:28–41, 1964.
43. Holman, B. L., D. F. Adams, D. Jewitt, P. Eldh, J. Idoine, P. F. Cohn, R. Gorlin, and S. J. Adelstein. Measuring regional myocardial blood flow with 133Xe and the Anger camera. Radiology, 112:99–107, 1974.
44. Ikeda, S., H. Duken, H. Tillmanns, and R. J. Bing. Coincidence counting and noncoincidence counting: a comparative study. J. Nucl. Med., 16:658–661, 1975.
45. Kamen, M.D. "Isotropic Tracers in Biology"; an introduction to tracer methodology. 3rd Ed., Academic Press, New York, 1957.
46. Cramer, R.D. and G.B. Kistiatowsky. The synthesis of radioactive lactic acid. J. Biol. Chem. 137:549, 1941.

47. Buchanan, J.M. and Hastings, A.B. The use of isotopically marked carbon in the study of intermediary metabolism. Physiol. Revs. 26:120–155, 1946.
48. Tobias, C.A., J.H. Lawrence, F.J.W. Roughton, W.S. Root, and M.I. Gregersen. The elimination of carbon monoxide from the human body with reference to the possible conversion of CO to CO_2. Am. J. Physiol. 145:253–263, 1945.
49. Ruben, S., W.Z. Hassid and M.D. Kamen. Radioactive carbon in the study of photosynthesis. J. Am. Chem. Soc. 61:661, 1939.
50. Ruben, S., M.D. Kamen, and W.Z. Hassid. Photosynthesis with radioactive carbon II chemical properties of the intermediates. J. Am. Chem. Soc. 62:3443–3449, 1940.
51. Ter-Pogossian, M.M. Positron Emission Tomography instrumentation. In: Positron Emission Tomography. New York, NY Alan R.Liss, Inc. 43–61, 1985.
52. Kennedy, C., M. Des Rosiers, M. Reivich, F. Sharp, J.W. Jehle, and L. Sokoloff. Mapping of functional neural pathways by autoradiographic survey of local metabolic rate with [^{14}C] deoxyglucose. Science 187:850–853, 1975.
53. Sokoloff, L., M. Reivich, C. Kennedy, M. Des Rosiers, H. Patlak, K.D. Pettigrew, O. Sakurada and M. Shinohara. The [^{14}C] deoxyglucose method for the measurement of local cerebral glucose utilization: Theory, procedure and normal values in the conscious and anesthetized albino rat. J. Neurochem 28:897–916, 1977.
54. Siri, W.E. "Isotropic Tracers and Nuclear Radiations" McGraw-Hill, New York, 1949.
55. Yano, Y. and H. O. Anger. Visualization of heart and kidneys in animals with ultrashort-lived 82Rb and the positron scintillation camera. J. Nucl. Med., 9:412–415, 1968.
56. Brownell, G.L. C.A. Burnham, B. Hoop and H. Kazemi. Positron scintigraphy with short-lived cyclotron-produced radiopharmaceuticals and a multicrystal positron camera, in Proc Symp Med Raioisotope Scintigraphy, Copenhagen, 1972, Vienna, IAEA, p. 313, 1973
57. Kuhl, D.E. and R.Q. Edwards. Image separation radioisotope scanning. Radiology 80:653–661, 1963.
58. Kuhl, D.E. and R.Q. Edwards. The Mark III scanner: A compact device for multiple view and section scanning of the brain. Radiology 96:563–570, 1970.
59. Rankowitz, S., J.S. Robertson and W.A. Higginbotham et al. Positron scanner for locating brain tumors. IRE Int. Conv Rec Pt 9:49–56, 1962.
60. Hounsfield, G.N. Computerized transverse axial scanning (tomography): Part I. Description of system. Br. J. Radiol 46:1016–1022, 1973.
61. Phelps, M.E., E.J. Hoffman, N.A. Mullan and M.M. Ter-Pogossian. Application of annihilation coincidence detection to transaxial reconstruction tomogrphay. J. Nucl. Med. 16:210–224, 1975.
62. Phelps, M.E., E.J. Hoffman, N.A. Mullani, C.S. Higgins and M.M. Ter-Pogossian. Design considerations for a positron emission transaxial tomograph (PETT III). IEEE Nucl. Sci. NS 23:516–522, 1976.
63. Phelps, M.E., E.J. Hoffman, S.C. Huang and D.E. Kuhl. ECAT: A new computerized tomographic imaging system for positron emmitting radiopharmacueticals. J. Nucl. Med. 19:635–647, 1978.
64. Ido, T., C-N. Wan, J.S. Casella, J.S. Fowler, A. Wolf, M. Reivich and D.E. Kuhl. Labeled 2-deoxy-D-glucose analogs: 18-F labeled 2-deoxy-2fluro-D-glucose,

2-deoxy-2-fluoro-D-mannose and [14]C-2 deoxy-2-fluoro-D-glucose. J. Lable Compds. Radiopharm. 14:175–183, 1978.

65. Reivich, M. D. Kuhl, A. Wolf, J. Greenberg, M.E. Phelps, T. Ido, V. Casella, E. Hoffman, A. Alavi and L. Sokoloff. The (^{18}F) fluorodeoxyglucose method for the measurement of local cerebral glucose utilization in man. Circ. Res. 44:127–137, 1979.

66. Phelps, M.E., S.C. Huang, E.J. Hoffman, C. Selin, L. Sokoloff and D.E. Kuhl. Tomographic measurement of local cerebral glucose metabolic rate in humans with (F-18) 2-fluoro-2-deoxy-D-glucose: validation of method. Ann. Neurol. 6:371–388, 1979.

67. Bernard, C. An introduction to the study of experimental medicine. Tr. by H. C. Green, New York, Macmillan, 1927.

Chapter 10

Myocardial Failure
Early History, Biochemistry, Receptors and Contractile Proteins

W. ABELMANN, A.M. KATZ AND R.J. BING

Heart failure is a pathologic state characterized by the inability of the heart to maintain a cardiac output sufficient to meet the metabolic requirements of the organ systems of the body at rest and during ordinary activity, at normal levels of ventricular filling pressures. A decline in ejection fraction (ratio of stroke volume to end-diastolic volume) is a more sensitive marker of cardiac performance then cardiac output. Heart failure is considered compensated when an adequate cardiac output can be maintained by virtue of the activation of compensatory mechanisms, albeit at elevated ventricular filling pressures. When accompanied by pulmonary and/or systemic congestion, or when physical activity is restricted by symptoms of pulmonary hypertension or fatigue secondary to inadequate systemic blood flow, heart failure may be considered decompensated.

In recent years, increasing attention has been given to alterations in diastolic function of the ventricles. Impaired diastolic function may result in elevated ventricular filling pressures associated with congestion in the presence of normal systolic function. The first portions of this chapter deal primarily with heart failure secondary to impaired systolic function, i.e. impairment of the pump function of the heart.

Although many manifestations of congestive heart failure were recognized early in the history of medicine, the modern concept of congestive heart failure had to await the understanding of the heart as as pump responsible for the circulation of the blood. Only with the recognition of the heart as a muscle could weakness or other impairment of this muscle be associated with failure of the pump and interference with the circulation of the blood.

The attribution of the manifestations of heart failure to this organ was made more difficult by the fact that—unlike disease or failure of other organs—these manifestations generally presented themselves elsewhere in the body, such as dyspnea implicating the lungs, ascites and edema implicating the liver, and oliguria attributed to the failure of the kidneys. Yet, even well before William Harvey's description of circulation, the study of the pulse and its variation in disease led many authorities to relate such changes to afflictions of the heart.

In the scholarly and comprehensive historical monograph on "The Concept of Heart Failure from Avicenna to Albertini" (1), Saul Jarcho analyses evolution of the understanding of the symptoms and signs of heart failure from the 11th to the 18th Century, from the description of dyspnea, orthopnea, ascites and edema, to the nascent recognition of clinicopathologic correlates, and finally to attribution of these manifestations to disease of the heart and/or circulations. Thus, Avicenna, also known as Ibn Sina (980-1037), in his extensive Canon of Medicine, clearly describes dyspnea and orthopnea, as well as pulmonary edema producing foam at the mouth and carrying a grave prognosis, but does not relate these manifestations to the heart (2).

In the chapter on dyspnea and dropsy of the lung in his text on the treatment of internal diseases published in 1619, Ludovicus Mercatus, a physician and teacher in Valladolid, Spain, was perhaps the first to list as one of the causes of dyspnea the suppression of urine, which he thought collected in the lung (3).

In 1618, Carolus Piso, Professor of Medicine at the University of Pont-à-Mousson, provided the most descriptive case history of an octogenarian nobleman with dyspnea and paroxysmal nocturnal dyspnea (4).

After he had first fallen asleep as usual, a suffocation would suddenly excite the old man and interrupt his sleep, so that against his will he was obliged to get out of bed and rush at once to the windows of his bedroom in order to breathe fresh air through dilated nostrils. The old man could be seen, with inflamed face, drawing breath deeply, and with his shoulders trembling. He could not remain quietly in one place and especially he could not stand the fireplace but exposed himself even in a severe winter. Gradually and insensibly as the day advanced he would be relieved of his oppression, especially in the afternoon, but during the next sleep the affection returned and troubled the excellent old man again...I concluded finally that the fluid which was occupying his bronchi and the lung itself, or which more probably was stagnating in the middle of his chest, was of the kind that at the time of sleep through return of the vital spirit flowing back into the precordia received a certain new fervor, so that while bubbling in this way it could not be kept within its own space as formerly and it would necessarily compress the lungs and block their free motion. However, when this fervor gradually became spontaneously quiescent and the spirit flowed again out of the precordia into the body generally, as is the case in persons who are awake, then the lungs could more freely regain their space and the patient could breathe without such great oppression. Further, the fluid could be aqueous or serous, as I had seen formerly and repeatedly in dissected cadavers. Therefore, the totality of my reasoning led at length to this conclusion: I decided in my own mind that the difficulty of breathing which troubled the patient night after night and remitted somewhat in the daytime was to be attributed to dropsy of the chest.

Yet, in neither the writings of Mercatus nor in those of Piso is there any attribution of the symptoms to disease of the heart. It should also be noted that Harvey's description of the circulation of the blood in his famous monograph *De Motu Cordis* (published in 1628) (5) did not contain any description of the effects of disease.

It remained for Marcello Malpighi to lay the foundation of cardiovascular pathophysiology. This great scientist took advantage of the unusual opportunities Northern Italy offered in the 17th century: he was a student of the famous anatomist Carlo Fracasati in Bologna, and as a professor in Pisa, his colleagues included the mathematician Giovanni Borelli and the physicist Galileo. It is not surprising, then, that Malpighi's work shows evidence of a quantitative bent, and that in his view of disorders of the circulation he may be considered the first hemodynamicist. Aside from two letters published in 1661 (6), in which he first described the pulmonary capillary circulation as well as the erythrocyte, Malpighi's contributions to cardiology are contained in 64 consultations, not published until 1747. In his second consultation (7), which deals with the illness of the King of Poland, who suffered from an irregular pulse, Malpighi postulated an altered entry of blood into the heart: "As a result the respiration and pulse are changed, for when blood in the lungs has been delayed, their weight is increased. This causes dyspnea."

In the third consultation, referring to the Queen of Poland, also suffering from intermission of the pulse, Malpighi states,

... when the passage of blood through the lungs is clogged by disease of the vessels, when the necessary amount of fluid is denied to the left auricle, the heart contracts but the impulse indeed is not transmitted through the arteries. Therefore, when the freedom of the pathways is impeded by convulsion of nerves or by a static coagulated object, or the diameter of the vessels has become altered, the pulse is varied and does not occur in the periphery of the body even though the heart does not desist from its motion, and indeed it may then be moved more often.

One must recall here that before the twentieth century the vast majority of heart disease was rheumatic heart disease, generally associated with atrial fibrillation.

The fourth consultation addresses a cardinal suffering from dropsy, which Malpighi explains by stating, "... the veins were not resorbing the fluids pushed forth by the arteries, stagnation necessarily followed." In the 31st consultation, orthopnea is explained as follows: "... the movement of the blood is slowed, the mass of the lungs becomes heavier..."

Jarcho (1) credits Giorgio Baglivi with the first clinical description of pulmonary edema (8). Describing "suffocative catarrh," Baglivi states: "In this catarrh the patient has a cold, pain in the chest, and difficulty in breathing; also interrupted speech, anxiety, cough, stertor, a widely space slow pulse, foam at the mouth, and the like." He also states that "An instant remedy for this disease during the paroxysm is repeated bloodletting."

With Raymond Vieussens (1636-1715), we see the beginning of delineation of heart disease by the method of clinco-pathologic correlation. At the St. Eloy Hospital in Montpellier, Vieussens was active clinically but stood out for performing autopsies personally or at least witnessing autopsies on many of the patients he had examined previously. Thus, he was able to describe both pericardial effusion and constrictive pericarditis, and he recognized that the latter "deprives (the heart) of part of its strength and of the liberty that it naturally must have in order to contract and expand (9)." In cardiology, Vieussens is best known for his description of mitral stenosis. An apothecary suffered from dyspnea, orthopnea and peripheral edema. His pulse was small. At autopsy,

> the lung was extraordinarily bulky and soft, because its entire tissue was drenched in watery lymphatic juices. The posterior part of the lobes on the left appeared inflamed. After having surveyed the condition of the lung, I pulled the heart, together with the common trunks of its blood vessels, out of the thoracic cavity in order to examine all its parts. Its size was so extraordinary as to approach that of an ox heart. The coronary veins and their branches were very greatly dilated. The cavity of the right ventricle and of the right auricle had become excessively large.

He noted that the columnae carneae of the right ventricle were thickened and that "... the common openings of this ventricle have been so greatly dilated that they became perceptible, and the membrane which covered them had become so greatly stretched that it allowed free passage to the blood that came out through them." He also described enlargement of the left auricle, and stated that "... the entrance of the left ventricle appeared to be extremely small and that it had an oblong oval shape. In looking for the cause of such a surprising fact I discovered that the triglossine (mitral) valves of this ventricle were truly bony." Vieussens further observed that "... some of the bundles of the fleshy ducts which formed the sides of the depression in this ventricle had lost much of their natural thickness because they did not receive as much blood as they were used to receiving before the triglossine valves had turned to bony matter." Hence, he concluded that

> ... the blood could not pass freely and as abundantly as it should into the cavity of this ventricle. As soon as the circulation became impeded by this, it began to expand to an extraordinary extent the trunk of the pulmonary vein, because the blood remained there too long and accumulated there in too large an amount. The blood had no sooner begun to stay too long in the trunk of this vein than it delayed the course of the blood in all the blood vessels of the lung, so that the branches of the pulmonary artery and vein, spread by all the tissue of this organ, were always too full of blood and hence so dilated.

Here then, we have a fairly complete description of congestive heart failure, including tricuspid insufficiency, secondary to mitral stenosis.

A 35 year old pauper with epilepsy was found to have a rapid and strong pulse which made resting on the left side most uncomfortable: "it seemed as if he was being beaten on the ribs with a hammer." At autopsy, the left ventricle was markedly dilated and "its semilunar valves were greatly stretched and cut off at the end. All the cut edges in them, which had a certain resemblance to the teeth of a saw, were truly stoney." Vieussens concluded that "... since the valves were slashed, their ends could never approach closely enough to leave no opening between them. This is why every time the aorta contracted it sent back into the left ventricle a part of the blood that it had just received." This, then, represents an early description of aortic regurgitation, with remarkable hemodynamic insight. Jarcho concludes that Vieussens should be credited with the first complete explanation of backward heart failure (1).

Vieussens thus described and understood congestive heart failure secondary to structural (anatomical) morbid processes of the heart and pericardium, with remarkable insight into the pathophysiology but no clear recognition of the heart as a muscle.

The Danish anatomist Nils Stenson (Nicolas Steno) (1638-1686) is credited with the first description of the heart as a muscle: "I am able to prove that there exists nothing in the heart that is not found also in a muscle (10)." (*See Chapter 4.*) Later recognition of the muscular nature of the heart was to be found in the work of Richard Lower in England in 1669 (11) and in Jean-Baptiste Senac's monumental textbook on cardiology published in 1749 (12). It was, however, the Swiss physician, naturalist, and poet Albrecht Von Haller, in 1736, who formulated the Myogenic Theory of Heart Action (13) and was most influential in its eventual acceptance.

It was Ippolito Francesco Albertini who in 1748 stated unequivocally "in actual fact the heart is a complex muscle (14)." He recognized that in disease this muscle might be weakened. Thus, he wrote,

> ... observations of patients and their autopsies have shown me that pericardial dropsy arising spontaneously and alone is differentiated at least partly from other lesions in sick persons. Usually it is associated with comparatively soft pulses, rather frequent and small, when the structure of the heart has begun to soften here and there in its fibers, a sluggish or merely watery fluid accumulating in the pericardium.

And again,

> I have found that edema, which at the start of an illness appears in the external parts of the body together with difficulty of breathing, also occurs in the internal organs and especially in the lungs. At such times much heavier and more difficult respiration is produced by a moderate amount of fluid collected in the interstices of the lungs than is produced by a much greater quantity poured out in the cavity of the chest.

Laennec (15) recognized what we now call cor pulmonale:

> All diseases which give rise to severe and long-continued dyspnoea produce, almost necessarily, hypertrophia or dilatation of the heart, through the constant efforts the organ is called on to perform, in order to propel the blood into the lungs against the resistance opposed to it by the cause of dyspnoea. It is in this manner that phthisis pulmonalis, empyema, chronic peripneumony, and emphysema of the lungs act in producing disease of the heart; and that those kinds of exercise which require great exertion, and thereby impede respiration, come to be the most common remote causes of these complaints.

The 17th and 18th centuries were the era of postmortem examination and correlation of the findings with clinical observations, the advances and insights of the 19th and 20th century were to be based to a great extent upon the assessment of normal and abnormal function by means of technical devices, permitting measurements, and by the devising and application of the experimental method, first to animals and then to man.

The Reverend Stephen Hales had measured blood pressure in animals by the direct method already in 1726 (16); the contributions of a long line of physiologists who studied circulation in the 19th century made possible the study of the circulation in disease in the 20th century. Thus, Claude Bernard (17), in 1844, carried out the first cardiac catheterization of both the right and left ventricles in a horse, to compare the temperatures in the two ventricles. The veterinarian Chaveau and the physician Marey in 1861 first measured intracardiac pressures by this approach (18), using a modification of the kymograph and recording manometer devised by the German physiologist Karl Ludwig (19).

Karl Vierordt is credited with the first application of graphic recording methods to the clinical study of the pulse in 1855 (20), and Samuel S.K. Von Basch (21), in 1883, with the development of the sphygmomanometer, upon which all subsequent clinical non-invasive measurements of blood pressure were to be based.

Based on graphic records, M. Potain in 1855 (22) postulated the following mechanism for gallop rhythm:

> The gallop sound is diastolic and caused by the rapid development of tension in the ventricular wall under the influence of the entry of blood into the cavity. It is the more pronounced the stiffer the wall, and this decrease of sclerotic thickening of the cardiac wall (hypertrophy due to Bright's disease) or of a change in muscular tone, with the result that the wall, having only its elasticity with which to resist the inflow of blood, will stiffen at the exact moment when the filling occurs (thyphoid fever, right ventricular dilatation of abdominal origin).

In 1870, Adolph Fick, a physicist and physiologist of broad interests, described the basic principles of measurement of cardiac output, although, because of a lack of instrumentation that would have allowed him to measure oxygen uptake and carbon dioxide excretion, he never made such a measurement himself (23). The pioneer work of this physiologist, however, as well as the demonstration by Werner Forssmann in 1929 that a urethral catheter could be introduced into the human right heart with impunity (24), enabled Cournand and Richards, in 1941, to develop cardiac catheterization in man (25), first as a tool for physiologic studies, but then rapidly applied to clinical studies of heart disease and heart failure. In 1956, Forssman, Cournand, and Richards were awarded the Nobel Prize. (*See Chapter 1.*)

Early in this century, Mackenzie (26), considered by some the first pure cardiologist in Great Britain (27), in his lectures and treatises stressed the effect of atrial fibrillation upon the heart's efficiency:

> There can be little doubt that the orderly action of the auricle in regulating the supply of blood to the ventricle, and in stimulating it in normal manner, results in a more efficient action of the ventricle than the variable and irregular stimulation to contraction. When the ventricle is rapidly and irregularly stimulated to contract, there results a gradual exhaustion of the strength of the ventricle, and evidences of heart failure supervene.

Although it would seem that Mackenzie, especially aided by graphic recordings with the polygraph he developed, recognized what we now call the "atrial kick," he did not seem to recognize the implications with regard to ventricular filling or the obligatory reduction of diastolic time which accompanies rapid tachycardias.

For many years the concept that congestive heart failure was due to backward pressure prevailed. We have seen this expressed in the writings of Vieussens (9), and Laennec (15), cited above, expressed perhaps most clearly in a treatise by James Hope in 1832 (28).

In 1913, Mackenzie challenged this theory, when he hypothesized the forward-failure concept which holds that the failing heart's inability to maintain a normal cardiac output is the main cause of congestive heart failure (29). When measurements of cardiac output in patients with congestive heart failure found this to be low (30), the latter theory appeared confirmed. On the other hand, hemodynamic studies soon revealed that cardiac output could be high, notwithstanding the presence of congestive heart failure, in conditions such as thyrotoxicosis, beriberi, and cor pulmonale. This led to the introduction of the terms "low output failure" and "high output failure" by McMichael (31). The concept of forward failure also derived support from the demonstration that in heart failure renal blood flow tends to be diminished, along with decreased excretion of sodium and water (32).

Seminal contributions to our understanding of cardiovascular physiology were made by Ernest Henry Starling and by Otto Frank. Frank studied with Carl Ludwig, and later moved to Munich where he succeeded Voit as Professor of Physiology and remained in this position until 1934. Frank was a great scientist and a very demanding teacher. He was thoroughly intolerant of mediocrity, which to his regret, he found prevalent amongst the young medical students who sat for the first medical examination. His work was carried out on the whole frog heart, perfused with diluted ox blood. By making continuous recordings throughout the cardiac cycle Frank was able to register intracardiac pressures as well as volumes and output. As he wrote "I discovered the following law concerning the dependence of the form of the isometric pressure curve, on the initial tension. The peaks (maxima) of the isometric pressure curve rise with increasing initial tension (filling). I call this part of the family of curves the first part. Beyond a certain level of filling the pressure peaks decline, the second part of the family of curves." He mentions Fick as co-discoverer of the same law for skeletal muscle. Frank also examined isotonic ventricular contractions, the ventricle ejecting blood into an elastic capsule; he found that the increased speed of pressure built up during early systole, increases with increased initial filling and the presence of residual blood at the end of systole increased with increased aortic resistance and increased diastolic filling (Circulation of the Blood, Men and Ideas, Oxford University Press, New York, 1964, edited by Alfred P. Fishman and Dickinson W. Richards, pages 111-113).

Ernest Starling of London's University College (1866-1927), trained in both physiology and medicine. His quantitative studies of ventricular volumes, stroke volumes, filling pressure and vascular resistance in the isolated perfused dog heart, begun in 1912, established that the output of a ventricle is determined by the amount of blood returned to it, and that an increase in filling results in an increase in filling pressure and stroke volume (33). These studies led to the enunciation of the "Law of the Heart." "The Law of the Heart is therefore the same as that of skeletal muscle, namely that the mechanical energy set free on passage from the resting to the contracted state depends on the area of 'chemically active surfaces,' i.e., on the length of the muscle fibres. This simple formula serves to 'explain' the whole behavior of the isolated mammalian heart... (34)."

Starling's work was extended in the studies of Stanley J. Sarnoff and Erik Berglund at the Harvard School of Public Health in the 1950s (35). These investigators, studying the intact circulation in the dog, constructed families of ventricular (Starling) curves and demonstrated that a descending limb of the Starling curve did not occur in the healthy heart, but that an alteration of myocardial contractility—e.g. myocardial failure—resulted in a shift of the normal function curve to a depressed function curve. Starling curves were to become a standard approach to the definition of effects of disease states and interventions upon myocardial function.

Studying the intact cat heart as well as the isolated cat papillary muscle, Sonnenblick and Downing (36) demonstrated that ventricular performance is determined not only by preload, i.e., the cardiac muscle length prior to initiation of contraction or shortening, but also by afterload, i.e., the arterial pressure. They concluded that "ventricular performance at a given constant inotropic state is the product of two largely independent variables, the preload (establishing initial muscle length) and the afterload (36)." This work was to form the basis of the later development of afterload reduction as a therapeutic approach to ventricular failure (37).

Further elucidation of the pathogenesis of heart failure had to await improved understanding of the mechanism of intrinsic contractility of the healthy heart. The early history of the evolution of our knowledge about the biochemical and biophysical mechanisms of contraction of heart muscle in the present century has been well reviewed by Wilfried FHM Mommaerts (38). Here again, major roles were played by methodologic developments such as the polarization and electron microscopes.

Myocardial metabolism has already been considered in Chapter 3 of the present volume. Much of what we know initially about heart muscle was derived not from studies of cardiac muscle, but from studies of skeletal muscle by pioneers such as A.V. Hill (39), who studied muscular contraction physiologically, and Szent-Györgyi (40) who recognized that the two contractile proteins actin and myosin combined to form actinomyosin and who delineated the role of ATP.

The nearly 50 years that have elapsed since the end of World War II have seen an explosion of research addressing the physiology and pathophysiology of the circulatory system, both in man and in experimental animals. These studies have been made possible by the development of new methods and concepts of modern cellular and molecular biology (41) as well as by the availability of a number of natural and experimental animal models of heart disease (42). Congestive heart failure is now recognized as a final more or less common pathway of many different forms of heart disease—congenital, valvular, ischemic, cardiomyopathic, metabolic—comprising abnormal cardiovascular structure, function of the myocardium, peripheral and pulmonary circulation and the humoral regulation of circulation. Considerable uncertainty exists as to the primary and possible causal changes and the secondary, perhaps compensatory effects. These advances have been summarized in a number of recent publications (43-46).

Historically, during the last fifty years clinical experience has been supplemented by fundamental studies which applied the tools furnished. This is particularly evident in the case of congestive heart failure. Protein chemistry, biological chemistry, physiology of circulation, fluid dynamics, even molecular genetics have helped to furnish a basis for the clinical phenomenon known as congestive heart failure. No definite answer appears to explain the total protean clinical picture, but some leads have emerged. They focus primarily on the contractile proteins and receptors.

Receptors

In 1948 an article which revolutionized cardiology and pharmacology appeared in the American Journal of Physiology "A study of the adrenotropic receptors" (47). The author was Raymond P. Ahlquist, from the Department of Pharmacology, University of Georgia School of Medicine (Figure 1). This paper had a curious history: in the first place, the project was undertaken to find a remedy for dysmenorrhea. A uterine muscle relaxant was therefore needed. In the second place, Ahlquist had difficulty in publishing his paper, and once published, it remained unnoticed for several years. He compared the effect of a series of sympathomimetic amines on uterine contraction, blood pressure, heart rate, myocardial contractility, peripheral vasoconstriction and dilatation, intestinal motility, ureteral contractility and nictitating membranes—at that time all standard tests for pharmacological analysis of catecholamines. Ahlquist found that a series of six sympathomimetic amines had an order of potency—1, 2, 3, 4, 5, 6—on the following functions: vaso-

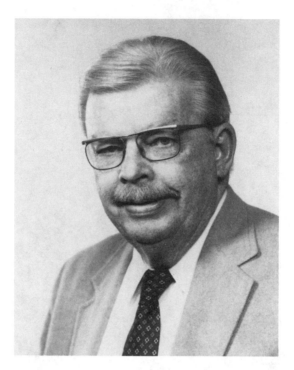

Figure 1. Raymond P. Ahlquist (*Courtesy of the New York Academy of Medicine*)

constriction, excitation of the uterus and ureters, contraction of the nictitating membrane, dilatation of the pupil, and inhibition of the gut. In contrast, the same series of amines has an entirely different order of potency on the following function: vasodilation, inhibition of the uterus, and myocardial stimulation. At the time Alhquist's article was written, pharmacology had already made peace in the dispute between "soup versus sparks," or chemical transmission versus transmission by electrical impulses (48). The arguments between Nachmanson in New York and Otto Loewi created much heat. In Loewi's experiments, supposedly inspired by a dream, he demonstrated that stimulation of the vagus nerve of a perfused frog heart produced a substance which slowed the heart rate of a second heart, and the work of the group around Henry H. Dale, such as J. Feldberg, Gaddum, H. Blaschko and others settled the argument in favor of chemical transmission (49).

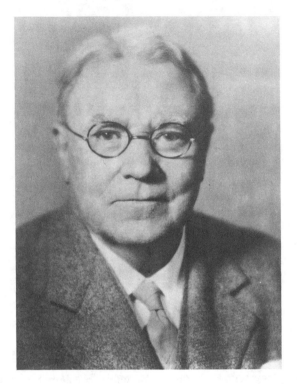

Figure 2.   Walter B. Cannon (*Courtesy of the New York Academy of Medicine*)

From the recognition of the importance of chemical transmission of nervous impulses, it was only a step to the discovery by U. Von Euler of the role of noradrenalin as the chemical transmittor (50). Walter B. Cannon and A. Rosenblueth, had postulated the role of two transmitter substances for adrenergic impulses, sympathin E and sympathin I (51). Cannon in a lecture given at the College of Physicians and Surgeons in 1936, made a good point for the difference between adrenaline and the sympathins (Figure 2). Stimulation of the hepatic sympathetic nerves released something into the blood with effect on the nictitating membrane different from adrenalin. Cannon and Rosenblueth therefore concluded that there are two kinds of sympathin, the excitatory (E) and the inhibitory (I). The heart muscle, so they thought, must discharge excitatory sympathin while the coronary circulation discharges inhibitory sympathin. This is a fine example of how uncertainties of different hypothetical transmitters substances, expounded with authority, can be taken as facts. It is not the transmitter which varies, but the receptors which are different. According to Ahlquist, at least two sets of adrenergic responses are present as judged by the comparative potencies of amines (47). His conclusion was that the differences must be due to two types of receptors: one set of responses—alpha receptors, the other—beta receptors. The receptor must be considered to be a part of the effector rather than of the nerve since surgical or pharmacological removal of the nerve does not abolish the effector response to the circulating transmitter. It is the receptor-effector complex rather than the transmitter that ultimately controls the response to stimulation. Ahlquist's concept ran into real difficulties (52,53,54). He mentioned that his new concept, arrived at by serendipity, "burst into print in 1948, was ignored for more than five years except when someone referred to the method used or the results obtained, but never to the concept (52)." The reasons for this are obvious: the concept did not fit with the ideas developed since the 1890's on the actions of epinephrine. Ahlquist had difficulties in publishing the paper; it was rejected by the Journal of Pharmacology and Experimental Therapeutics, was a loser in the Abel Award Competition, and only could be published in the American Journal of Physiology due to his personal friendship with W.F. Hamilton, the editor. He compares his fate with that of other pioneers of science, for example, to that of Avery who, in 1944, proved that DNA and not protein was the genetic carrier. It was not until 1950 that its correct structure was found, and still later when Watson and Crick showed the double helix. Ahlquist wrote, "Few remember or credit Avery for his concept (52)." In 1977 in the Post-Graduate Medical Journal, J.W. Black paid Ahlquist the credit which was his due; "looking back, his paper can be seen to have been hidden in the long shadows cast by two giants—Dale in England and Cannon in the United States (55; Figure 3)."

Looking into the past, we find that the idea of a receptor did not originate with Ahlquist, but earlier with J.N. Langley, Professor of Physiology in Cambridge, England. His paper in the Journal of Physiology, in 1905, is entitled, "On the reactions of cells and of nerve endings to certain poisons, chiefly as regards the reaction of striated muscle to nicotine and curari (56)." Reading Langley's paper, which comprises 39 pages, one can only reflect with nostalgia at those happy times when a writer had plenty of space available and when the editors did not object to lengthy introductions, detailed descriptions of the experiments, nor to a splendid free style of the English language; alas, our scientific language has become ossified in order to be acceptable. Langley reasoned as follows: "Since curari prevents nerve stimulation from having an effect, but does not itself cause muscular contraction,

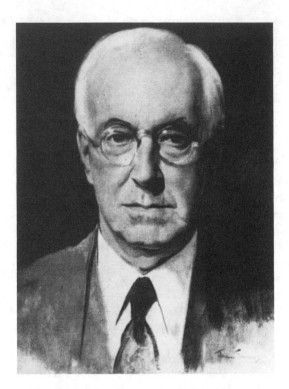

Figure 3.   Sir Henry H. Dale (*Courtesy of the New York Academy of Medicine*)

and nicotine, although preventing nerve stimulation from having an effect, does cause muscular contraction, it seems possible that the latter might act on some substance or structure placed more peripherally than that on which the former acts (56)." The Professor from Cambridge concluded that

> ... two poisons, nicotine, and curari, act on the same protoplasmic substance or substances. With this proviso, I take it that the action consists in a combination of the alkaloid with the protoplasm. Curari in combining leads to diminished excitability and does not stimulate; nicotine in combining also leads to diminished excitability, but it stimulates in combining.

And then he continues in the discussion,

> Since this accessory substance is the recipient of stimuli which it transfers to the contractile material, we may speak of it as the receptive substance of the

muscle." Langley went further, this being the time of Paul Ehrlich, "The relation between the receptive and the contractile substance is clearly very close and on the general lines of Ehrlich's immunity theory, it might be supposed that a receptive substance is a side chain molecule of the molecules of contractile substance, but at present there does not seem to me to be any advantage in attempting to refer the phenomena to molecular arrangement. I conclude then that in all cells two constituents at least must be distinguished 1) substances concerned with carrying out the chief functions of the cells, and 2) receptive substances especially liable to change and capable of setting the chief substance in action.

These were the golden years of English physiology. When and where else would it have been possible that, in 1905, in the Journal of Physiology, a student in physiology could write a 66 page article on the action of adrenaline which foreshadows future experiments on chemical transmission of nervous impulses by comparing the action of adrenaline to that of the sympathetic nervous system (57)? That medical student was Thomas Renton Elliott, who four years after he became a student at University College in London, was appointed to the staff, and became the first unit director at London University (Figure 4). A very British wish was expressed to Professor Elliott on the occasion of his retirement, "We hope he will long remain an active player when he goes north to his newly built home among the grouse moors of Scotland." The contribution of other great British physiologists and pharmacologists, like Henry Dale and others are not mentioned here since they contributed only indirectly to the concept of receptors.

Despite the fact that Ahlquist's 1948 paper was ignored for five years, a time came when it was finally noticed, primarily because of the confirmation of his work by C. E. Powell, I. H. Slater, and Black (58,59). Powell and Slater, working at the Lilly Research Laboratories, published an article in 1957 entitled, "Blocking of Inhibitory Adrenergic Receptors By A Dichloro Analog Of Isoproterenol (58)." It was found that in the anesthetized dog dichloro-isoproterenol did not constrict blood vessels, nor produce a pressor response, nor cause decongestion. Instead it produced vasodilation, a depressor response, and tachycardia. As Ahlquist explained in Perspectives in Biology and Medicine, "This anomalous behaviour was most difficult to explain to medical students (52)." Powell and Slater's discovery in 1958 provided the turning point in the acceptance of the idea of dual receptor mechanism (58). They found that this dichloro analog of isoproterenol selectively blocked some inhibitory effects of ephinephrine and isoproterenol. In addition, the pressor actions of isoproterenol and the secondary depressor action of ephinephrine were inhibited by the dichloro analog which of itself had at most caused a transient fall in blood pressure.

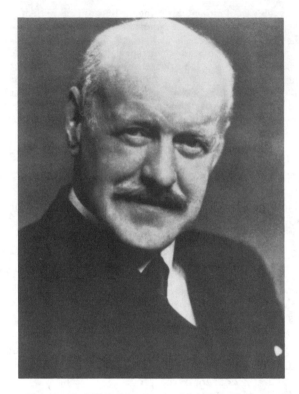

Figure 4.   Thomas R. Elliott (*Courtesy of the New York Academy of Medicine*)

The concluding sentence of the paper is worth noting in the line of Ahlquist's work, "It seemed probably that 20522 (the dichloro analog of isoproterenol) was combining with certain adrenergic inhibitory receptor sites and failed to trigger the series of reactions that lead to typical inhibitory effects (58)." In 1964, Black, working with the Imperial Chemical Industries at the Medical Unit of St. Georges Hospital, in London, synthetized a new adrenergic beta-receptor antagonist, pronethalol, a specific adrenergic beta-antagonist which was relatively free from sympathomimetic activity on the cardiovascular system (59). He had searched for this compound because of his interest in the treatment of angina pectoris. Unfortunately the compound had some undesirable effects and for this reason Black published his results on a new compound InderalR, which has been found to satisfy all the criteria of a beta blocker. Soon this compound was used not only for the treatment of angina pectoris but also for hypertension. Since that time a large series of beta blockers has been synthetized, some with primarily cardiac receptors (beta 1), and those with primarily smooth muscle receptors (beta 2).

Looking over this enormously fruitful field of cardiovascular pharmacology, one is struck by the observation that the truth had been delayed by authoritarian thoughts and dogma some originating from a high authority. In science, authority can be as much of a hindrance to progress as ignorance.

The importance of receptors in myocardial failure became apparent in 1977 when it was discovered that after several days the inotropic response to norepinepherine and isoproterenol became markedly depressed in dogs in congestive heart failure, while chronotropic and blood pressure response remained unaltered (60). At the same time it was shown that a reduction in norephinephrine stores in the heart muscle was associated with a depressed inotropic response to tyramine in papillary muscle from patients with heart failure. Later it was found that the injection of dobutamine, a beta-1 agonist, resulted in development of tolerance to long term infusion; tolerance became significant at 72 and 96 hours (61). This suggested that beta adrenergic receptors are "desensitized in the failing human heart", possibly by norepinephrine (62). This desensitization was not restricted to the heart muscle alone. Colucci for example found that density of beta-adrenergic receptors on lymphocytes of patients treated with a beta-adrenergic agonist, was significantly depressed as compared with that of untreated patients with heart failure of comparable severity. Apparently tolerance can develop in areas other than heart muscle. It is likely that clinically relevant concentrations of administered sympathomimetic agents can affect beta-adrenergic receptor density (63). Other reports soon confirmed this. Obviously the burden of proof is on the beta-adrenergic receptor which through combination with hormone agonists stimulates the enzyme adenylate cyclase to form cyclic AMP which in turn promotes transmembrane calcium flux. In 1986 a selective down grading of beta-1 as compared to beta-2 receptors was found in the failing ventricle (64).

The question arose as to the cause of this selective down regulation. Increased exposure to norepinephrine which has a very high affinity for beta receptors may be resonsible for selective beta-1 down grading. It is known that the failing human heart is exposed to a high concentration of norepinephrine and that selective myocardial beta-1 receptor down regulation is a mark of the degree of prior norepinephrine exposure (65). The reduction in the number of beta-adrenergic receptors appears to be chamber specific; patients with primary right ventricular failure show a greater reduction in beta-receptor number in the right ventricle than in the left, whereas patients with biventricular failure show equivalent degree of beta-adrenergic receptor down regulation in both ventricles (65,66). Post-synaptic myocardial alpha-1 receptors exist in most mammalian species including humans. They mediate a positive inotropic response without notably affecting heart rate (65). This positive inotropic mechanism is not related to the accumulation of cyclic AMP and the stimulation of adenylate cyclase. Selective myocardial alpha-1 adrenergic stimulation may provide effective inotropic support in congestive heart failure even if beta receptors density is markedly reduced (67). Enhanced vasocontriction which is a hallmark of congestive heart failure may result in part from increased alpha-1 adrenoceptor activity in peripheral arterial smooth muscle (68). The mechanism by which cardiac alpha-1 adrenergic receptors increase the force of myocardial contraction is not completely understood, but their inotropic effect may be mediated by receptor-mediated hydrolysis of phosphoinositides to diacylglyceride (69) or more important by inositol triphosphate, which opens intracellular calcium channels. It has been speculated that the loss of inhibition of norepinephrine release in congestive heart failure contributes to the elevation in synaptic and plasma catecholamines levels in congestive heart failure.

From a clinical viewpoint it seemed logical to counteract the down grading of beta-1 receptor in the myocardium by treatment with beta-1 adrenergic agonists. Several beta-agonists have been proposed which might accomplish this goal. But treatment of down grading of beta-receptor with beta-1 adrenergic blockers appears more promising; there have been reports that beta-adrenergic blocking agents are of benefit in congestive heart failure. Treatment with beta-1 blockers such as propranolol in patients with congestive heart failure appears to increase the number of beta-1 receptors (70).

Biochemistry of Myocardial Failure and Contractile Proteins

The preceding discussion indicated that studies dealing with congestive heart failure were primarily descriptive or clinical. At the beginning of this century, there occurred a definite shift: knowledge from the fundamental sciences, physics, chemistry, and molecular biology, biochemistry, electromicroscopy began to influence the approaches to myocardial failure (71).

Coronary sinus catheterization begun in the middle 1940s, was among the early studies on myocardial failure (71). By introducing a catheter in the coronary sinus and simultaneously sampling of arterial and coronary sinus blood, the coronary arteriovenous differences not only of oxygen, but also of nutrients such as glucose, lactate, pyruvates, amino acids, ketone bodies and fatty acids could be determined. Congestive heart failure was thought to be a disturbance of energy production rather than energy utilization since there was no change in myocardial extraction of either oxygen or substrates.

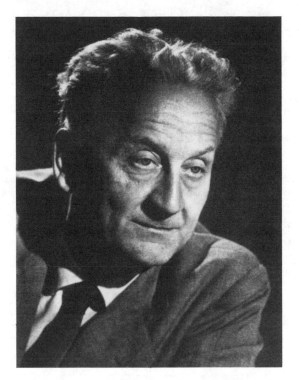

Figure 5.   Albert Szent–Györgyi (*Courtesy of the New York Academy of Medicine*)

It is not the subject of a historical review to detail current knowledge of the biochemical basis of heart function and contractile failure. The reader is referred to recent reviews on this subject (71,72,73,74).

Recent development in fundmental knowledge of myocardial failure are concerned with 1) calcium movements, membrane function of mitochondria, subcellular organelles (cyctoplasmic reticulum) and 2) Contractile machinery of the heart, the contractile proteins.

The pioneering figure in the field of contractile proteins is Albert Szent-Györgyi (Fig. 5). Szent-Györgyi received the Nobel Prize in medicine and physiology for his discoveries in connection with the biological combustion process and the catalysis of fumaric acid, leading to the discovery of vitamin C. Unquestionably Szent-Györgyi was one of the most colorful and creative scientists of our age. He was born in 1893 in Budapest, Hungary and his early career was intimately connected with the fate of his native land. He published an autobiographical note in the Annual Review of Biochemistry (75).

> I finished school in feudal Hungary as the son of a wealthy land owner and I had no worries about my future. A few years later I find myself working in Hamburg, Germany with a slight hunger edema. In 1942 I find myself in Istanbul involved in secret diplomatic activity, with a setting fit for a cheap and exciting spy story. Shortly after, I get a warning that Hitler had ordered the Governor of Hungary to appear before him, screaming my name at the top of his voice and demanding my delivery. Arrest warrants were passed out even against members of my family. In my pocket I find a Swedish passport, having been made a full Swedish citizen on the order of the King of Sweden—I am "Mr. Swenson," my wife, "Mrs. Swenson". Sometime later I find myself in Moscow being treated in the most royal fashion by the government (with caviar three times per day), but it does not take long before I am declared a "traitor of the people" and I play the role of the villain. At the same time I am refused entrance to the USA for my Soviet sympathies. Eventually, I find peace at Woodshole, Massachusetts, USA working in a solitary corner of the Marine Biological Laboratory. After some nerve-wrecking complications, due to McCarthy, things straighten out, but the internal struggle is not completely over. I am troubled by grave doubts about the usefulness of scientific endeavor and have a whole drawer filled with treatises on politics and their relation to science, written for myself with the sole purpose of clarifying my mind completely and finding an answer to the question: will science lead to the elevation or destruction of man, and has my scientific endeavor made any sense?

What may lend additional interest to his story is that it reflects the turbulence of our days. This is not very different from the story of Copernicus who lived in the sixteenth century and whose life was influenced and darkened by the turmoil of his times. Szent-Györgyi was a rebel and an unruly genius. In science he fought what he called "accepting things without evidence" and he believed that we were living in the middle of the transition from the prescientific to the scientific thinking, hence the "tumult." As a child he described himself as dull and his uncle, a noted histologist believed that he was not promising enough to go on to medical school, but suggested that he go into cosmetics. Later his uncle admitted the possibility of his becoming a proctologist. So his first scientific paper written in the first year of medical studies, dealt with the epithelium of the anus. As he says, "I started science at the wrong end, but soon I shifted to the vitreous body." Later in his career he became fascinated by the succino and citrocodehydrogenase. He believed that these enzymes should have some general catalytic role and he demonstrated that once the succinodehydrogenase was inactivated which could be done by malonic acid, respiration stopped. This proved that succinic acid and citric acid had some general catalytic activity and could not be simple metabolites as thought before. This idea was later confirmed by Krebs and became the foundation of the so-called "Krebs cycle." It was partly this discovery of the C4 dicarboxylic acid catalysis for which Szent-Györgyi was honored by the Nobel prize.

At the same time Szent-Györgyi became interested in vegetable respiration because as he expressed it, "there is no basic difference between man and the grass he mows". Eventually, he was able to isolate a reducing agent crystallized from oranges, lemons, cabbages, and the adrenal glands. He knew that it was related to sugars, but he did not know which. He called this compound "Ignose". The editor of the biochemical journal to whom he submitted the article reprimanded him for being flippant. Thereupon Szent-Györgyi changed the name of this sugar to "Godnose", but this was not more successful. Finally he called the new substance hexuronic acid since it had six carbons and was acid. To get more material he moved to the Mayo Clinic where there was ample adrenal tissue available. Returning back to Hungary and the University of Szeged, he found that hexuronic acid was identical to Vitamin C. As he wrote "we (that is Hayworth and I) rebaptized hexuronic acid to ascorbic acid." (75)

Szent-Györgyi then turned to the biochemistry of muscle. As he wrote "with its valiant, physical, chemical and dimensional changes, muscle is an ideal material to study." With his associates he discovered a new protein "actin" which was isolated by his pupil Straub. By complexing actin and myosin he found a contractile protein actomyosin which contracted upon the addition of adenosine triphosphatc (ATP). As Szent-Györgyi wrote "to see these fibers contract for the first time, and to have reproduced in vitro one of the oldest signs of life, motion, was perhaps the most thrilling moment of my life." Szent-Györgyi concludes his autobiographical sketch:

> to me, science in the first place is the society of men which knows no limits in time and space. I am living in such a community, in which Lavoisier and Newton are my daily companions; an Indian or Chinese scientist is closer to me than my own milkman. The basic moral rule of this society is simple: Mutual respect, intellecutal honesty, and good will. (75).

Based on Albert Szent-Györgyi's discovery, the knowledge of the role of contractile proteins in normal and failing hearts has expanded (72,73). It has been found that reconstituted actomyosin exhibits the salient properties of muscle. It was Huxley who first proposed the sliding model, in which actin and myosin molecules slide by each other during shortening of the muscle (76). Actin has been found to consist of two portions F and G actin. Tropomyosin and troponin are found with actin on the thin filament (77). In the myofibril, the thin filament surrounds the thick filament and interacts by overlapping. Actin forms a macromolecule to comprise a thin filament (72). Troponin and trypomyosin are known to play a regulatory role in the interaction of actin and myosin and an additional protein, (C-protein) has also been identified in cardiac muscle (72). Actin-myosin forms cross-bridges and shorten against mechanical load at the expense of the chemical energy contained in the high energy phosphate bond in ATP. The tropomyosin and troponin proteins confirm calcium sensitivity on the contractile machinery. Troponin-C is the subunit which binds Ca^{2+} and troponin I (72,73,74).

Another important development also concerns the phosphorylation of cardiac contractile proteins (78). Phosphorylation of proteins by protein kinase is a reversible process. Aside from the regulation of cardiac contractility through changes in intracellular concentration of calcium ions, phosphorylation of cardiac contractile proteins also plays a considerable role. When hearts are stimulated with catecholamines, troponin-I and C protein are rapidly phosphorylated in response to increased intracellular concentration of cyclic AMP.

Molecular biology has also been applied in an attempt to understand myocardial failure. It is now apparent that the well-known changes in gross and histological structure, and in the ultrastructure of the failing heart, extend to the molecular level. Hypertrophy of the overloaded myocardium is accompanied by complex changes in the expression of the genes that encode key myocardial proteins. For example, in the pressure-overloaded rodent ventricle, preferential synthesis of a "slow" isoform of the myosin heavy chain helps ventricular function adapt to a chronic increase in the rate of energy expenditure. This occurs because the slow myosin reduces the rate of energy expenditure while, at the same time, increasing efficiency (77). While these abnormalities are not seen in the human ventricle, changes in myosin gene expression similar to those in the rat ventricle have been documented in overloaded human atria (79,80).

The changes in myosin described above represent but one example of a growing number of alterations in the composition of the overloaded, hypertrophied heart (81). A reduction in the density of calcium pump ATPase molecules in the sarcoplasmic reticulum of the hypertrophied human heart has also been described (82), in this case, without a change in the protein itself.

A pattern that emerges is that there is a preferential synthesis of fetal isoforms of several proteins in the failing heart. This appearance of fetal isoforms may be related to the accelerated growth that occurs in cardiac hypertrophy. It is well known that the cells of the adult myocardium, which are unable to divide, normally synthesize protein at only a very slow rate. In order for the overloaded myocardium to initiate rapid protein synthesis, it appears that isoforms of many newly synthesized proteins revert to those seen earlier in development, during fetal life. The functional significance of this reversion to primitive isoforms is not well understood, but may result in myocardial cells that "wear out" at an accelerated rate, and so may contribute to the deterioration of the myocardium that is largely responsible for the poor prognosis in patients with heart failure.

REFERENCES

1. Jarcho, S. The Concept of Heart Failure from Avicenna to Albertini. Cambridge, MA, Harvard University Press 1980, pp 407.
2. Husain ibn 'Abd Allah, (Abu 'Ali) called Ibn Sina or Avicenna. On the Signs [of Suffocation and Angina] (book 3, Gen 9 treatise 1, chapter 9) Quoted by Saul Jarcho 91) op cit p.4.
3. Mercatus, L. (Luiz Mercado). De internorum morborum curatoine. Frankfurt: Palthemius 1619-1620, Bk 2, chap 1, pp 160-161, Quoted by Saul Jarcho op cit (1) p. 91.
4. Piso, C. (Charles le Pois). Selectiorum observationum et consiliorum de praetervisis hactenus morbis affectibusque praeter naturam, ab aqua seu serosa colluviae et diluvie ortis Pont-à-Mousson 1618. Quoted by Saul Jarcho (1) op cit p. 113.
5. Harvey, W., Exercitatio anatomica de motu cordis et sanguinis in animalibus. Francoforti, Sumpt. Guilielmi Fitzeri, 1628.
6. Malpighi, M. De pulmonibus. Bologna, 1661.
7. Malpighi, M. et Jo. Mariae Lancisii. Consultationum medicorum, Venezia, Corona, 1747, Translated, in part, by Saul Jarcho (1), op cit pp 190-209.
8. Baglivi, G. Opera omnia medico-practica, et anatomica. Lugduni, Anisson, J. Posuel, 1704.
9. Vieussens, R., Traite nouveau de la structure et des causes du mouvement naturel du coeur. Toulouse; Guillemette, 1715. Quoted by Jarcho (1) op cit p. 243 (1).
10. Sten, N. De musculis et glandulis observationum specimen Cum epistolis duabus anatomicis. Ludg. Batav., 1683. Hafniae, Lit. Matt. Godicchenii, 1664 [OT].
11. Lower, R. Tractatus de corde. London, J. Allestry 1669.
12. Senac, J.B. Traité de la structure du coeur, de son action, et de ses maladies. 2 vols. Paris. Chez Braisson 1749 pp 1246.
13. Haller, A. Deux mémoires sur le mouvement du sang; et sur les effets de la saignée; fondes sur des expériences faites sur des animaux. Lausanne, Mark-Mic Bousquet Comp 1756, pp 342.
14. Albertini, I. F. Animadversiones super quibusdam difficilis respirationis vitiis a laesa cordis et praecordiorum structura pendentibus. In De Bononiensi Scientiarum et Artium Instituo atque Academia Commentarii 1:382-404, 1731, reprinted in 1748. Translated in (1).
15. Laennec, R.T.H. A Treatise on the Diseases of the Chest in which they are Described According to their Anatomical Characters and their Diagnosis Estab-

lished as a New Priniciple Means of Acoustic Instrument. Book 3, Chapter 1, Section 290. Translated by John Forbes. Philadelphia, Janus Webster, 1823.

16. Hales, S. Statical essays, containing haemostaticks. Vol. 2 London. W. Innys and R. Manby, 1733.
17. Bernard, C. Lecons sur la chaleur Animale. Bailliere, Paris, 1876.
18. Chaveau, A. and Marey, J. Determination graphique des rapports du choc du coeur avec les mouvements des oreillettes et des ventricules: experience faite a l'aide d'un appareil enregistreur (syphygmographe). C.R. Acad. Sci. (Paris) 53:622-625, 1861.
19. Ludwig, C. Beiträge zur Kenntnis des Einflusses der Respirationsbewegungen auf den Blutlauf im Aortensysteme. Arch. Anat. Physiol. Wiss. Med. 242-302, 1847.
20. Vierodt, K. Die bildliche Darstellung des menschlichen Arterienpulses. Arch Physiol. Heilk. 13:284-287, 1854.
21. Basch, S.S. von. Ein Metall-Sphygmomanometer. Wien. Med. Wschr. 33:673-675, 1883.
22. Potain, M. Theorie du bruit de galop. C.R. de L'Assoc. Francaise pour L'Avancement des Sciences, pt 1, 14:201-203, 1885.
23. Fick, A. Über die Messung des Blutquantums in den Herzventrikeln. S.B. Phys. Med. Ges. Würzburg 16, 1870.
24. Forssmann, W., Die Sondierung des rechten Herzens. Klin. Wschr. 8:2085-2087, 1929.
25. Cournand, A. Cardiac catheterization. Development of the technique, its contributions to clinical medicine and its initial applications in man. Acta. Med. Scand. Suppl. 579, 1975.
26. Mackenzie, J. Abnormal inception of the cardiac rhythm. Quart. J. Med. 1:39, 1907.
27. Krikler, D.M.: Sir James MacKenzie. Clin. Cardiol. 11:193-194, 1988.
28. Hope, J. A treatise on the diseases of the heart and great vessels. Kidd, London 1832.
29. Mackenzie, J. Diseases of the Heart. 3rd ed. London, Henry Frowde, 1913.
30. Stead, E.A. Jr., Warren, J.V. and Brannon, E.S. Cardiac output in congestive heart failure. An analysis of the reason for lack of close correlation between the symptom of heart failure and the resting cardiac output. Am. Heart J. 35:529-541, 1948.
31. McMichael, J. Circulatory failure studied by means of venous catheterization. Adv. Intern Med. 2:64-101, 1947.
32. Merrill, A.J. Edema and decreased renal blood flow in patients with chronic congestive heart failure. Evidence of "forward failure" as the primary cause of edema. J. Clin. Invest. 25:389-400, 1946.
33. Patterson, S.W. and Starling, E.H. On the mechanical factors which determine the output of the ventricles. J. Physiol. 48:357-279, 1914.
34. Patterson, S.W., Piper, H. and Starling, E.H. The regulation of the heart beat. J. Physiol. 48:465-513, 1914.
35. Sarnoff, S.J. and Berglund, E. Ventricular function. I. Starling's law of the heart studied by means of simultaneous right and left ventricular function curves in the dog. Circulation 9:706-718, 1954.

36. Sonnenblick, E.H. and Downing, S.E. Afterload as a primary determinant of ventricular performance. Am. J. Physiol. 204:604-610, 1963.
37. Franciosa, J.A., Guiha, N.H., Limas, C.J., Rodriguerqa, E. and Cohn, J.N. Improved left ventricular function during nitroprusside infusion in acute myocardial infarction. Lancet 1:650-654, 1972.
38. Mommaerts, W.F.J.M. Chapter III Heart muscle. In: Circulation of the blood: men and ideas, A.P. Fishman and D.E. Richards, Eds, New York, Oxford University Press, 1964, pp 127-198.
39. Hill, A.V. The design of muscles. Brit. Med. Bull. 12:165-166, 1956.
40. Szent-Györgyi, A. Chemical physiology of contraction in body and heart muscle. New York, Academic Press, 1953.
41. Fozzard, H.A., Haber, E., Hennings, R.B., Katz, A.N. and Morgan, H.E., eds. The Heart and cardiovascular System: scientific foundation. New York, Raven Press, 1986.
42. Abelmann, W.H. The dilated cardiomyopathies: experimental aspects. Cardiol. Clin. 6:219-231, 1988.
43. Katz, A.M. Regulation of myocardial contractility, 1958-1983: An Odyssey. J. Am. Coll. Cardiol. 1:42-51, 1983.
44. Parmley, W.W. Pathophysiology and current therapy of congestive heart failure. J. Am Coll. Cardiol. 13:771-785, 1989.
45. Wever, K.T., ed. Heart Failure: current concepts and management. Cardiol. Clin 7, 1989.
46. Williams, J.F., Jr. Evolving concepts in congestive heart failure. Mod. Concepts Cardiovasc. Dis. 59:43-48, and 49-53, 1990.
47. Alhquist, R.P. A study of the adrenotropic receptors. Am. J. Physiol., 153;586-600, 1948.
48. Koelle, G.B. Reflections on the pioneers of neurohumoral transmission. Perspect. Biol. Med., 28:434-439, 1985.
49. Blaschko, J. Dihydroxyphenylscrine (DOPS) as a therapeutic agent: reflections on pure and applied science. J. Appl. Cardiol. 3:429-432, 1988.
50. Von Euler, U.S. A specific sympothomimetic ergone in adrenergic nerve fibers (sympathin) in its relations to adrenaline and noradrenealine. Acta Physiol. Scand., 12:73-97, 1946.
51. Cannon, W., and A. Rosenblueth. Studies on conditons of activity in endocrine organs; XXIX. Sympathin E and Sympathin I. Am. J. Physiol., 104:557-574, 1933.
52. Ahlquist, R.P. Adrenergic receptors: a personal and practical view. Perspect. Biol. Med., 17:119-122, 1973.
53. Ahlquist, R.P. Present state of alpha and beta adrenergic drugs II. The adrenergic blocking agents. Am. Heart J., 92:804-807, 1976.
54. Ahlquist, R.P. Development of the concept of alpha and beta adrenotropic receptors. Ann. N.Y. Acad. Sci., 139:549-552, 1967.
55. Black, J.W. Ahlquist and the development of beta-adrenoreceptor antagonists. Postgrad. Med. J., 52(Suppl. 4):11-13, 1976.
56. Langley, J.N. On the reaction of cells and of nerve-endings to certain poisons, chiefly as regards the reaction of striated muscle to nicotine and to curari. J. Physiol., 33:374-413, 1905/6.

57. Elliott, T.R. The action of adrenalin. J. Physiol., 32:401-467, 1905.
58. Powell, C.E., and I.H. Slater. Blocking of inhibitory adrenergic receptors by a dichloro analog of isoproterenol. J. Pharm. Exp. Ther., 122:480-488, 1958.
59. Black, J.W., A.F.Crowther, T.G. Shanks, L.H. Smith, and A.C. Dornhost. A new adrenergic beta-receptor antagonist. Lancet, 1:1080-1081, 1964.
60. Newman, Walter H. A depressed response to left ventricular contractile force to isoproterenol and norepinephrine in dogs with congestive heart failure, Am. Heart J. 93:216-221, 1977.
61. Unverferth, D.V., Blanford, M., Kates, R.E., and Leier, C.V. Tolerance to dobutamine after a 72 hour continuous infusion. Am. J. Med. 69:262-266, 1980.
62. Thomas, J.A. and Marks, B.H. Plasma norepinephrine in congestive heart failure. Am. J. Cardiol. 41:233-243, 1978.
63. Colucci, W.S., Alexander, W., Williams, G.H., Rude, R.E., Holman, B.L., Konstam, M.A., Wynne, H., Mudge G.H., Jr., and Braunwald, E. Decreased lymphocyte beta-adrenergic-receptor density in patients with heart failure and tolerance to the beta-adrenergic agonist pirbuterol. N. Engl. J. Med. 305:185-190, 1981.
64. Bristow, M.R., Ginsburg, R., Umans, V., Fowler, M., Minobe, W., Rasmussen, R., Zera, P., Menlove, R., Shah, P., Jamieson, S., and Stinson E. β-1 and β-2-Adrenergic receptor subpopulations in nonfailing and failing human ventricular myocardium: coupling of both receptor subtypes to muscle contraction and selective β-1-receptor down-regulation in heart failure. Circ. Res. 59:297-309, 1986.
65. Ruffolo, R.R., Jr. and Kopia, G.A. Importance of receptor regulation in the pathophysiology and therapy of congestive failure. Am. J. Med. 80:67-72, 1986.
66. Bristow, M.R., Ginsburg, R., Minobe W.A., Harrison D.C., Reitz, B.A. and Stinson, E.B. Beta-adrenergic receptor measurements in normal and failing human right and left ventricle (abstr). Circulation Suppl. II207, 1982.
67. Chang, H.Y., Klein, R.M., and Kunos, G. Selective desensitization of cardiac beta receptors by prolonged in vivo infusion of catecholamines in rats. J. Pharmacol. Exp. Ther. 221:784-789, 1982.
68. Forster, C. Carter, S.L. and Armstrong P.W. α-1-Adrenoreceptor activity in arterial smooth muscle following congestive heart failure. Can J. Phys. and Pharmacol, 67:110-115, 1989.
69. Wald, M., Borda, E.S. and Sterin-Borda, L. α-Adrenergic supersensitivity and decreased number of α-adrenoceptors in heart from acute diabetic rats. Can. J. Phys. Pharm. 66:1154-1157, 1988.
70. Bristow, M.R., Laser, J.A., Minobe W., Gisburg R., Fowler M.B. and Rasmussen, R. Selective down regulation of beta-adrenergic receptors in failing human heart abstract Circulation Suppl. II-67, 1974.
71. Bing, R.J. Metabolism of the heart. Harvey Lectures. 50:27-70, 1954-1955.
72. Dhalla, N.S., Dixon, I.M.C., Beamish, R.E. Biochemical basis of heart functions and contractile failure. J. Am. Col. Cardiol. 6:7, 1991.
73. Katz, Arnold M. Physiology of the Heart. Raven Press, New York, NY 1977. 2nd Ed. 1992.
74. Kako, K. and Bing, R.J. Contractility of actomyosin bands prepared from normal and failing human hearts. J. Clin. Invest. 37:465-470, 1958.

75. Szent-Györgyi, A. Lost in the twentieth century. Annual Review of Biochemistry 32:1-14, 1963,
76. Huxley, A.F.. Muscular contraction. J. Physiol. 243:1-43, 1974.
77. Hamrell, B.,B., Alpert, N.A. Cellular basis of the mechanical properties of hypertrophied myocardium In: The Heart and Cardiovascular System, Eds: Fozzard, H., Haber, E., Katz, A., Jennings, R., Morgan, H.E. New York: Raven Press, 1986.
78. England, P.J. Phosphorylation of cardiac contractile proteins. Chapter 16. Handbook of Physiology, Baltimore, Williams and Wilkens, 1977.
79. Tsuchimochi-H., Sugi, M., Kuroo, M., Ueda, S., Takau, F, Furuta, S., Shirai, T. and Yazaki, Y. Isozymic changes in myosin of human atrial myocardium induced by overload. Immunohistochemical study using monoclonal antibodies. J. Clin. Invest. 74:662-665, 1984.
80. Mercadier, J.J, dela-Bastie, D, Menasche, P, N-Guyen-Van-Cao, A., Bouveret, P., Lorente, P. Piwnica, A., Slama, R. and Schwartz, K. Alpha-myosin heavy chain isoform and atrial size in patients with various types of mitral valve dysfunction: a quantitative study. J. Am. Coll. Cardiol. 9:1024-1030, 1987.
81. Katz, A.M. Cardiomyopathy of overload. A major determinant of prognosis in congestive heart failure. N. Engl. J. Med. 322:100-110, 1990.
82. Mercadier, J.J., Lompre, A.M., Duc, P., Boheler, K.R., Fraysse, J.B., Wisnewsky, C., Allen, P.D. Komajda, M. and Schwartz, K. Altered sarcoplasmic reticulum Ca^{2+}-ATPase gene expression in the human ventricle during end stage heart failure. J. Clin. Invest. 85:305-309, 1990.

Chapter 11

Valvular Surgery

R. HEIMBECKER, T. DAVID AND R.J. BING

Cardiopulmonary bypass was the long path that made valvular surgery effective. A look at the history of medicine with the retrospectroscope reveals costly, often futile, slow graspings for solutions until a breakthrough drastically changes the situation. This happened in surgery of cardiac valves with the introduction of cardiopulmonary bypass. It is easy for a Monday morning quarterback to judge yesterday's football game; it is difficult for the players in the midst of a game to foresee if and when a touchdown will occur. Players must painfully advance yard by yard until a sudden spurt by a particular player brings victory. Nevertheless, there is heroism in the steady plodding, pioneering work with difficult inch by inch advance.

The history of valvular surgery started with a suggestion concerning treatment of mitral stenosis. Sir Lauder Brunton, in 1902, was motivated like many others by a particular patient's suffering (1; Fig.1). He wrote, "mitral stenosis is not only one of the most distressing forms of cardiac disease, but in its severe form it resists all treatment by medicine." He continued,

I was much impressed by the case of a man under middle age whom I had under my care at St. Bartholomew's hospital. For no fault of his own, but simply because of his disease, this man was really exiled from his family, one might almost say imprisoned for life in as much as he could only live in a hospital ward or a work house infirmary. It occurred to me that it was worthwhile for such a patient to run a risk and even a greater risk in order to obtain such improvement as might enable him at least to stay at home. But no one would be justified in attempting such a dangerous operation as dividing a mitral stenosis on a fel-

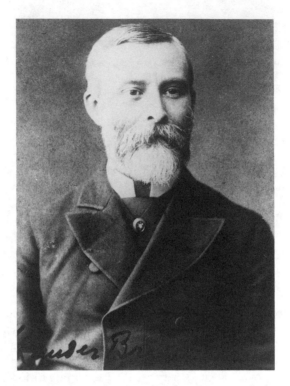

Figure 1.   Sir Lauder Brunton (*Courtesy of The New York Academy of Medicine*)

low-creature without having first tested its practicability and perfected its technique by previous trials on animals.

Brunton accordingly performed experiments of dividing stenosed valves in diseased hearts from the post-mortem theatre, and operated on the hearts of cats, and also tried operations on the dead animal. He continued,

> I therefore think that it may be worthwhile to write the preliminary note, especially as, after all, if the operation is to be done in man it will be surgeons who will do it and they must of course make their own preliminary experiments, however fully the operation may be described by others and each must find out for himself the methods which he will employ in each particular case.

Brunton suggested use of a tenotomy knife "but some which I had made of ladies bonnet pins, were too thin and flexible for stenosed valves, although they were sufficiently strong to divide the normal valves in the hearts of cats." He mentioned that the main part of the valve can be divided with comparative ease, but the thickened edge resists the knife. He wrote that he had not yet decided on the best form of knife and he believed that this would depend on whether or not the surgeon approaches the valve from the atrium or the ventricle. He suggested that in the living heart the knife should be used during diastole only, as one is less likely to wound the opposite wall of the ventricle. One sentence in particular is worth noting: "The good results that have been obtained by surgical treatment of wounds in the heart emboldens one to hope that before very long similar good results may be obtained in cases of mitral stenosis."

Brunton's fame does not rest entirely on his suggestion for operation on the mitral valve. Introduction of the use of amylnitrite in the treatment of angina pectoris was certainly another important Brunton contribution to medicine. In 1876, he also reported results of his studies on the use of nitroglycerin in animal experiments. But he found the headache induced by nitroglycerin so severe in man that he delayed its use. It was Murrell who first advocated the use of nitroglycerin in patients with angina pectoris (1a).

In 1908, Harvey Cushing and J.R.B. Branch, from the Johns Hopkins Hospital in Baltimore, published some notes on the experimental and clinical approach to chronic valvular lesion in the dog and the possible relation to future surgery of the cardiac valves (2; Fig.2). (This was prior to Cushing's main interest in neurosurgery). In his paper in the Journal of Medical Research, Cushing described the clinical history and the autopsy finding on animals with valvular heart disease. He mentions that "Our interest in these observations was researched in the spring of this year by the admission to the laboratory of another animal with symptoms the counterpart of those which were present in the patient whose malady first suggested these investigations." A large Newfoundland dog brought to the Hunterian Laboratory of the Johns Hopkins Hospital in 1905 suffering with general anasarca, ascites, and other sequelae of passive congestion due to tricuspid insufficiency with compensatory failure, resulting in advanced chronic endocarditis. Autopsy on that animal disclosed a thickened mitral valve, a dilated and hypertrophied heart showing tricuspid insufficiency, together with an unusually marked degree of venous congestion. Being interested in experimental surgery, Cushing then proceeded to produce this condition experimentally (2).

Cushing's was the first successful attempt to produce valvular lesion by an intrathoracic exposure of the heart with subsequent recoveries. He pays particular attention to anesthesia and mentions the fact that the desired intrapulmonary pressure could be readily achieved by inflation of the lung through

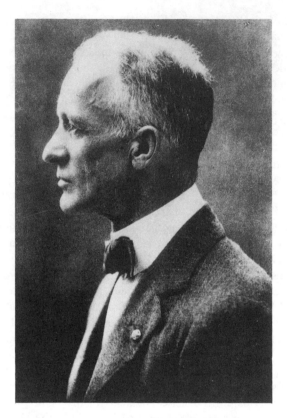

Figure 2.   Harvey Cushing (*Courtesy of The New York Academy of Medicine*)

an opening in the trachea as commonly used in a physiological laboratory. He wrote, "I have twice in a human subject given artificial respiration by this method with immediate closure of the tracheal wound without drainage. These were cases of temporary respiratory failure due to an intracranial pressure. Both patients recovered and in both the cervical wound healed without reaction."

Cushing used a valvulotome to produce mitral insufficiency by dividing one mitral valve leaflet with a cutting hoop, introducing the instrument through the apex of the left ventricle. He mentions the difficulty of producing serious mitral insufficiency in the dog since the heart is able to compensate rapidly for the lesion; he thought it might be necessary for the operation to be done in successive stages in order to reproduce conditions of compensatory failure such as occurs in chronic endocarditis resulting from disease of the valves. "During the course of our observation our attention was called by Futcher to a recent note in the Lancet by Sir Lauder Brunton which puts the matter from a physician's point of view so forcibly that his words may well be used to express our own feeling in regard to these measures should it ever prove justifiable to transfer the experiments to man."

From the same John's Hopkins laboratory, B.M. Bernheim repeated most of Cushing's experiments confirming that, "We have not as yet been able to reproduce the typical presystolic murmur of the usual symptoms characteristic of the 'button hole' stenosis in man (3)." Cushing and his group believed that in order to proceed with the surgical treatment of valvular disease the condition had to first be reproduced in the dog.

In 1914 in New York, a particularly ingenious approach to the treatment of pulmonary stenosis was introduced by the French surgeons Theodore Tuffier and Alexis Carrel of the Rockfeller Institute for Medical Research (4). (Carrel's pioneering work has been repeatedly noted in these pages, particularly in regard to blood vessel surgery.) Carrel and Tuffier sought to develop a technique to enlarge the pulmonary orifice. The operation involved suturing a venous patch to the anterior side of the pulmonary orifice permitting an increase in the circumference of the orifice after the arterial wall had been incised. Eight experiments on dogs were carried out. The authors concluded that it is possible to perform an operation aimed at increasing the circumference of the pulmonary orifice, without involving much danger to the life of the animal. The pulmonary valve itself was incised by the long blade of specially constructed scissors. Once the instrument had been used and the valve incised, the surgeon compressed the flap against the opening, thus arresting hemorrhage. Then the lower side of the flap was rapidly united to the cardiac wall by means of continuous suture. Tuffier and Carrel predicted that operations of this type might be employed in the treatment of pulmonary artery stenosis in man. In 1913, Tuffier operated on a 26 year old man with severe aortic stenosis. The patient surived and was reported to be improved and alive 12 years later (5). As Lindblom writes, "This must be regarded as the first successful surgical approach to valvular heart disease (6)." Another attempt, by Allen and Graham, using a cardioscope with a knife attachment for widening the orifice of cardiac valves was destined for failure (7). One wonders about the use of the cardioscope since obviously visualization of the valve through the cardioscope did not contribute to the technique's success. Allen and Graham's method was a valiant attempt, but the big step forward was operation under direct vision made possible by cardiopulmonary bypass.

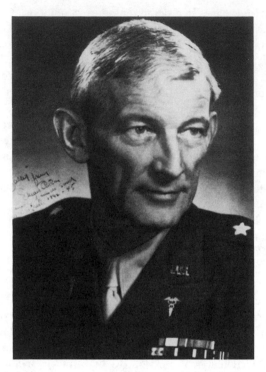

Figure 3.   Elliott C. Cutler (*Courtesy of The New York Academy of Medicine*)

In the 1920s the idea of incising the valve by an appropriate instrument was vigorously pursued by Elliot Cutler and his group from the Harvard Medical School (Fig.3). In the Boston Medical and Surgical journal of 1923, Cutler and S.A. Levine described the first operation on a patient, carried out on May 20, 1923 (8). A valvulotome, an instrument which they likened to a tenotome or a slightly curved tonsil knife, was plunged into the left ventricle at a point about one inch from the apex and away from the branches of the descending coronary artery. The knife was then pushed upward about two and one-half inches until it encountered "what seems to us, must be the mitral orifice." Two cuts were then made on opposite sides of the valve. Cutler was so proud of the results that "the patient was brought to the large amphitheatre and presented before the reunion group of doctors and nurses the fourth day after the operation."

Alas, this success could not be duplicated. Cutler and C.S. Beck, (Beck would later make important contributions to cardiac surgery) reported such

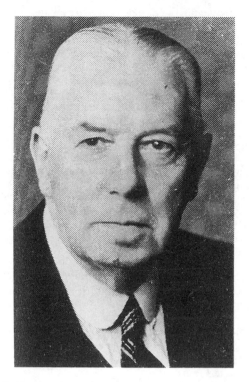

Figure 4.   H.S. Souttar (*Courtesy of The New York Academy of Medicine*)

operations on a total of seven patients at the Peter Bent Brigham Hospital in Boston (9). Only one patient survived; six died following the operation. In another paper by Beck and Cutler, the cutting instrument was described in detail (10). The instrument actually excised a segment from the mitral orifice and removed this from the blood stream.

The persistence and optimism of these pioneers is to be admired. The situation was not dissimilar to that at the onset of cardiac transplantation when the mortality rate was also extremely high.

In 1925, a great step forward was made by H.S. Souttar at the London hospital using a method noteworthy for its simplicity and directness. (11; Fig.4). Souttar had the good sense not to employ sharp cutting instruments, but merely his finger to open the mitral valve. He furthermore used the atrial approach and applied a curved clamp, strikingly similar to the Pott's clamp, to occlude the atrial appendage. The clamp was then withdrawn and the appendage was drawn over the finger like a glove by means of sutures. As Souttar wrote,

> ...the whole inside of the left auricle could now be explored with facility. It was immediately evident from the rush of blood against the finger that gross regurgitation was taking place, but there was not so much thickening of the valves as had been expected. The finger was passed into the ventricle through the orifice of the mitral valve without encountering resistance and the cusp of the valve could be easily felt and the condition estimated.

How much simpler this was than the use of a cardioscope. He continued,

> As however the stenosis was of such moderate degree, and was accompanied as a little thickening of the valves, it was decided not to cut out the valve section which had been arranged, but to limit intervention to such dilatation as could be carried out by the finger. It was felt that an actual section of the valve might only make matters worse by increasing the degree of regurgitation, while the breaking down of adhesions by the finger might improve the condition as regards to both regurgitation and stenosis.

The patient made an uneventful recovery, being kept in bed for six weeks according to the surgical practice at that time. Souttar concluded his article in the British Medical Journal,

> It appears to me that the method of digital exploration through the auricular appendage cannot be surpassed for simplicity and directness. I could not help being impressed by the mechanical nature of these lesions and by the practicability of their surgical relief (11).

Souttar was an extraordinary surgeon (12). He participated in World War I as Surgeon in Chief of a field ambulance and wrote a book on his experience, "A Surgeon in Belgium." He mentions how, at a time when things were in complete chaos in Belgium, he felt reassured when he saw the First Lord of the Admiralty, Winston Churchill quietly eating breakfast at a local hotel.

Souttar was particularly interested in physics which helped him to play a leading part in the development of radium therapy. When radium was first discovered. he travelled to Paris to meet the Curies and he may have been the first Englishman to see the new element radium. His obituary, published in Lancet in 1964, mentions that his interest may well have been further stimulated by meeting Madame Curie during his war work in Belgium (12). Souttar's interest in physics extended to construction of a private planetarium. Souttar who died at the age of eighty-eight in 1964 was evidently twenty years ahead of his time. Twenty years passed before Charles P. Bailey of Philadelphia, using Souttar's atrial approach, divided the mitral valve at the fused commissures under digital control, a procedure which he called "commissurotomy (13; Fig. 5)."

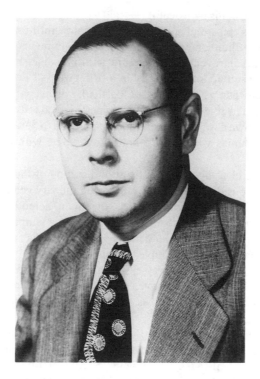

Figure 5. Charles Bailey (*Courtesy of The New York Academy of Medicine*)

In 1948, Horace G. Smithy from Charleston, South Carolina had attempted a surgical approach to aortic stenosis with an aortic valvulotome (14,15,16,17). His failure to successfully treat this condition was particularly tragic since Smithy himself succumbed to this disease. In 1950, Smithy persuaded Alfred Blalock, from the Johns Hopkins Hospital, to operate on him using his method. Smithy's method consisted of division of one or more valvular leaflets by approaching the valve through the wall of the left ventricle, using a valvulotome. Like most other attempts with valvulotomes, this one also failed. Smithy described the operative results in seven patients with a high mortality (16). In one of the patients the aortic valve apparently had not been cut at all.

In most of his papers, Smithy was concerned with the frequency of arrhythmias which occurred in these patients during the operation (15). This also was the cause of his own death! He tried various means to overcome this difficulty, such as epicardial application of procaine, infiltration of procaine beneath the epicardium and into the myocardium, intravenous procaine, or infiltration of the intraventricular septum with procaine. He also administered quinidine sulfate intravenously in a fifth group of experimental animals. These procedures were not of particular value when it came to operation on aortic valves with markedly hypertrophied left ventricles. As it happened in his own case, a transventricular approach to the aortic valve created fatal arrhythmias which could not be overcome with antiarrhythmic compounds.

It had become clear by that time that blind cutting of the cardiac valves carries with it a considerable mortality. Since pulmonary venous congestion and pulmonary artery hypertension are the main hemodynamic consequences of mitral stenosis, it seemed appropriate to attempt to decompress pulmonary veins by creating a shunt between these vessels and the low pressure venous circulation, for example, the superior vena cava or the azygos vein. The first such operation was experimentally performed on dogs by Henry Swan in 1948 (18). He proved that in dogs the shunt is technically feasible if an end to end anastomosis of the azygos and pulmonary veins is carried out using a vitallium tube.

R.H. Sweet, working with E.F. Bland, carried the shunt idea further by constructing an anastomosis between the dorsal segment branch of the right inferior pulmonary vein to the azygos vein (19,20). The first report described the results in five patients (19). Considerable improvement in the first three patients was noted. The authors admit that this operation is "a compromise and not a cure." In another report, in 1949 Sweet and Bland presented their findings to the American Surgical Association (20). The report published in the Journal of Thoracic Surgery contains an interesting discussion by Blalock. He also mentioned the possibility of creating a shunt between left atrium and ventricle thus bypassing the stenotic mitral valve using a vein graft. Another suggestion made was the creation of an intraatrial defect already accomplished by him and Hanlon several years before.

John H. Gibbon's pioneering work was the breakthrough in cardiac surgery that made blind approaches to the cardiac valves obsolete. Gibbon wrote a paper with J.Y. Templeton in 1944 (21) concerned with the future when "eventually a practical method of oxygenating large quantities of blood outside the body will permit operation in the open human heart." He undertook experiments to determine whether grafted tissue could be used to replace a portion of the cardiac valve. A cusp of the tricuspid valve of dogs was replaced by grafts of vein or pericardium sutured in position. The results were good, seven of the dogs survived in apparent good health. Several years later, in 1950, Murray, from Toronto, transplanted an aortic-valve segment as replacement of a diseased aortic valve with good results (22).

In the late 1940s, considerable progress was made toward the treatment of cardiac valvular disease by C.P. Bailey and Dwight E. Harken. These improvements made prior to the introduction of cardiopulmonary bypass, remained limited in scope.

In 1949, Bailey presented his procedure of surgical treatment of mitral stenosis before the American College of Chest Physicians (23). After briefly referring to the success of manual dilatation of the valve reported by Souttar, Bailey presented his conclusions on the surgical treatment of mitral stenosis: approach through the left atrial appendage is the most satisfactory with less chance of arrhythmias, greater ease of entering the valve, and greater ease of controlling hemorrhage; extensive cutting of the anterior cusp of the mitral valve is dangerous since it results in the production of mitral insufficiency which is poorly tolerated; the accurate placement of an instrument to divide a mitral valve depends upon actually palpating the valve from within at the time of operation. A considerable variety of instruments may be employed for commissurotomy. We, so he wrote, "now prefer a backward cutting punch and a scalpel with a hooked blade." In contrast to others who had used cutting instruments, one of Bailey's approaches was to attach the commissurotomy knife to the right index finger between two layers of gloves.

Bailey presented several operative cases; some cases of mitral stenosis showed gratifying postoperative results. He concluded that the operation of commissurotomy has great value in certain cases of mitral stenosis. Later in 1954, Bailey and co-workers presented procedures for the treatment of mitral insufficiency by grafting pericardial tissue to the valve orifice (24).

Bailey also tackled the problem of surgical treatment of aortic insufficiency and aortic stenosis. He quoted two papers of Hufnagel in his bibliography. Following the example of Hufnagel, Bailey's paper also describes a valvular prosthesis which was made of nylon and silicon rubber. Bailey concluded that the rather remarkable immediate improvement obtained in some of his patients encouraged him to feel that he was at least on the right course. Perhaps, he wrote, it will soon be possible to add aortic insufficiency to the growing list of cardiac lesions readily responsive to surgical intervention.

Concerning the treatment of aortic stenosis, Bailey mentioned that his interest in this disease was aroused by a discussion he had with Smithy in June 1958. Bailey applied the principle of commissurotomy which he had successfully used in the treatment of mitral stenosis to the problem confronting him in aortic stenosis (25). He wrote that it is occasionally necessary to bend or redirect a guidewire inserted through a valve. Initially, the actual mortality

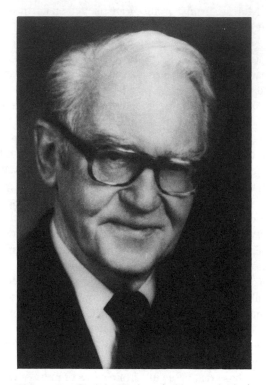

Figure 6.   Dwight Harken (*with permission*)

rate was high. There was no further mortality in nine patients, using the new instrument. Six of these patients were subjected to simultaneous commissurotomy procedures for coexisting mitral stenosis.

In 1948, Harken and his group published a report in which they described their approach to the surgery of mitral stenosis by a procedure which they called "valvuloplasty" (26; Fig. 6). The main principles were: access of the mitral valve should be from the atrial side; surgical enlargement of the stenotic orifice should be planned so that there is minimal burden from the associated regurgitation and maximum restoration of valvular function by "valvuloplasty" and, undue acceleration of the heart rate should be prevented.

Harken and Black expanded on this theme in 1955 (27). They wrote that a technique now available assures complete separation of the commissures out to the annulus, together with mobilized valve leaflet by freeing restricting fused chordae and papillary muscles. Harken did not shy away from using the finger alone, if a fracture of the valve could easily be obtained (28).

Harken and co-workers also addressed the problem of mitral and aortic insufficiency. For the treatment of mitral insufficiency, they used a lucite prosthesis in the shape of bottle to be inserted into the orifice of an incompetent valve (29). Twenty-four terminal patients with proven mitral insufficiency were operated using this procedure, with seven post operative and seven late deaths. The high mortality was explained to be correlated with inconsistency of the position of the baffle. Harken believed he could overcome this mortality using a spindle baffle by anchoring both ends of the baffle.

For the treatment of aortic insufficiency, Harken and his group used a circumcluding suture to reduce the aortic valve area (30). Of eleven patients, five survived and were improved. Later, after the introduction of cardiopulmonary bypass, Harken and co-workers used as a prosthesis a caged ball valve (31). By that time the breakthrough perfection of cardio-pulmonary bypass had been made.

The new era of cardiac valvular surgery dawned with the introduction of cardio-pulmonary bypass by Gibbons, followed by the work of C. Walton Lillehei and others. The first patient operated on by Gibbons had an atrial septal defect. Lillehei used cardiopulmonary bypass for the operation on aortic stenosis (1956), and on mitral stenosis (1958) (32).

With the introduction of cardio-pulmonary bypass, the aspects of valvular surgery changed. New issues arose, for example whether to produce cardiac arrest, or to retroperfuse the coronary sinus, or initiate hypothermia to avoid global myocardial ischemia, or utilize techniques of reconstructing diseased valves, or replace diseased valves with prosthesis.

Lillehei and co-workers pioneered in the field using a simple heart lung machine for cardio-pulmonary bypass (Fig.7) (*See Chapter 3*). They operated on patients with aortic and mitral stenosis and aortic and mitral insufficiency. A particularly difficult problem was the initiation and maintenance of cardiac arrest. Lillihei used both potassium chloride and acetylcholine; acetylcholine was finally preferred. For the treatment of mitral insufficiency, they used what they called annuloplasty, consisting in part of selective suturing of the annulus fibrosus to reduce its circumference, reminiscent of the efforts of Bailey and of Harken. Direct vision of the valve rendered cutting by valvulotomes unnecessary. Lillehei attempted aortic valve replacement in aortic insufficiency with a prosthesis. As he wrote, "clearly the abnormal leaflet had to be replaced by a space-occupying prosthesis, which would provide sufficient substance." The procedures consisted of a compressed polyvinyl plastic sponge (ivalon) together with one annuloplasty stitch.

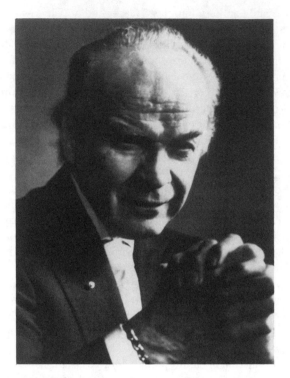

Figure 7. C. Walton Lillehei (*Courtesy of The New York Academy of Medicine*)

A major step forward was the introduction of a prosthetic valve by Charles Hufnagel in 1952. He performed the first implantation of an artificial heart valve in a patient with severe aortic regurgitation. The prosthesis was a caged-ball valve implanted in the descending aorta, thus preventing some regurgitation. Hufnagel (1914 to 1989) was a remarkably inventive surgeon. The son of a physician surgeon, he graduated from Harvard with the M.D.degree in 1941 and received his surgical training at the Peter Bent Brigham Hospital and a year at Children's Hospital under Robert Gross. He participated with Gross in the early pioneering work on coarctation of the aorta.

In 1944, Hufnagel was appointed director of the surgical research laboratory at Harvard where his investigation of vascular replacement with plastic material originated. Another pioneering venture in which he participated was the first kidney transplant in 1947 by David Hume. He assisted in this epochal operation at the Brigham Hospital (33). Hufnagel thus participated in and witnessed two truly history making events: the surgical treatment of coarctation of the aorta and the first human kidney transplant; the latter work resulted in a Nobel Prize more than forty years later.

In 1950, Hufnagel was appointed Professor of Experimental Surgery at Georgetown University where he became associated with cardiologist Proctor Harvey who furnished clinical expertise to the team. The first insertion of a valve in the descending aorta was carried out on a thirty year old patient with advanced aortic regurgitation. She recovered promptly after the operation and returned to an active life. An unfortunate byproduct of plastic ball valve was a disturbing click, particularly when the patient opened her mouth. This was soon controlled by altering the composition of the valve. In addition, Hufnagel anchored the prosthesis in the aorta by use of multiple perforations, eliminating the use of sutures. The procedure could be carried out at that time because it did not necessitate use of a cardiopulmonary bypass. The valve was further modified, eventually leading to a tri-leaflet type and later to a disc valve. Hufnagel implanted the valve in more than two hundred individuals. The valve, on display at the Smithsonian Institute, is part of an exhibit on the development of heart surgery.

Hufnagel also followed Alexis Carrel's example by developing methods of preserving arterial grafts by freezing and use of orlon prosthesis. It is not surprising that he had a particular interest in cataloging and editing papers by Alexis Carrel which are stored in a special portion of the Georgetown library. Another vignette in the life of Hufnagel was his appointment by Judge Sirica of Watergate fame to examine former President Richard Nixon, to determine whether Nixon was medically fit to testify at the Watergate trial. (The former President was considered to be medically unfit to appear.) Hufnagel died of heart disease and renal failure, two of the areas of his main research interest.

The caged ball concept was later developed by Harken and Birtwell. This resulted in the first clinically used caged ball valve on March 10, 1960, and the second on June 6, 1960. The first patient, Mary Richardson lived for 30 years finally succumbing to carcinoma of the esophagus. The second patient also survived to succumb recently to another cardiac operation for mitral valve disease. Of importance is the fact that the same dimensions that were defined in those valves for the height of the cage and for the ratio of the ball to the annulus, set the standards in the development of subsequent caged ball valves (33).

Albert Starr, also building on the work of Hufnagel, in association with M. Lowell Edwards (an engineer) developed the Starr/Edwards prosthetic cardiac valves that are, even today, the "gold standard" of valve prostheses.

Starr later became the Chairman of the Division of Thoracic Surgery at the University of Oregon, organized and performed the necessary research and practical applications of these valves. In 1960, Starr published his mitral valve replacement experiments in animals, and one year later reported his clinical work in patients (34). It is remarkable that he was successful since the canine is prone to hypercoagulation. Starr tried many replacement variations and decided that the model using a ball valve was the best. He developed the technique of valve replacement and fixation in the heart; he recognized the problem of thrombosis. "Thrombosis is a major problem; it first appears at the zone of fixation to the mitral annulus and extends over the valve ring despite changes in the materials used and despite anticoagulant drugs. This always interferes with leaflet function but is less likely to interfere with a ball valve (34)."

Albert Starr's clinical success with mitral valve replacement was remarkable. "While early satisfactory results were obtained in some patients, survival beyond three months has not been reported to now (35)." He reported twelve cases with one operative and three late deaths due to infection.

During the last three decades, numerous prosthetic heart valves were developed, used and discarded. With them vanished the hope for an easy solution. The Starr-Edwards silastic ball valve has proven to be the most durable. Pyrolitic carbon disc valves are most often chosen by surgeons today as a mechanical valve for valve replacement. Currently, the St. Jude Medical bi-leaflet valve is the most frequently implanted mechanical valve in the United States. Other currently available mechanical valves are the Medtronic-Hall, the Omniscience, the monostrut Bjork-Shiley, and the bi-leaflet Carbomedics (the latter two were not yet available in the United States at time of publication).

Of the well-known late complications of mechanical valve implantation, perhaps the convexo-concave 70° tilt valve of Bjork-Shiley was associated with the most dramatic events. It was developed in 1976 (36) with a larger opening angle to 70° as a means of reducing the transvalvular gradient. The high incidence of devastating late strut fractures caused it be withdrawn from the market. Since then the Bjork-Shiley monostrut valve has been developed. By 1989 there were more than 53,000 such implants world-wide without a single mechanical complication (37). All the other advantages of such a valve have been retained.

Aortic valve replacement with antibiotic sterilized aortic valve homografts was described by Donald Ross from England in 1962 (38), and Sir Brian Barrat-Boyes from New Zealand in 1964 (39). Raymond Heimbecker of Canada had previously reported the replacement of the mitral valve by an antibiotic sterilized aortic valve homograft (40). Some enthusiasm for this procedure was generated after these reports, but it became popular in only a few centers around the world. With the development of cryopreservation for aortic valve homografts and the encouraging report from Mark O'Brien from Australia (41) however, interest in this operation grew to such a degree that an adequate supply of homografts became the limiting factor in its increased usage. Cryopreservation keeps the aortic valve fibroblasts viable but it is still not known whether they remain alive after implantation.

Glutaraldehyde-preserved porcine aortic bioprostheses were introduced in the late 1960's by Alain Carpentier from France. Henry Hancock made them commercially available in 1970. This type of bioprosthesis has been extensively used for replacement of the aortic, mitral, and tricuspid valve. Thromboembolism is uncommon with this type of bioprosthesis (42). The main problem with this valve is tissue degeneration; at the end of ten years, 20 to 25 percent of patients required reoperation because of structural failure (42). A larger percentage of valves are probably already calcified at ten years. Tissue degeneration occurs very rapidly in children and slowly in elderly patients. Mechanical stress plays an important role in the degeneration of tissue valves. It has been shown that the durability of the aortic valve homograft is significantly shortened when it is mounted in an artificial stent before being implanted in a patient (43). Based on this clinical observation and other experimental information, Tirone David from Canada postulated that the aortic root was the best stent for aortic valve leaflets, a concept that formed the basis of the development of his stentless glutaraldehyde preserved porcine aortic valve replacement (44).

The anatomy and function of the mitral valve and of the left ventricle are interrelated. Interactions between these two structures are complex and not yet entirely understood. The attachments between the mitral annulus and the ventricular wall are important for left ventricular geometry and function. Lillehei and colleagues were the first to point out the importance of preserving the chordae tendineae during mitral valve replacement (45). This method of mitral valve replacement did not become popular until David and associates published their data on the importance of the mitral apparatus in left ventricular function (46,47). Understanding of the interactions between the mitral valve and the left ventricle has been greatly improved by the work of Craig Miller from Stanford University (48). Miller and his group established the fact that the papillary muscles with their chordae tendineae not only prevent leaflet prolapse and mitral regurgitation during systole, but also serve as a working structural element of the contractile ventricle to enhance left ventricular systolic pump performance.

Carpentier's contributions in reconstructive procedures of the mitral valve have been considerable (49). Carpentier made mitral valve repair a logical and reproducible operation. Mitral valve reconstruction has been particularly successful in patients with mitral incompetence due to degenerative disease of the mitral valve. Patients with pure mitral stenosis due to rheumatic heart disease may have their valves repaired surgically or by percutaneous balloon valvuloplasty. Intraoperative Doppler echocardiography has allowed surgeons to assess the mitral valve after repair in the operating room.

Reconstruction of the aortic valve is possible in only a small percentage of patients who need aortic valve surgery. The senile calcific aortic stenosis in the older population can sometimes be successfully debrided and the results are excellent in properly selected patients. Reconstruction of the incompetent aortic valve is also possible, particularly when the leaflets are normal and distortion of the aortic sinuses is the cause of valve dysfunction. Aortic valve repair is not as easily reproducible as mitral valve repair and should be judiciously performed.

Until the perfect artificial heart valve is created, the diseased native valve should be repaired—but only as long as the results are better than with valve replacement!

The decade of the 1980's was a time of further consolidation and maturation of devices and techniques. Heart transplantation under cyclosporin has been a very worthwhile answer in advanced multivalvular disease with associated myocardial damage. Many centers, including Stanford, Pittsburgh, London (Canada), report a five year survival rate of over 80 percent with a return to a normal way of life (50,51).

A new development has been the introduction of valvuloplasty. The classical paper by Charles T. Dotter and Melvin P. Judkins was published in 1964. In their original work, the authors did not use balloon equipped catheters but successfully dilated atherosclerotic obstructive lesions of the femoral and popliteal arteries using catheters of increasing diameter, the largest about .2 inches (outer diameter). A spring catheter guide was first inserted.

Dotter and Judkins were able to successfully treat six of eleven patients with marked occlusion of the femoral artery. In all their patients amputation had been the only remaining option. They wrote "we are satisfied that percutaneous transluminal recanalization is the treatment of choice for many lesions of the femoral and popliteal arteries ... no doubt the interest and ingenuity of others will lead to refinements of technique as well as the clarification of the role of this attack on arteriosclerotic obstruction" (52). They answered the criticism of some surgeons that coexistent disease in distal branches may defeat the purpose of the procedure by stating that "even a

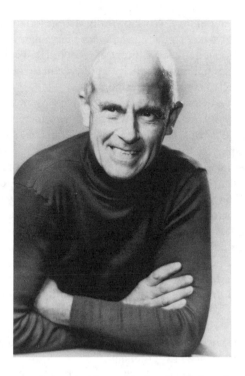

Figure 8. Charles Dotter (*with permission the University of Oregon, Portland OR*)

rusty sprinkler may prove capable of doing a creditable job once the faucet is fully opened."

This pioneering venture lead to the development of a new technical specialty for nonoperative treatment of obstructive vascular disease including coronary disease. In European countries the procedure of transluminal recanalization of an artery is often referred to as "Dotterize".

Charles Dotter (1920-1985) was a true pioneer in the field of the use of balloon equipped catheter to dilate vascular obstructive lesions (Figure 8). Other procedures also originated from his fertile mind, among them the technique for percutaneous catheterization which was introduced in 1958, and the use of guide wires which he developed jointly with Bill Cook and the safety J-tipped guide wire (52). Dotter also first described a flow-guided catheter, an overlooked predecessor of the Swan-Ganz catheter, and a transvascular catheter biopsy. Working with Melvin Judkins, Dotter helped to develop today's standard techniques for coronary angiography. Like Mason Sones, Charles Dotter used a direct approach. He went straight to the heart of a problem, applying simplicity and directness. Neither Sones nor Dotter could be called sophisticated scientists.

Balloon mitral valvoplasty has been attempted by many authors (53). Transluminal dilatation for example, was of primary interest to many urologists. The first use of a balloon catheter was by Guthrie in 1834 when a catgut balloon was employed to dilate the urethra (54). It is interesting that Gruentzig in 1974 used a similar instrument. Abele was one of the first to define the theoretical basis underlying balloon dilatation, by defining "dilating force" and basing it on the law of LaPlace (55). This law defined the extension of a balloon to stretch and separation at its circumference when inside pressure was applied. Identical pressures will produce more force in larger balloons than in smaller ones. For identical pressures, the dilating force is proportional to the radius. Abele related the dilating force to the balloon pressure, stenosis size, degree of stenosis, material used, and to balloon length. Finally, he related burst pressure to the inflation time. Abele's conclusion based on Poiseuille's Law was that in a tight stenosis, a very small difference in size can make a very large difference in flow. He suggested that it is preferable to dilate to the physiological requirement under conditions of reactive or pharmacologically induced hyperemia.

Following Dotter's original publication in 1964 it took more than fifteen years to apply his principle to various stenosed vascular beds. Tegtmeyer applied balloon dilatation to the renal artery (56), Gruentzig to the coronary artery (57), Lock to the pulmonary arteries (58) and to coarctation of the aorta (59). Kan used percutaneous transluminal dilatation for congenital pulmonary stenosis (60). McKay and Palacios used this method in the treatment of calcified mitral stenosis (61,62). McKay also treated calcific aortic stenosis with this technique (63). Lababidi (64) and Cribier (65) applied it to the stenosed aortic valve. The first percutaneous balloon valvulotomy of a stenosed triscupid valve was reported by Zaibag (66). For mitral valve surgery J.E. Lock (67) used the antegrade transeptal approach while U.U. Babic et al. (53) used a long guide wire transversing the vascular system from femoral vein to femoral artery to control the position of the balloon catheter advanced retrogradely across the mitral valve. In 1990, C. Stefanadis et al. reported success in 10 adult patients (68). All patients had a significant reduction in valve gradient together with an increase in valve area and were without serious complications. This encouraging report must be judged against the fact that many mitral commissures are heavily scarred and can be very difficult to split even under direct vision and even with a very foreceful surgical transventricular dilator. Obviously careful selection of cases is of paramount importance. Fatal ventricular perforation is the most feared of the many complications of the procedure (69).

Pulmonary valve stenosis is another area in which there has been considerable success beginning with Serub et al. in 1979 and further developed by Kan in 1982. The field has since grown with a low morbidity and mortality so that some centers now report that 10 percent of all catheterizations are for the correction of pulmonary stenosis (70).

Aortic stenosis has been similarily managed in pediatric group cases beginning with Lababidi in 1983. S. Perry et al. report (71) 111 balloon valvotomies for congenital aortic stenosis ranging from one day to 39 years of age. In neonates it is considered an urgent palliative procedure, with a mortality of six in 16. In the 93 other patients, the majority achieved a 60% increase in valve area, only a minority developed severe regurgitation which required open heart surgery.

REFERENCES

1. Brunton, Sir Lauder: Preliminary note on the possibility of treating mitral stenosis by surgical methods. Lancet, I:352, 1902.
1a. Murrell, W. Nitroglycerine as a remedy for angina pectoris. Lancet I:80,113, 151, 225, 1879.
2. Cushing, Harvey and J.R. Branch. Experimental and clinical notes on chronic valvular lesions in the dog and their possible relation to a future surgery of the cardiac valves. J. Med. Res 17:471–486, 1908.
3. Bernheim, B. Experimental surgery of the mitral valve. Johns Hopkins Hosp. Bull., 20:107–110, 1909.
4. Tuffier, T. and A. Carrel. Patching and section of the pulmonary orifice of the heart. J. Exp. Med. 20:3–8, 1914.
5. Tuffier, T., Etat actuel de la chirurgie intrathoracique. Trans. XVII Int. Cong. Med., Section VII:316–317, London 1913.
6. Lindblom, D., Heredity and mortality after heart valve replacement. Carolinska Medico Chiruska Instituted, Stockholm, 1987.
7. Allen, D., and E. Graham. Intracardiac surgery - A new method. J. Am. Med. Assoc., 79:1028–1030, 1922.
8. Cutler, E. and S. A. Levine. Cardiotomy and valvulotomy for mitral stenosis. Experimental observations and clinical notes concerning an operated case with recovery. Boston Med. Surg. J. 188:1023–1027, 1923.
9. Cutler, E. and C. Beck. The present status of the surgical procedures in chronic valvular disease of the heart. Arch. Surg., 18:403–416, 1929.
10. Beck, C.S. and E. Cutler E. A cardiovalvulotome. Jour. Exp. Med., 40:375–379, 1924.

11. Souttar, H.S. The surgical treatment of mitral stenosis. Br. Med. Jour. 2:603-606, 1925.
12. Greenwood, J. Obituary Notices. Br. Med. J. 2:1335–1336, 1964.
13. Bailey, C.P. The surgical treatment of mitral stenosis (mitral commissurotomy). Diseases of the Chest. 15(4):377–397, 1949.
14. Smithy, H.G., H.R. Pratt-Thomas and H.P. Deyerle. Aortic valvulotomy experimental methods and early results. Sur. Gynecol. Obstet. 86:513–523, 1948.
15. Smithy, H.G. The control of arrhythmias occurring during operation upon the valves of the heart: experimental and clinical observations. The Southern Surgeon. 14:611–618, 1948.
16. Smithy, H.G., J.A. Boone and J.M. Stallworth. Surgical treatment of constrictive valvular disease of the heart. Sur. Gynecol. Obstet.
17. Smithy, H.G. and E.F. Parker. Experimental aortic valvulotomy. Sur. Gynecol. Obstet. 84:625–628, 1947.
18. Swan, H. Mitral stenosis: an experimental study of pulmonary-azygos venous anastomosis. Am. Heart. J. 367–375, 1948.
19. Bland, E.F. and R.H. Sweet. A venous shunt for advanced mitral stenosis. J. Am. Med. Assoc. 140:1259–1265, 1949.
20. Sweet, R.H. and E.F. Bland. The surgical relief of congestion in the pulmonary circulation in cases of severe mitral stenosis. Ann. Surg. 130:384–397, 1949.
21. Templeton, J.Y., III and J.H. Gibbon, Jr. Experimental reconstruction of cardiac valves by venous and pericardial grafts. Ann. Surg. 129:161–176, 1949.
22. Murray, G. Homologous aortic valve segment transplants as surgical treatment for aortic and mitral insufficiency. Angiology 7:466–471, 1956.
23. Bailey, C.P. and Likoff, W. The surgical treatment of aortic insufficiency. Ann Int. Med., 42:388–416, 1955.
24. Bailey, C.P. W.L. Jamison, A.E. Bakst, H.E. Bolton, H.T. Nichols and W. Gemeinhardt. The surgical correction of mitral insufficiency by the use of pericardial grafts. J. Thor. Surg. 28:551–603, 1954.
25. Bailey, C.P., R. Ramirez and H.B. Larzelere. Surgical treatment of aortic stenosis. J. Am. Med. Assoc. 150:1647–1652, 1952.
26. Harken, D.E., L.B. Ellis, P.F. Ware and L.R. Notman. The surgical treatment of mitral stenosis. I. Valvuloplasty. N. England J. Med., 239:801–809, 1948.
27. Harken D.E. and H. Black. Improved valvuloplasty for mitral stenosis. N. Engl. J. Med., 253:669–678, 1955.
28. Ellis, L.B. and D.E. Harken. Closed valvuloplasty for mitral stenosis. N. Engl. J. Med., 270:643–650, 1964.
29. Harken, D.E., H. Black, L.B. Ellis and L. Dexter. The surgical correction of mitral insufficiency. J. Thor. Surg. 28:604–627, 1954.
30. Taylor, W.J., W.B. Thrower, H. Black and D.E. Harken. The surgical correction of insufficiency by circumclusion. J. Thor. Surg. 35:192–205, 1958.
31. Harken, D.E. H.S. Soroff, W.J. Taylor, A.A. Lefemine, S.K. Gupta and S. Lunzer. Partial and complete prostheses in aortic insufficiency. J. Thor. Cardiovasc. Surg., 40:744–762, 1960.
32. Lillehei, C. W., V. L. Gott, R. A. DeWall, and R. L. Varco. The surgical treatment of stenotic or regurgitant lesions of the mitral and aortic valves by direct vision utilizing a pump-oxygenator. J. Thor. Surg., 35:154–190, 1958.

33. Hufnagel, C.A. Basic concepts of cardiac and vascular reconstruction. Georgetown Med Bull 14:88–96, 1988.
34. Starr, A. Total mitral valve replacement: fixation and thrombosis. Surg. Forum, 11:258–260, 1960.
35. Starr, A. and M.L. Edwards. Mitral replacement: clinical experience with a ball-valve prosthesis. Ann. Surg., 154:725–740, 1961.
36. Björk, V.O. The improved Bjork-Shiley tilting disc valve prosthesis. Scand. J. Thorac. Cardiovasc. Surg., 12:81–84, 1978.
37. Björk, V.O. Development of mechanical heart valves: Past, present and future. Can J. Cardiol., 5:64–73, 1989.
38. Ross, D.N. Homograft replacement of the aortic valve. Lancet, II:487, 1962.
39. Barrat-Boyes, B.G. Homograft aortic valve replacement in incompetence and stenosis. Thorax, 19:131–150, 1964.
40. Heimbecker, R.O., R.J. Baird, T.Z. Lajos, A.T. Varga, and W.F. Greenwood. Homograft replacement of the human mitral valve. Can. Med. Assoc. J., 86:805–809, 1962.
41. O'Brien, M.F., E.G. Stafford, M.A.H. Gardner, P.G. Pohlner, and D.C. McGiffin. A comparison of aortic valve replacement with viable cryopreserved and fresh allograft valves, with a note on chromosomal studies. J. Thorac. Cardiovasc. Surg., 94:812–823, 1987.
42. Magilligan, D.J., M.W. Lewis, P. Stein, and M. Alam. The porcine bioprosthetic heart valve: experience at 15 years. Ann. Thorac. Surg., 48:324–330, 1989.
43. Angell, W.W., J.H. Oury, J.J. Lamberti, and J. Koziol. Durability of the viable aortic allograft. J. Thorac. Cardiovasc. Surg., 98:48–56, 1989.
44. David, T.E., C. Pollick, and J. Bos. Aortic valve replacement with stentless porcine aortic bioprosthesis. J. Thorac. Surg., 99:113–118, 1990.
45. Lillehei, C.W., M.J. Levy, and R.C. Bonnabeau. Mitral valve replacement with preservation of papillary muscles and chordae tendineae. J. Thorac. Cardiovasc. Surg., 47:532–543, 1964.
46. David, T.E., D.H. Strauss, E. Mesher, M.J. Anderson, J.L. MacDonald, and A.J. Buda. Is it important to preserve the chordae tendineae and the papillary muscles during mitral valve replacement? Can. J. Surg., 24:236–239, 1981.
47. David, T.E., D.E. Uden, and H.D. Strauss. The importance of the mitral apparatus in left ventricular function after correction of mitral regurgitation. Circulation, 68 (Suppl. II):II76–II82, 1983.
48. Sarris, G.E., J.I. Fann, M.A. Niczyporuk, G.C. Derby, C.E. Handen, and D.C Miller. Global and regional left ventricular systolic performance in the in situ ejecting canine heart. Importance of the mitral apparatus. Circulation, 80 (Supp. I):I24–I42, 1989.
49. Carpentier, A. Cardiac valve surgery: the "French Connection". J. Thorac. Cardiovasc. Surg. 86:323–337, 1983.
50. Devineni, R., R.N. McKenzie, W.J. Kostuk, and R.O. Heimbecker, et al. Cyclosporine in cardiac transplantation: Observations on immunological monitoring, cardiac histology and cardiac function. Heart Transplantation, Vol. 11, 3–219, May 1983.
51. Heimbecker, R.O., McKenzie, N., C. Stiller, W.J. Kostuk, and M.D. Silver. Heart and Lung Transplantation. Heart & Lung: J. of Critical Care, 13:11–4, 1984.

52. Riosch, J., Abrams, H.L. and Cook, W. Charles Theodore Dotter Memorials Am. J. Roentgenol. 144:1321–1323, 1985.
53. Babic, U.U., P. Pejcic, and Z. Djurisic, et al. Percutaneous transarterial balloon valvuloplasty for mitral valve stenosis. Am. J. Cardiol., 57:1101–1104, 1986.
54. Guthrie, G.J. On the anatomy and diseases of the neck of the bladder and the urethra. London: Burgess and Hill, 1834.
55. Abele, J.E. Balloon catheters and transluminal dilatation: technical considerations. Am. J. Roentgenol., 135:901–906, 1980.
56. Tegtmeyer, C.J., R. Dyer, C.D. Teates, R.M. Carey, H.A. Wellons, L.W. Stanton. Percutaneous transluminal dilatation of the renal arteries: techniques and results. Radiology, 135:589–599, 1980.
57. Gruentzig A.R., A. Senning, W.E. Siegenthaler. Nonoperative dilatation of coronary artery stenosis: percutaneous transluminal angioplasty. N. Engl J. Med, 301:61–68, 1979.
58. Lock, J.E., W.R. Castaneda-Zuniga, B.P. Fuhrman, J.L. Bass. Balloon dilatation angioplasty of hypoplastic and stenotic pulmonary arteries. Circulation, 67:962–967, 1983.
59. Lock J.E., T. Niemi, B.A. Burke, S. Einzig, W.R. Castaneda-Zuniga. Transcutaneous angioplasty of experimental aortic coarctation. Circulation 66:1280–1285, 1982.
60. Kan JS, R.I. White, S.E. Mitchell, T.J. Gardner. Percutaneous balloon valvuloplasty: a new method for treating congenital pulmonary artery stenosis. N Engl J Med, 307:540–542, 1982.
61. McKay RG, J.E. Lock, J.F. Keane, R.D. Safian, J.M. Aroesty. Percutaneous mitral valvuloplasty in an adult patient with calcific rheumatic mitral stenosis. J Am Coll Cardiol 7:1410–1415, 1986.
62. Palacios I.F., J.E. Lock, J.F. Keane, P.C. Block. Percutaneous tranvenous balloon valvotomy in a patient with severe calcific mitral stenosis. J Am Coll Cardiol 7:1416, 1986.
63. McKay R.G, R.D. Safian, J.E. Locke, V.S. Mandell, R.L. Thurer, S.J. Schnitt and W. Grossman. Ballon dilatation of calcific aortic stenosis in elderly patients: postmortem, intraoperative, and percutaneous valvuloplast studies. Circulation 74:119–124, 1986.
64. Lababidi Z, W. Jiunn-Ren, J.T. Walls. Percutaneous balloon aortic valvuloplasty; results in 23 patients. Am J. Cardiol, 53:194–197, 1984.
65. Cribier A, T. Savin, N. Sauudi, P. Rocha, J. Berland and B. Letac. Percutaneous transluminal valvuloplasty of acquired aortic stenosis in elderly patients: an alternative to valve replacement? Lancet, 1:63–67, 1986.
66. Zaibag A.L., M.. Ribeiro, S.A. Al-Kasab. Percutaneous balloon valvotomy in triscupid stenosis. Br. Hrt. J. 57:51–53, 1987.
67. Lock, J.E., M. Khalilullah, S. Shrivastavca and J.F. Keane. Percutaneous catheter commissurotomy in rheumatic mitral stenosis. N. Eng. J. Med., 313:1515–1518, 1985.
68. Stefanadis, C., C. Kourouklis, C. Stratos, C. Pitsavos, C. Tentolouris, and P. Toutouzas. Percutaneous balloon mitral valvuloplasty by retrograde left atrial catheterization. Am. J. Cardiol., 65:650–654, 1990.
69. Butany, J., G. D'Amati, D. Charlesworth, L. Schwartz, L. Daniel, A. Adelmen,

and M. Silver. Fatal left ventricular perforation following balloon mitral valvuloplasty. Can. J. Cardiol. 6:343–347, 1990.

70. Beekman, R.H., A.P. Rocchini, and A. Rosenthal. Therapeutic cardiac
catheterization for pulmonary valve and pulmonary artery stenosis. Cardiology
Clinics, 7:331–340, May 1989.

71. Perry, S.B., B. Zeevi, J.F. Keane, and J.E. Lock. Interventional catheterization of
left heart lesions, including aortic and mitral valve stenosis and coarctation of the
aorta. Cardiol. Clin., 7:341–347, 1989.

Chapter 12

Electrophysiology, Electrocardiography, Cardiopulmonary Resuscitation

H. HELLERSTEIN

Chance has played an important role in the development of electrophysiology as in all fields of science. Chance was particularly influential in Galvani's discovery of bioelectricity.

Electricity had become the popular topic of the day for hypotheses and speculation when Luigi Galvani (1737–1798) performed the first of his classic experiments. Galvani's career was a mixture of triumph and frustration (1). His initial great discoveries were followed by years of tumultuous controversy during which he strove in vain to uphold a mistaken hypothesis. Born in Bologna in September 1737, he became a doctor and soon after married the daughter of Professor Galeazzi. He had great success in comparative anatomy, made 90 dissections of birds, and published an article on the urinary apparatus of birds... (1). Appointed a lecturer at the University of Bologna at the age of 25 (1762), he was later appointed Professor of Anatomy.

Interest in electrical phenomena was based on knowledge derived from four sources: the electric ray or torpedo fish, rubbed amber, the lodestone and terrestrial lightning (2–5a). The interrelationships between these four sources were established over a total period of nearly 200 years. One of the sciences created out of this conjunction was electrophysiology.

Interest in animal electricity was widespread in the early part of the 18th Century; electricity and electrical experiments were the fashion of the day. The numbing power of the torpedo fish had begun to arouse the interest of experimenters at the end of the 17th Century. Bancroft in 1676 suggested that the active discharge of the torpedo fish might be electrical in origin. Almost 100 years later, John Walsh reported that the shock of the torpedoes was due to the release of compressed electrical fluid. At the same time, John Hunter confirmed Walsh's anatomic and physiologic findings. Catastrophic effects on animals tissues of powerful electrical discharges from electric machines (friction) and Leyden jars (condensers) had been noted. The uses of electricity were manifold, for example, to kill small animals, to shock large numbers of persons connected to one another by wire, etc. In one notable case, lightning was lethal to Professor Richmann in St. Petersburg, Russia, when he repeated Benjamin Franklin's famous kite experiment, unfortunately, with an improperly insulated rod. In 1756, Leopoldo Caldani, a former student of Morgagni, demonstrated excitation of an isolated nerve and muscle by discharge from a Leyden jar. Luigi Galvani was a student of Caldani at that time.

Electricity had also become fascinating for clinical practitioners and anatomists. Electricity was not only in the air; it was also fashionable. The identity of lightning and electricity had been established. Leyden jars, electric machines (friction machines), and other machines were the fashion in science. This vogue flourished because of the considerable number of scholars, students, and experimentalists who were receptive to new and attractive ideas. It was so prevalent that it was not unusual that an obstetrician, an eminent practitioner and Professor of Anatomy at the University of Bologna, Luigi Galvani should possess electrical machines and use them in scientific investigations. These experiments are now listed in the annals of history. The following is a quotation from Galvani, as translated by Foley in 1953 (6,7):

> The course of the work has progressed in the following way. I dissected a frog and prepared it ... Having in mind other things, I placed the frog on the same table as an electrical machine... so that the animal was completely separated from and removed at a considerable distance from the machine's conductor. When one of my assistants by chance lightly applied the point of a scalpel to the inner crural nerve of the frog, suddenly all the muscles from the limbs were seen so to contract that they appeared to have fallen into violent tonic convulsions. Another assistant observed that this phenomenon occurred when a spark was discharged from the conductor of the electrical machine... Marvelling at this, he immediately brought the unusual phenomenon to my attention when I was completely engrossed in contemplating other things. Hereupon, I became

extremely enthusiastic and eager to repeat the experiment so to clarify the ob-
scure phenomenon and make it known. I, myself, therefore, applied the point
of the scalpel first to one and then to the other crural nerve, while at the same
time some one of the assistants produced a spark. The phenomenon repeated
itself in precisely the same manner as before. Violent contractions were induced in the individual muscles of the limbs, and the prepared animal reacted
just as though it were seized with tetanus at the very moment when the sparks
were discharged.

This *fortuitous* observation of twitching of frog legs under the action of
electric current, together with an alert, communicative assistant, was the beginning of many experiments by which Galvani tried to prove the importance
of electricity in physiological phenomena (Figures 1,2). A somewhat different account of this event was presented by P. Sue in 1902 (6) as follows:

One evening, Galvani was in his laboratory doing some experiments with
some friends and with one of his nephews, Camille, of whom he was particularly fond. By chance, some skinned frogs out of which they were going to
make soup had been placed on a table where there was an electric machine: the
frogs were separated from the conductor by a certain space. One of the men
who was helping in the experiments put, by accident, the point of a scalpel
close to the internal crural nerve of one of the animals; immediately, all the
muscles of the members underwent strong convulsions. Galvani's wife was
present: she was struck with the novelty of the phenomenon; she believed that
she noticed that it coincided with the release of the electric spark. She ran to tell
her husband, who decided immediately to verify this extraordinary fact. Having as a consequence brought the point of the scalpel a second time close to the
crural nerves of the frogs while a spark from the electric machine was released,
the contractions began to take place. They could be attributed simply to the
contact of the scalpel which served as a stimulus rather than to the release of
the spark. To clarify this doubt, Galvani touched the same nerves on other
frogs while the electric machine was inactive; then, the contraction did not take
place: the experiment was repeated often and was constantly followed by the
same results. (*Doubts have been raised whether the good Luigi would have
been preparing this delicacy in the laboratory rather than in the kitchen. The
fact remains, however, that his wife was ill, and she died one year before the
publication of his manuscript.*)

Influenced by Franklin, Galvani hoped to demonstrate that lightning
flashes acted upon the limbs in an identical fashion when similar electrical
connections were made for it. The next experiment proved also to be the
source of the great Galvani-Volta controversy. One day, presumably on November 6, 1786 (or September 20, 1786 according to Garrison), being interested in testing the influence of atmospheric electricity on the muscles of
frogs, Galvani hung up a number of skinned frogs, possibly with their legs on
the balcony of a terrace of his home (iron lattice in his garden).

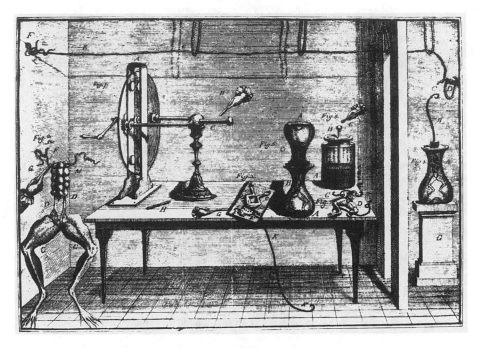

Figure 1.   Galvani's friction machine (*The Burndy Library, Norwalk, CT*)

He "hooked the hind legs to the iron of the balcony by a copper wire which passed under the lumbar (crural) nerves. Galvani noted with surprise that every time the feet touched the balcony, the frogs' limbs contracted even though at that moment there were no signs of a stormy cloud and, therefore, no particular influence of the atmosphere. At first, he thought this was due to the escape to the earth of some atmospheric electricity accumulated in the frog. Stimulation occurred when both metals (copper and iron) were in contact with some part of the body. Galvani pursued this new line of investigation with vigor and enthusiasm. He recreated the same conditions indoors. Placing the frog on an iron plate and pressing a brass hook against it produced similar muscular contractions. Other combinations of metal or even a circuit through his own body or homogenous wire, with which he made a conducting arc between nerve and muscle, had the same effects, but insulators did not."

Thus, Galvani believed that there was a cumulative electricity inside a muscle which could be discharged by the dissimilar metals and, thereby, cause electrical stimulation. The influence of vogue is shown by the comparison

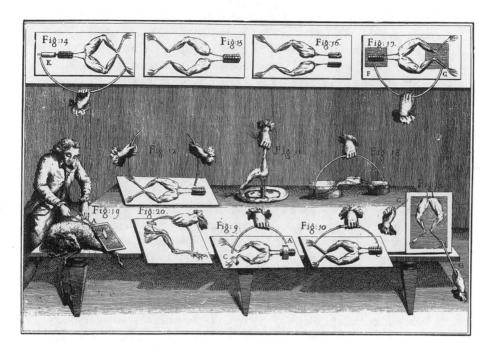

Figure 2. Galvani's experiments to show animal electricity (*The Burndy Library, Norwalk, CT*)

Galvani made between muscular contraction in frogs and other animals and the commotions produced by the discharge of a Leyden jar. Galvani's classic monograph in 1791, "De Viribus Electricitatus in Motu Musculari Commentarius" (7), was his only major communication.

Alessandro Volta (1745–1827), then Professor of Natural Philosophy at Pavia, at first accepted Galvani's own explanation and hailed these discoveries as being of epochal value, equivalent to those of Franklin. However, within a year he uncovered facts which forced him to differ from Galvani. Volta proved there was a contact between dissimilar metals which produced electricity, one of the metals being charged with positive and the other with negative electrification. These charges combined to traverse the muscle and nerve. Volta, thus, showed that the behavior of muscle described by Galvani was not caused by animal electricity but, rather, by the action of physical electricity between two different metals.

Galvani was spurred on by Volta's objections, and with further experiments he was able to produce, in 1794, contractions without metals (8). Subsequently, he studied the nature of the electrical circuits more carefully and found that some metals were less effective in the conducting arc; liquids could be used; and a single conductor was less effective than one side of two metals. Galvani was unimpressed by the importance of the bimetallic circuit because convulsions were obtained with a single conductor. He was convinced that the conducting arc was an ordinary conductor of electricity since he had earlier excluded Leyden jars, electric machines, thunderstorms, and other familiar sources of electricity as stimuli in his experiments. Since it appeared that mere metal connection of the nerve and muscle was able to produce the same contraction as the application of electrical stimulus, he assumed that the stimulus given by a nerve to a muscle was electrical.

He postulated that the electricity was prepared in the brain and distributed by the nerves; and that the principle reservoirs of this electricity are the muscles, each fiber of which may be considered as having two surfaces and therefore two types of electricity, positive and negative, each of them representing a small Leyden jar, of which the nerves are the conductors. This animal electricity entered the muscles and caused them to contract. Galvani postulated his theory of animal electricity on the basis of many meticulous experiments repeated over and over again in the next five years. His complete theory was summarized by DuBois-Reymond in a later generation (9):

(1) Animals have an electricity peculiar to themselves which is called Animal Electricity.
(2) The organs to which this Animal Electricity has the greatest affinity, and [to] which it is distributed, are the nerves, and the most important organ of its secretion is the brain.

The principal value of Galvani's work was the interest generated by the discovery of bioelectricity. It led to the proper explanation of his experiments, development of the battery, electrometers, and eventually demonstration of bioelectricity present in his preparations.

In 1797, von Humboldt demonstrated bioelectricity when he bridged the freshly cut section of a muscle and its undamaged surface with the sciatic nerve and caused contraction. Von Humboldt repeated the experiments of Galvani and of Volta and recognized that both had discovered real phenomena. After numerous experiments, he concluded that Galvani had made two genuine discoveries, viz. bimetallic and intrinsic electricity (10). Galvani had not discovered a new example of animal electricity but had "invented" a new electrical instrument and a source of electricity in motion—the bimetallic conductor of his later experiments.

The conflict between the two celebrated scientists particularly between Galvani's followers and those of Volta enriched science with a plethora of new facts. Volta's objections prompted Galvani to continue with new experiments for years. In 1794, Galvani could show contractions even without metals, with confirming experiments by von Humboldt, Matteucci, and others.

Electricity emerged as a science, from phenomena originally studied for their physiologic significance, then reinterpreted by physicists, and finally analyzed by chemists. For the next 20 years, the chemical manifestation of electricity dominated research with the work of Oersted (11) and Faraday, when the mechanical effects of current electricity, provided by the voltaic battery, attracted attention. All this was the fruit of one crucial invention of the voltaic pile, the battery to which Volta was led systematically from the first *chance* observations of Galvani. Volta, as the inventor, gave electrical experimenters a constant source of current of nonbiologic origin for the first time.

The development of batteries led also to new concepts, such as electromagnetism. With the development of more sensitive galvanometers, the electric phenomena of muscle, nerve, and other tissues including the heart could be identified and measured.

Understanding the electrophysiology of the heart was facilitated by development of the mercury capillary electrometer of Lippmann (12); its use by Waller in intact animals and man (13); the development of the string galvanometer by Ader (1897) (14); its improvement by Einthoven in 1903 (15); and its application as a diagnostic and investigative tool, etc. With the development of the practical usable galvanometer for recording electrocardiograms and with the advances in knowledge of the anatomy of the conducting system, a great outburst of work in electrocardiography developed which has continued to the present.

The chance production and observation of contraction of frog's muscle was made by Galvani, whose mind was prepared for new interpretations interrelating ancient observations of electrical phenomena to animal electricity. His chance observation catalyzed important developments in the subsequent 200 years, which have continued to the present.

MODERN ELECTROCARDIOGRAPHY

The era of the modern electrocardiogram was opened by Ader who, in 1897, invented a new type of galvanometer known as the string galvanometer. "This galvanometer works on the principle that a current generates a magnetic field acting at right angles to its course, which varies with the strength of the current and which may, thus, exert a varying attraction or repulsion

upon a second magnetic field in its vicinity.".". William Einthoven, Professor
of Physiology in the University of Leiden, and founder of modern electrocardiography, recognized the potential value of Ader's new, elegant galvanometer. Einthoven's construction of an improved and more sensitive
galvanometer superseded all others throughout the scientific world at that
time (for example the clinical polygraph, the capillary electrometer) and provided a practical tool for electrocardiography.

Einthoven recognized the vast potential importance of the electrocardiogram as a diagnostic and investigative tool.

THE HEART VECTOR AND THE FIELD: CONTRIBUTIONS OF
WALLER, EINTHOVEN AND WILSON

The fact that the heart lies within the animal body which is in essence a three
dimensional solid conductor, was known to Waller in 1889 (13) and a subject
of theoretical analysis by Einthoven. "In such a solid conductor, an electrical
field can be envisioned, and the electrical currents created by the heart can be
considered as fluctuating vectorial force subject to mathematical analysis."
(16).

The heart vector may be defined as a manifest potential difference in the
medium surrounding the heart resulting from its electrical activity. Drastic
changes have occurred in the concept and manner of measuring the magnitude and direction of this vector quantity, following Waller's original presentation in 1887 and 1889 (13,17).

The laws governing the distribution of potential differences within solid
conductors were evidently known to Waller in 1889. In that year, he presented but did not explain the basis for a schematic drawing of the trunk with
a series of isopotential lines, seen in cross section, drawn about the heart.
Waller was aware that the entire mass of ventricles did not contract simultaneously. He believed that the wave of excitation began at the apex and lasted
longer at the bases. He was convinced that the myocardium of the ventricles
could be considered electrically as a single unit. He represented the isopotential surface as if the apex of the heart could be treated as the negative pole and
the base as the positive pole, the source of the potential differences produced
by the ventricles. Waller used this diagram to present "the current axis of the
heart" in order to explain why some leads yielded favorable larger deflection
and others did not. He recognized the relationship of the position of the heart
in the body to the mode of distribution of its potential and presented his findings of a human subject with situs inversus viscerum (13) with the heart tilted
to the right. Thus, he was also aware of the influence of the position of the
human heart upon the form of the electrocardiogram. Waller noted that the

dog heart has an electrical median position behind the sternum (vertical in modern terminology). He used lead combinations to reflect the vertical, horizontal, and sagittal (front to back of the chest) components of the heart vectors. For clinical studies, he later presented the electrical field as a four-sided figure, a "tetrahedron," his own term, formed by the mouth, right arm, left arm, and left leg, from which he obtained five leads. He decried the omission of leads from the mouth, since he considered they afforded the most convenient demonstration of the difference between the right and left sides and, in certain cases, information not obtained from observations of the right and left lateral leads.

In 1913, Einthoven, Fahr, and DeWaert (16) made a seminal contribution to the new science of electrocardiography when they described their methods of determining the direction and "the manifest value" of the potential difference produced by the heartbeat at any given instant in the cardiac cycle. This contribution has been the source of inspiration, controversy, misunderstanding and misinterpretation.

The principles and assumptions on which their methods were based were clearly stated but generally not appreciated. It is regrettable that more valuable effort and thought were not expended in the extension of the theory based on these postulates than on testing the validity of the assumptions.

Einthoven and associates were concerned with the effect of the position of the heart upon the form of the electrocardiogram. "... One understands easily that if, by a chance of position of this organ, an alteration in the form of the curve has been produced, difficulty would be encountered in deciding about the activity of the heart by means of this form. This difficulty can be best resolved if one has previously learned to recognize exactly the influence of position." (16). Being thoroughly familiar with electric theory and with mathematical physics, but apparently not with the reciprocity theorem of Helmholtz (18), Einthoven made several assumptions in order to establish certain relationships between leads based upon the assumed geometry of the body. In answering the question, "How, from the tracings taken in the three leads, is one to determine the actual direction of the potential difference in the body?" Einthoven stated that one obtains the goal in the simplest way by schematizing the human body. The following schema, which can be well designated as the schema of the equilateral triangle, is readily recognized as being especially useful. Herein, the body is represented as a flat, homogenous plate in the form of an equilateral triangle (right, left, and foot). Current is led off to the galvanometer from the corners, R representing the right arm, L to the left arm, and F representing the potential of both feet. A lead from R and L correspond, therefore, to lead I, from R to F to lead II, and from L to F to lead III. A small spot, H, in the middle of the triangle, represents the heart.

The difference of potential between the two points on the surface of the heart was proportional to the cosine of the angle formed by the line of derivation of the adis of the electrical force. The value of the potential of each lead at a given moment was represented by the geometric projection of the assumed heart vector on the corresponding side of the triangle (19).

Einthoven and associates made the assumptions that the heart lies as a material point in a homogeneous mass and that the distance of the heart from the three leads and also the resistances concerned are equally great and that the three leads form an equilateral triangle. They assumed that the electromotive forces of the heart in the frontal plane may be represented as a single vector in the center of an equilateral triangle (19).

Einthoven's assumptions (19) may be restated as follows:

(1) The body is a large conducting medium;
(2) The medium is homogeneous and resistive;
(3) The source of the potential is a dipole;
(4) The dipole is at the center of the medium (the three electrodes are symmetrically located about a centrally placed equivalent dipole whose positive and negative poles are close together, compared to the equal distance between the center of the dipole and the three electrodes);
(5) the dipole undergoes no change in position (location) during the cardiac cycle.

These assumptions were made for practical purposes, and there can be no doubt that they have made it possible for the young plant of electrocardiography to bear an amazingly large amount of fruit in accordance with Einthoven's expectation. Einthoven himself realized very well that this method yielded only an approximation of the truth.

Unfortunately, the basic assumptions were lost sight of in the later developments, especially when the subject was taken over by enthusiastic and worshipful disciples. Having established a point of view, investigators often continue to expand it until the superstructure of the theory becomes too heavy for the narrow pivot of fact upon which it rests. Attempts to make the interpretation of the data yield more precise quantitative information than is justified by the true initial assumption is in many instances the basic fault.

For the third of a century following the postulation of Einthoven's triangle and his assumptions, students of electrocardiography were confronted by a barrage of publications expanding theory based on their validity and often disputing or confirming the validity of these postulates.

Wilson, in the 1930s, gave a needed but not altogether painless introduction to the complication of volume conductors to which Helmholtz, Einthoven, and others had contributed for the benefits of electrocardiography. Wilson and his associates learnedly described the laws which govern the distribution of electromotive forces in solid conductors, assuming the conductor to be infinite, homogeneous, and the source to be a single, fixed dipole, and showed that these laws pertaining to the flow of current in volume conductors applied to electrocardiography (20). These findings were confirmatory of Craib's studies employing strips of cardiac and skeletal muscle and medullated nerve fibers (21,22). These laws were considered to be important for the scientific analysis of chest leads in which one electrode is placed near the heart and the others in the analysis occurring by direct leads.

From these theoretic extensions based on Einthoven's postulates, V leads and, later, augmented unipolar leads (the so-called unipolar limb leads), and the central terminal with a resistive network were developed and received widespread clinical acceptance. It was believed possible to determine the potential variations produced by the heartbeat at any point of the body and on or near the heart, free from the influence exerted by potential variations at the distant, supposedly indifferent electrode. These laws were applied to the distribution of the currents of action and myocardial injury.

Experiments were designed to test this new extension of Einthoven's hypothesis. They included cadaver and immersion experiments (tubs, swimming pools, lakes, cylinders, spheres). The potential of the central terminal was found not to be zero but approximately minus 0.2 to 0.3 mv and less than other reference electrode proffered by non-Wilsonians (23–25).

The error of Wilson's central terminal may be ascribed to the Z component (dorsoventral component) of the heart's field. The predictable difference between CF (chest to left leg), CH (chest to right arm) or the CL (chest to left arm) leads and the V (central terminal) lead were clarified. It soon became the fashion to use the Wilson central terminal as the indifferent electrode for chest leads and to use a form of his unipolar leads, later replaced by Goldberger's arrangement, which augmented the size of the deflection.

In the early 1940s, the practicing cardiologist was soon imbued with the feeling that the interpretation of the electrocardiogram was scientific because it was based on a theory which could be expressed mathematically and, hence, was superior to one which was admittedly empirical. The fact that he, the clinician, could not comprehend the mathematics disturbed him not at all. This attitude is typified by the following note by Francis F. Rosenbaum, regarding Wilson's presentation of a learned paper at the meeting of the Association of American Physicians in Atlantic City in May 1941 (26).

The late Doctor Soma Weiss, who was at that time the Hershey Professor of Medicine at Harvard and a man of wide interests in cardiovascular disease, passed me in the audience as he was leaving the hall. I had left his service at the Peter Bent Brigham, and he knew that I was associated with Doctor Wilson. He said to me, "I hope you understand what your Chief was saying because I certainly didn't."

This did not imply, of course, that Soma Weiss accepted the Wilsonian dogmas but merely emphasized the atmosphere prevailing in clinical circles.

At the very time when the dominance of the system based on Einthoven's postulates began, the groundwork was being laid for its replacement by a better system. Many voices were raised against the "authoritarianism" of the equilateral triangle. The use of Wilson's central terminal as an indifferent electrode was investigated and debated vigorously and in many ways (24,25,27–29).

It was soon well established that although the potential of the central terminal is less than that of other reference electrodes (the right arm, the left arm or the left foot), it is not absolutely at zero, and it shows significant fluctuations during the heart cycle. Inaccuracy introduced by the potential variations of the central terminal (0.2 to 0.3 mv) had not however impaired its practical clinical usefulness. It is interesting that despite the differences in electrocardiograms obtained with the central terminal or other indifferent reference electrodes, similar diagnoses were made by the various proponents of the various reference leads.

THE IMPACT OF HC BURGER

A more realistic triangle and approach to the cardiac vector was provided by H.C. Burger and his associates (30–32). Burger, a relative newcomer to the subject, was a theoretical physicist with experience in handling problems involving boundary conditions. I (H.H.) gained insight into how a theoretical physicist became involved in this field by a prolonged interview with him in the fall of 1958 in Brussels, Belgium. Professor Burger stated that his involvement began in 1939 when he saw by chance a schematic representation of Einthoven's concept (Figure 3) in a book by E. Koch-Momm which was sent to him by his brother, O.O.E. Burger, a physician with the Philips Company in Holland. He recalled that he was struck by the absurdity (33) of a diagram of a man with outstretched hands with extended fingers and left foot forming an equilateral triangle. This was similar to Leonardo da Vinci's proportion of the human figure. Burger and his associates then began to study, using models and making measurements.

Burger was convinced that "the basis of the physical foundation had to be analytical (or algebraic) and not geometrical." He doubted from the very beginning that "the special case of the equilateral triangle was a good approximation." He looked for a way to solve the equation of the heart vector by the

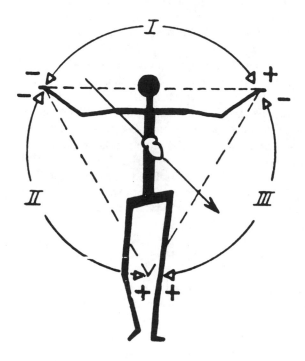

Figure 3.   Diagram of the equilateral triangle. The extended fingers and left foot are represented as forming an equilateral triangle (*with permission*)

use of realistic phantoms, rather than by equations. From the onset, he saw that the body was heterogeneous and not homogeneous and that there was no reason to believe that he would find the field to be an equilateral triangle. He measured the electrical conductivity of human tissues, including his own. He found that the voltages obtained from a dipole placed in glass models of a body were not in accord with Einthoven's hypothesis and, thus, he was stimulated to find a "true" quantitative relationship.

Burger's background in physics, although not directed originally toward solving problems in medicine, enabled him to make an important contribution. He had been well prepared to approach unknown problems in pure research in theoretical physics such as the study of the intensity of spectral lines. Although interested in medicine since youth, Burger decided to enter the field of physics even though he lacked background in Latin or Greek then required for the study of physics but not for medicine. He was attracted by the more exact and quantitative character of this science. Although he first became aware of the dipole concept from Koch-Momm's book (33) and had never worked with volume conductors, he had, however, learned to solve problems of boundary conditions in his work with Koll and Ornstein. Burger stated that he also had another advantage, that is, of "ignorance." He was not aware, either of the differences of opinions that raged and existed, particularly in the American literature, about the validity of Einthoven's assumptions, nor was he aware of torso, cadaver, and immersion experiments by Wilson and others at that time! His professor, Ornstein, had often expounded the theoretical aspects of experimentation and had admonished him not to be influenced by established thought: "Don't read too much; investigate it yourself." ... words of advice still valuable today. Burger volunteered that Einthoven's postulates were originally accepted because his hypotheses were so simple and therewith attractive, and because of the prestigious value of Einthoven's name.

Unfamiliar with either the prevailing controversy about the validity of Einthoven's assumptions or with the recent experiment in favor of these assumptions (22,34), Burger began his own investigation using models and making measurements.

By means of innovative experiments, Burger and van Milaan developed in the period of 1939 to 1946 the concept of "the lead vector" and image space, in an effort to eliminate the need for most of the restrictive assumptions upon which the Einthoven triangle was founded (33). They studied the electrical field generated by an artificial dipole in a model of the human body and constructed a triangle by measuring the potential difference between electrodes corresponding in location to the limb electrodes used in clinical electrocardiography. They considered the "deflection in a given lead as the scalar product of two vectors, one of which represents that lead and the other the electromotor force responsible for the field." The dot product (the product of two vectors) is a scalar quantity. "The value of this expression is obtained by multiplying the product of the length of the two vectors by the cosine of the angle between the positive direction of the one and the positive direction of the other. This amounts to the same thing as multiplying the length of one vector by the projection of the other upon it." (30).

Burger and van Milaan placed bags filled with sand in appropriate sites of the human model to represent the lungs and liver and bags filled with cork to represent the spinal column. They showed that the distribution of currents is considerably modified by the bags in the position of the lungs and spinal column and the current density was much greater at the left arm than at the right. As a consequence, that triangle representing current flow is not an equilateral triangle, but is scalene; and besides, lead I is considerably shortened as is lead II, to a lesser amount. "So-called unipolar and augmented unipolar leads were shown by means of lead fields to be essentially the same genre as bipolar leads and, thus, may be relegated to their proper role in the scheme of things." (30). The lead fields supplanted and generalized the so-called solid angle concept.

The significance of the above refutation was soon recognized and widely accepted, both by believers and nonbelievers of Einthoven's hypothesis. In 1946, Hill (28) went so far as to state, "It is not too much to say that the whole doctrine of electrical axes resultant in component currents, right and left preponderance, summation of currents of equilateral triangles, etc. is quite untenable and must be abandoned. The direction of an electrical current is determined solely by the conducting paths available and has no relation to the orientation of the battery in space." Moreover, the refutation acted as a spur to new thinking and experimentation.

In 1949, Wilson, Bryant, and Johnson reported a method (still clinically impractical) for constructing an accurate Einthoven triangle for a given subject (35). When these investigators began their study they were not aware of the work of Burger and van Milaan of Utrech (30), who for several years had been studying electrical fields generated in a model of the human body which they had built. Since becoming familiar with their publications, Wilson and associates were "considerably influenced by their ideas, and particularly by their elegant method of constructing a triangle which summarizes all the information concerning the nature of the electrical field and their model, obtainable by measuring the potential differences between electrodes corresponding in location to the limb leads used in clinical electrocardiography." (35). For the first time in Wilson's scientific publication, reference was made in 1949 to the reciprocity theorem of Helmholtz (18).

Wilson and associates used the method of Burger and van Milaan to construct a triangle for a given subject. In general the triangle was oblique rather than equilateral (35).

Wilson et al. concluded that

> there may be little value in computing the exact position of the electrical axis of the heart by Einthoven's method, but there can be no question that the Einthoven triangle has made it possible to recognize with considerable facility peculiarities in the form of the electrocardiogram that result from rotation of the heart about a sagittal axis... It has seemed to us that it is desirable to place all methods concerned with the study of the electrical axis of the heart upon a

foundation more secure that that upon which they now rest by a thorough experimental study of the distribution in the body of currents similar to those associated with the heart beat. (35).

The skepticism of the empiricists was justified when they decried the tendency to characterize the electrocardiogram in terms of mathematical, precise quanta derived from unproven postulates.

Burger's concept of lead field was the revival of the reciprocity theorem proved by Helmholtz as a young man of 32 years in 1853 (18) to apply for both homogeneous and heterogeneous volume conductors.

According to this theorem, "every single element of an electromotive surface will produce a flow of the same quantity of electricity through the galvanometer as with flow through that element itself if its electromotive force were impressed on the galvanometer wire. If one adds the effects of all the electromotive surface elements, the effects of each of which are found in the manner described, he will have the value of the total current through the galvanometer." (36).

Burger seemed amused when he told the author (H.H.) that the theoretical knowledge about the reciprocity theorem with which he was familiar had been present for over 50 years at the time of Einthoven who, if he had been familiar with it, would not have made the restrictive assumptions. Apparently, this information also escaped the attention of Waller, Lewis, Wilson, and many other investigators (37).

The lead field concept best provided a simple and powerful tool not only to explain how any type of lead will function, but even more important to indicate what type of electrodes or electrode systems should be employed to obtain leads that are ideal for specific purposes. The lead field concept clarified the type of field that must exist in the heart if a lead is to be ideal for vectorcardiography.

The superiority of the Burger triangle was confirmed by experiments by several groups of investigators (38,39). The orthogonal correction coefficient determined from different models by various investigators were alike in magnitude. With the empirical development of correction factors for the eccentricity of the heart and for the nonhomogenity of the body, meaningful electrocardiography and vector analysis became possible. Both mathematical and experimental approaches using intracardiac and esophageal lead dipoles, cancellation techniques, models, etc. have substantially favored the concept that the electromotive force generated by the heart is equivalent at any moment of the cardiac cycle to a single, fixed dipole (38); however, in exploring leads near the heart, especially if abnormal, local effects may predominate, and the heart cannot truly be considered as a single, fixed dipole.

The concept of the fixed position on the equivalent dipole in the chest has also come under scrutiny. Evidence has developed that the position of the dipole does vary.

In brief, the theoretical knowledge which would have made so many restrictive assumptions unnecessary had already been available for 50 years at the time of Einthoven (40).

CARDIOPULMONARY RESUSCITATION: HISTORICAL BACKGROUND

In 1926, Consolidated Electric Company of New York City, concerned by the increasing number of electric shock accidents and deaths, sought advice from the consultants of the Rockefeller Institute. Five working groups were established, and one chaired by Professor Howell was given the task of studying the effects of electric shock on physiological parameters." (41). In 1928, the Consolidated Edison, a New York power company, gave Johns Hopkins University a $10,000 grant to investigate the effects of electricity on the body, because many linemen were dying from electrical shock. Professor W.H. Howell elected a number of scientists amongst them Kouwenhoven to begin these studies (42). The increasing mortality rate from accidental electrocution by faulty electric appliances had led to a conference on electric shock and to the appointment of a Committee on Physiology for its study.

Carl J. Wiggers was in a receptive frame of mind to go into a new direction of research when Howell invited him in 1929 to join with Donald R. Hooker in research into possible ways of resuscitating hearts from fibrillation induced by electric currents (43; Figure 4).

Both Hooker and Wiggers felt honored to be selected as responsible investigators in their respective institutions, namely, Johns Hopkins and the School of Medicine at Western Reserve University. Funds placed at the disposal of Howell were limited yet sufficient to organize new teams in both schools. Wiggers indicated that this was important for it expanded the research programs of his department without interfering with other existing projects (43). Wiggers admitted in his memoirs that "the most I could hope for, however, was some discovery that might reduce the mortality rate of experimental animals." (43). "Our early attempts to abrogate fibrillation were not motivated by hopes that the method might ever prove useful in man..." (44). At that time, he had little concept of how important the findings of these research efforts would be for clinical application. Wiggers had been focusing his research particularly on special hemodynamic problems.

During his early studies on the hemodynamics of hemorrhage, Wiggers realized that available pressure recorders were not reliable for quantitative

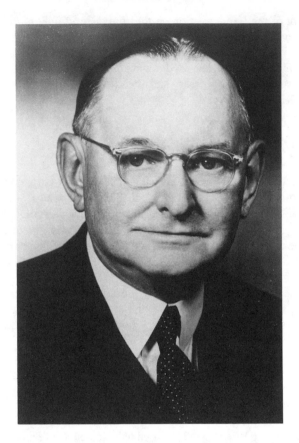

Figure 4.   Carl J. Wiggers (*Courtesy of the Case Western Reserve University Library*)

readings of systolic and diastolic pressures (43). He realized the relative inadequacy of MacKenzie's method to study the pulse and, for this reason, was eager to be exposed to the discipline and techniques developed by Otto Frank at his institute in Munich. Frank had devised new types of manometers. The brief period of training with Frank in 1912 and later visits in 1923 and 1926 gave him an opportunity to obtain a first-hand acquaintance with optically recording instruments.

An understanding of the principles of their construction enabled him to make modifications in the design of Frank's instruments, including optical manometers, capsules and recording flow meters. The period of 1912 to 1929 was extremely fruitful, with an outpouring of research on hemodynamics, on central and peripheral arterial pulses, on pressure pulses in various parts of the cardiovascular system including the venous side, the atria and ventricles, and the hemodynamics of normal and experimental dysfunctional valves. He summarized these primary observations in *"Pressures Pulses in the Cardiovascular System"* in 1929 (45).

The invitation in 1929 from Howell to join with Hooker and others in research to resuscitate hearts from ventricular fibrillation was unexpected but most opportune and welcome. Howell had taken an interest in Wiggers' career and had stimulated his interest in physiology by recommending his membership in the American Physiologic Society in 1907, by "kindly providing comments on his presentation of papers, and by mentioning 'my minor contributions' in his textbooks." (43). Howell had successively become Professor of Physiology and Histology at the University of Michigan from 1889-1892, Associate Professor of Physiology at Harvard in 1892-1893, Professor of Physiology in the Medical School at Johns Hopkins University in 1893-1917, and later in the School of Hygiene at Johns Hopkins in 1917-1931, remaining Professor Emeritus 1931-1945 to his death.

Interest in defibrillation by countershock was stimulated by Howell in 1930 when he suggested to the investigators at both institutions that they reinvestigate the claims of Prevost and Battelli who in 1899 (46) reported that strong currents do not produce ventricular fibrillation but may even abrogate it when it does exist. They described a technique for defibrillating the heart of a dog using a charged capacitor. Wiggers stated, "The idea seemed so fantastic that I read their reports in a biased and unfriendly frame of mind and concluded that their experimental evidence fell short of their claims. At any event, I did not deem a reinvestigation of their claims worthy of the time, effort or expense it would involve." (43).

Hooker, in association with Kouwenhoven and Langworthy, did accept the challenge to test the countershock method for fibrillation. A preliminary report of its success was made in 1932 and a more detailed paper a year later (47). Wiggers and his associates then repeated the procedure and confirmed its effectiveness. In the meantime, Ferris and his associates confirmed the observation that a single strong shock applied during the vulnerable period induced ventricular fibrillation and that this can be abolished by immediate application of a strong current to the chest wall (48).

Research efforts of the two groups, at Western Reserve University and at Johns Hopkins, followed different roads but ultimately came together. Wiggers and his associates focused upon the countershock directly on the exposed heart and the Johns Hopkins group on the closed chest, the latter because of their commitment to solve the problem of defibrillation of line-men exposed to high tension (41,43).

Countershock directly to the heart or to the intact chest was found by both groups to be effective in restoring normal heartbeats only when applied within two or three minutes after induction of fibrillation (49,50). This period was so short that countershock proved a useful defibrillating method in animal experiments only when electrodes had been applied to the heart previous to the onset of ventricular fibrillation and when the equipment for furnishing shocks of appropriate strength was immediately available. Consequently, efforts were made to extend the period of revival during which countershock would be effective after the development of fibrillation. The inability to restore normal action of the heart by applying countershock after more than five minutes was usually not due to failure to abrogate it but rather the failure of the ventricles to develop vigorous beats.

Wiggers and associates recognized that the fibrillating ventricles lose their power of effective contraction after two to three minutes because they are deprived of a supply of oxygenated blood. Two approaches were developed to restore the vigor of myocardial contraction after countershock: Wiggers used cardiac massage, and Hooker and associates used central carotid injections of saline with adrenaline and calcium (41,51).

It was apparent to Wiggers that the remedy needed was a supply of oxygen for the myocardium before application of countershock. If oxygen were provided, muscular contractions would become vigorous the moment incoordination was abolished by countershock (51). In 1936, Wiggers recommended that cardiac massage be started as quickly as possible and continued until fibrous fibrillatory movements were re-established. (51). Wiggers described a method of cardiac massage as consisting of "gentle manual compression of the ventricles about 40 times per minute, thereby raising aortic pressure to 50 or 60 mm Hg. This pressure proved sufficient to supply the heart with oxygenated blood, restore vigorous fibrillatory movements, and incidentally maintained the viability of the central nervous system. An electric shock applied after this procedure usually resulted in prompt redevelopment of the coordinated ventricular beats." (51). Wiggers reported, "I have personally witnessed over 1,000 revivals in all kinds of fibrillation in dogs weighing up to 18 kg through use of this method." (43).

Wiggers' major contribution to the problem which ultimately had clinical application by Beck and others was the development of experimental methods to extend the period of revival.

Defibrillation was occasionally difficult in dogs with large hearts because the current used was not strong enough to penetrate all parts of the myocardium. Wiggers and associates developed a technique called serial defibrillations, consisting of three to five brief shocks at approximately two second intervals, which was found to be effective in abolishing ventricular fibrillation (52). Beck and associates also occasionally encountered difficulty in successful defibrillation in the laboratory and sought a modification for use on the human heart "if it should be necessary at the time of operation."(53). Mautz, Beck's associate, demonstrated that procaine or metycaine applied directly to the fibrillating heart reduced the irritability of the myocardium and that electric shock would uniformly stop ventricular fibrillation (54). Soon, Mautz (55) adopted Wiggers' modification of the countershock method (massage, serial shocks if necessary) and found that injections of a small amount of procaine into the ventricular cavity prior to the use of massage and countershock was helpful in abolishing residual areas of fibrillation.

OPEN-CHEST CARDIAC RESUSCITATION.
APPLICATION TO HUMANS.

Wiggers produced ventricular fibrillation in animals with electrical currents as well as by ligation of the coronary arteries. He found that the coronary ligatures had to be removed before he could defibrillate a dog's heart (51). Because of this, he seriously questioned whether ventricular fibrillation could be corrected electrically after coronary thrombosis. "The normal dog's heart can rarely be revived unless the occlusion is removed, and this is impossible in man." (51).

Beck appeared to share a similar view in 1937, when he wrote, "I should like to make this statement, that any heart that stops beating in the operating room can be revived provided there is no intrinsic disease of the heart. Of course, a heart that is poisoned by bacterial toxin or a heart that is poorly vascularized because of coronary artery disease cannot be expected to recover. Patients who die suddenly and who have good hearts constitute a group that can be saved if we are trained to grasp the occasion as it arises." (56). (Figure 5; *See chapter 8 Coronary Artery Surgery, Figure 1*).

In 1937 and thereafter, with messianic zeal, Beck disseminated widely with lectures, articles, demonstrations, and motion pictures, his procedure for defibrillation of the ventricles in the operating room (57). Beck and Mautz presented a motion picture of fibrillation and defibrillation to the American Surgical Association in 1937. Unfortunately, the audience was not appreciative of the possible clinical application (57,58,59).

Beck's recommended procedure was as follows:

Adequate aeration of the lungs. This is possible only through an intratracheal tube and intermittent insufflation with air and oxygen. This is the first step to

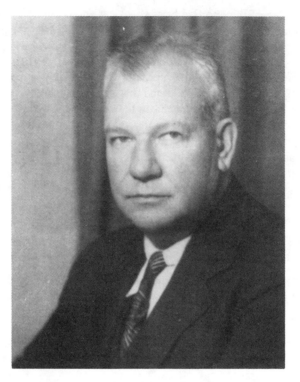

Figure 5. Claude S. Beck (*Courtesy Dr. Mary Ellen Wohl, Brookline, MA*)

be taken and requires preparation. Exposure of the heart and massage of the ventricles about 50 times per minute. This will raise arterial pressure to 40 to 60 mm of mercury. It must not be so vigorous as to bruise the myocardium. The central nervous system is now being oxygenated and reflexes return. Restoration of the coronary circulation brings oxygenated blood to the myocardium. Restoration of circulation with oxygenated blood to the brain and to the myocardium is essential. As long as it is carried out, recovery is a possibility, even though the ventricles continue to fibrillate. It is possible to continue this artificial circulation over a period long enough to wash out an overdose of anesthetic and long enough for drug effects to disappear... Before the next step is taken two things must be accomplished by the massage. First, the dilation of the heart must be overcome completely. This is important for success because a dilated heart must have a good color. A cyanotic heart is also prone to keep on fibrillating. When both of these objects are accomplished by aeration and massage, the heart will show slow and coarse fibrillatory movements. An electrode, preferably of silver, measuring about 25 square centimeters in area, is placed on each side of the heart and an electric current is sent through the ventricles. The electrodes need not be padded to prevent burning if there is a large area of contact with the heart. The current is an ordinary alternating current of 60 cycles and 1 to 1.5 amperes. The duration of the current is short, from 0.5 to about two seconds.

If the shock fails to stop fibrillation, the use of procaine is indicated. Two cubic centimeters of 5 percent solution are dripped upon the auricles and the ventricles. Massage as before until dilation disappears. Electric shock is usually successful in stopping fibrillation. If it is not, 2 cc. of procaine in 10 cc. of physiologic solution of sodium chloride are injected into the right ventricular cavity. Massage until dilation disappears. Electric shock now will stop the fibrillation routinely in dogs.

Every vestige of fibrillatory movement must disappear before there is any hope of success. After fibrillation has been abolished and the heart is at a standstill, massage is used. This usually starts a coordinated rhythm. At this place in the procedure, epinephrine may be useful.

After using procaine or metycaine upon the heart, ventricular fibrillation may be converted into ventricular standstill by the current without restoration of any signs of contractibility. In this event massage is continued, and a solution of calcium chloride is injected into the right ventricle...

It is needless to say that throughout the entire procedure, massage of the ventricles is absolutely necessary to preserve the viability of the brain and the myocardium. We have succeeded in reviving hearts that were in ventricular fibrillation or standstill for periods as long as 30 minutes. During this entire period an arterial pressure was maintained by massage of the heart...

Defibrillators were placed by Beck and his associates in the accident room and various operating rooms of the University Hospitals of Cleveland. Lectures and laboratory demonstrations were frequently made. The staff was alerted. Beck defibrillated a human heart in 1938 and another in 1939, but these patients died sometime later from damage to the brain (53).

THE ERA OF OPEN-CHEST CARDIAC DEFIBRILLATION

The first successful defibrillation in the operating room with complete neurologic recovery was reported by Beck et al. in 1947 (58).

The patient was 14 year old boy who was being operated upon to relieve extreme sternal depression. When the wound was being closed, the heart suddenly stopped. The wound was reopened, and cardiac massage was started. The mechanical respirator was attached to an intra-tracheal tube, and cardiac massage was continued for 35 minutes, at the end of which time the electrocardiogram continued to show ventricular fibrillation. The first electric shock did not cause any change in the mechanism. Procaine hydrochloride was injected into the right auricle, and the heart was massaged. A second series of electric shocks was given, producing complete cardiac standstill, following which cardiac contractions were observed, and while it was still in sinus rhythm, the heart was massaged for five minutes, at which time the contractions were coordinated and vigorous. Electrocardiogram at that time showed supraventricular tachycardia at a rate of 175. At no time was cyanosis or pupillary dilation present. This demonstrated that cardiac massage had maintained an adequate cerebral circulation. This case of a healthy boy with a depressed sternum was presented in which ventricular fibrillation developed during a thoracic surgical procedure and was present during one hour and ten minutes when manual massage of the heart was necessary to maintain life. For 35 minutes of this time, electrocardiographic tracings showed the presence of ventricular fibrillation.By electric shock, applied directly to the exposed heart, ventricular fibrillation was abolished and supraventricular rhythm was restored (Figures 6,7a). "The patient made

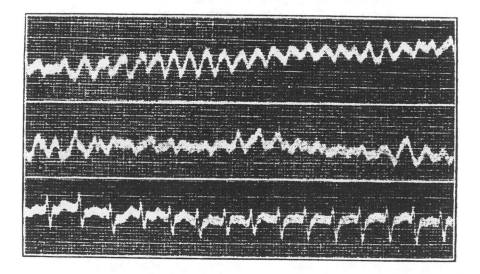

Figure 6.   Electrocardiogram of a 14 year old patient, the first documented patient with ventricular fibrillation who recovered, with open chest cardiac massage, and defibrillation in 1947. The upper two rows show ventricular fibrillation.   The bottom row shows supra–ventricular tachycardia which occurred after direct electrical 110 volts alternating current countershocks. (*Courtesy of the Journal of the American Medical Association, 135:985–986, copyright 1947*).

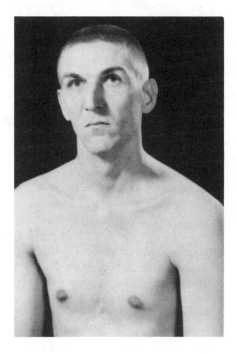

Figure 7a. Photograph of a survivor of open chest direct cardiac massage and defibrillation, without neurological impairment (*Courtesy of the Archives of the University Hospitals of Cleveland, OH.*)

a complete recovery without detectable neurologic or cardiac damage" (58) and lived 22 years (59).

RESUSCITATION PROCEDURES STARTED IN A PATIENT'S ROOM

Resuscitation was started on a patient who fibrillated while in bed in her room in a medical area in 1956. "The chest was opened by the medical resident; the heart was pumped by hand, and the lungs were oxygenated. This consumed 15 minutes. The oxygen-system was maintained in transit to the operating room and this consumed 10 minutes. The chest was draped. The heart was defibrillated. The patient made an uneventful recovery." (60).

Resuscitation Outside the Hospital

As a result of the successful recovery of the patient in 1947, Beck renewed his efforts to spread the "gospel" of "Hearts Too Good to Die," (53) with the development of a policy statement for the Veteran's Administration and with the establishment of post-graduate courses for nurses and physicians on the prevention and management of cardiac arrest. He dared to recommend that the procedure be done on victims who had "fatal" heart attack outside the hospital. This involved opening the chest. The Dean of the Medical School of Western Reserve University stated that Beck "was not a safe man to have on the faculty." (53). Nevertheless, the concept of "Hearts Too Good to Die" was disseminated with hands-on experience in Beck's surgical laboratory and qualification of the medical students of Western Reserve University School of Medicine, of the resident physicians in training, and of over 3,500 physicians and nurses in two day courses of instruction each month from 1950 to 1965 (53,61,62). Some participants of the last group came from Britain, France, Sweden and other countries. Soon reports of successful open chest resuscitation outside of the hospital appeared in a great variety of venues, in the hallways of hospitals, darkrooms, in the offices of physicians and dentists, on the golf course, at athletic contests, etc.

In 1950, Beck provided the Veteran's Administration Technical Bulletin TB 10-65, on the Treatment of Cardiac Arrest (62). This became policy throughout the Veteran's Administration. There was emphasis upon the restoration of the oxygen system, restoration of the heartbeat, methods of application of drugs in asystole and ventricular fibrillation, and closure of the chest.

Beck emphasized the restoration of the oxygen system,

> Two things must be accomplished: oxygen must be delivered to the blood, and the oxygenated blood must be circulated. The surgeon and anesthetist have three to five minutes to place this system in operation. If a longer period of time is taken, irreversible damage to the brain may have occurred, and complete recovery may not be possible. The existence of this time limit is the cause of most failures. As soon as it is realized that either respiration or the heart has stopped, the surgeon and anesthetist must realize that a crisis is at hand. No moment of time can be lost. ... Before beginning the positive steps to be taken, it might be advisable to state what steps should not be taken. The most important thing to avoid is to take time in order to make sure that the patient is dead. Do not listen for a faint heart sound which may or may not be present. The surgeon need not be fearful that he will open the chest and then find a vigorously beating heart. If there is no palpable pulse, no blood pressure, and if the respiration has ceased, he can be certain that any slight movement of the heart which may still be present is of no consequence. Do not wait for an electrocardiogram. Do not try inject epinephrine through the chest wall into the heart. Do

not try to give mechanical respiration by compression of the chest. Do not give a blood transfusion. Do not give an intra-arterial transfusion. The time taken to carry out these steps will preclude success in almost all cases.

The 1950 bulletin is summarized as follows:

(1) A procedure for resuscitation in the operating room is described which, under certain conditions, may be successful. The requirements for success are discussed.
(2) The importance of separating the procedure into two components is stressed. Restoration of the oxygen system is the emergency act. Restoration of the heartbeat can be accomplished minutes or hours after the oxygen system has been restored.
(3) Valuable training in the procedure may be gained by practice on the dog heart. A special postgraduate course in resuscitation would appear to be desirable and is being planned." This was accomplished beginning in 1950 and continued for 15 years, until its replacement by the closed chest technique of Kouwenhoven and associates (62).

Birth and development of coronary care ward was another byproduct of the concept of "Hearts Too Good To Die." "The birth occurrred in the University Hospitals of Cleveland in 1958 with Doctor David Leighninger (Doctor Beck's associate) gave round-the-clock care to a patient stricken with coronary occlusion." (53). The patient was a Professor of Pediatrics who had developed cardiac standstill while rushing up several flights of stairs. Blows to the precardium by a medical resident initiated a heartbeat. The patient was transported to a private hospital room and connected to a direct writing electrocardiograph for continuous monitoring. Leighninger slept in an adjacent room and was made available over a period of seven days. In 1962, Hughes A. Day established the first physical unit to provide this specialized care to the coronary patient. (*See also Chapter 7, page 164.*) A letter to Beck from Day, Bethany Hospital in Kansas City,Kansas, September 12, 1969, follows:

During the six years I served as Director of the Unit from 1962 to 1968, a total of 530 proven myocardial infarcts were treated. There were 98 deaths. Ventricular fibrillation occurred in 59. Of these, 44 were resuscitated for a salvage rate of 74 percent. Similar results are occurring in other coronary care units across the country. My first two articles were published in *Lancet*, 1962 and 1963. They were published in *Lancet* for the simple reason that I could not get any national journal to publish them. One editor wrote me that "the article on Cardiac Resuscitation was nothing new and everything had been written about cardiac resuscitation that was worthwhile." (63).

At the present time, almost every large hospital has a coronary care unit. In 1967, and after Beck retired, one was finally established in the hospital (University Hospitals of Cleveland) where the idea was born.

CHANGING ATTITUDE TOWARD REVIVAL OF A HEART WITH INTRINSIC DISEASE "HEART TOO GOOD TO DIE"—EVEN WITH CORONARY DISEASE

In 1956 the prevalent view that open chest resuscitation of patients without "intrinsic" heart disease should be restricted to the operating room was changed dramatically by the sucessful resuscitation of a patient with ventricular fibrillation (due to an acute myocardial infarction) which occurred outside the operating room.

Case Report (64)

A patient with ventricular fibrillation after a heart attack was successfully defibrillated by a countershock at the University Hospitals of Cleveland in June 1955, and lived until February 1984 (53). "The patient was a 65 year old practicing physician and staff member who fell over at the back entrance of the hospital. He was quickly taken to the emergency ward, where he remained unconscious, pulseless, apneic, and cyanotic. He had no heart sounds, and his pupils became dilated. (This was five years before the introduction of closed chest cardiac massage.) Thoracotomy was done without skin preparation. The ventricles were fibrillating. Intermittent ventricular compression was carried out by hand over a protracted period until an electrical defibrillator was brought from Beck's animal laboratory. (This laboratory defibrillator consisted of a row of electric light bulbs used for resistance.) The third shock, consisting of 3 amperes for two seconds (110 AC) was successful," without neurologic deficit. The patient left the hospital 11 days later, returned to practice for awhile, and then retired to Florida. He died on February 2, 1984 at the age of 93 years (65) (Figure 7b). He had 28-1/2 good years of life after conversion to normal ventricular rhythm (65). Beck later opined: "Had he (the patient) taken a few steps out of the hospital, his body would have been taken to the morgue. Why should a few steps make the difference between life and death?" (65).

In their 1955 report, Beck, Weckesser, and Barry speculated on the future application of open heart cardiac resuscitation:

> Resuscitation is indicated in these victims of coronary artery disease who die from electrical instability. Resuscitation is feasible when the victim dies in the hospital, provided supplies and personnel trained in resuscitation methods are available as soon as the patient dies. Preparation for resuscitation must be made before death occurs. It is suggested that trained resuscitation teams take over when a patient dies from an acute heart attack. No doubt some lives will be saved by such action. When death occurs on the golf course, in the office, or in the home, resuscitation cannot be done unles equipment and trained person-

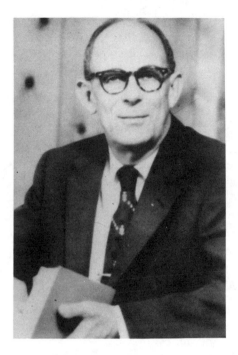

Figure 7b. Photograph of a 65 year old physician with long term survival, who was the first documented case of acute myocardial infarction successfully resuscitated outside of the operating room by open chest cardiac massage and defibrillation. He survived 28 years. (*Courtesy of the Archives of the University Hospitals of Cleveland, OH*)

nel are immediately available. These problems are not insurmountable. *Any intelligent man or woman can be taught to do resuscitation.* A medical or nursing degree is not a prerequisite to learn resuscitation, nor is it impossible to provide resuscitation kits to be opened for emergency; these could be located in selected areas and be serviced whenever necessary. The veil of mystery is being lifted from heart conditions, and the dead are being brought back to life. (64).

Once again, Beck's advocacy of cardiac resuscitation by properly trained lay personnel created a storm of protest, followed by ridicule, vigorous condemnation of this "outrageous recommendation," and rejection by the medical profession and by agencies approached for funds for training purposes.

Beck's concept of "Hearts Too Good to Die" finally was appreciated and vindicated by the development of the closed chest cardiac method and its successfull application, not only in the hospital but also outside of the hospital. Zoll was the true pioneer in these endeavors (66). The general public has become involved in the initial management of patients with cardiac arrest and with the development of cardipulmonary resuscitation training programs of the lay public teaching both mouth-to-mouth ventilation and external cardiac compression. The annual rate of successful resuscitation "in the pre-hospital scene and discharge home has continued to rise based upon the increased involvement by citizen CRPR and more rapid response by trained lay personnel capable of delivering definitive therapy." (67).

The method of open chest cardiac massage and defibrillation was not suitable for the electric industry to use in the field, since it entailed a major operation to open the chest.

DEVELOPMENT OF CLOSED CHEST CARDIAC MASSAGE AND DEFIBRILLATION

The saga of the development of closed chest cardiac massage and defibrillation has its beginning at The Johns Hopkins University, where earlier investigators of accidental electrocution had been responsible for the involvement of Western Reserve University scientists in this problem and, ultimately, their successful technique of direct open chest cardiac massage and resuscitation.

The present author (H.H.) became aware of the importance of several chance encounters of scientists of the two institutions in the development of closed chest cardiac massage when he presented a lecture in 1958 on rehabilitation and resuscitation to an audience in Hurd Hall at Johns Hopkins Medical School, at the invitation of E. Cowles Andrus, then recently Past President of the American Heart Assocation from 1954 to 1955. In the course of my presentation on cardiac rehabilitation, which was becoming a very topical and somewhat new approach in the 1950s to treatment and managemnt of patients with heart disease, I mentioned our difficulties in returning people to work especially after they had undergone open chest cardiac resuscitation. This approach to sudden cardiac death was quite the vogue in Cleveland, Ohio, thanks to the pioneering work of Wiggers, a physiologist, and Beck. Beck et al had reported in 1947 the first case of a human with ventricular fibrillation who recovered completely with no neurological residual (58). Having matriculated at Western Reserve University School of Medicine in 1941, and being familiar with the work of Wiggers and his associates on ventricular fibrillation and having studied the terminal electrocardiogram in humans and methods to deal with cessation of ciculation due to cardiac standstill or ventricular fibrillation I had become familiar with the pioneering contributions of the investigators at Johns Hopkins, especially Hooker and Kouwenhoven.

At the end of my lecture, an elderly gentleman approximately 68 inches tall, balding, and with a pipe in hand, made his way from the back row of the amphitheatre, and to my great surprise, he asked, "How's Carl and how's Claude?" He obviously was referring to Claude Beck and Carl J. Wiggers. Not allowing time for response and with an obvious glint in his eyes, he continued, "I guess it's about time to set things straight once again and to redirect their research in the proper way." He identified himself as William Bennett Kouwenhoven (Professor Emeritus of Electrical Engineering since 1954.) (Figure 8). He proceded to regale me with a story of how interactions be-

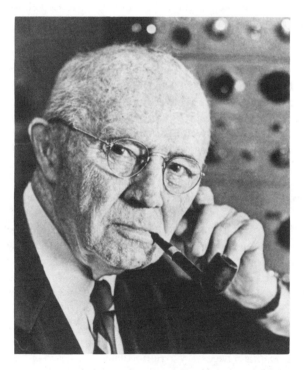

Figure 8.   Photograph of William B. Kouwenhoven in 1973 when he received the Albert and Mary Lasker Foundation Award for Clinical Medical Research (*Courtesy of the Lasker Foundation, New York*)

tween investigators at The Johns Hopkins University and Western Reserve University and "chance" observations promised in 1958 to make open chest cardiac resuscitation obsolete. He gently urged me to be sure to take this message back to Cleveland. The following pages reflect Kouwenhoven's account and unique perspective and insight into cardiopulmonary resuscitation, essentially in accord with the preceding narration.

Kouwenhoven indicated that as a result of contacts with Howell at Johns Hopkins in 1929, Wiggers shifted his energies and focus away from pulse curves and hemodynamics to the problem of ventricular fibrillation and the importance of finding solutions. As a result of this "chance" encounter in 1929, Wiggers devoted the next six or more years to a study of ventricular fibrillation in the dog, the nature of its genesis, method of control, and successful management and survival, using the open chest cardiac approach (49,51). While Wiggers and associates focused upon a direct approach to the open chest experimental model, Kouwenhoven and his Johns Hopkins group, because of contractual interest, focused upon closed chest defibrillation, and developed a simple electrical apparatus for closed chest ventricular defibrillation of humans (41,50) survival depended upon the termination of ventricular fibrillation within one or two minutes of its onset. Wiggers established that cardiac massage with restoration of some coronary perfusion was essential *before* countershock (51), and Kouwenhoven and his group continued to be unable to produce recovery with restoration despite successful closed chest defibrillation (abrogation of ventricular fibrillation) unless it were applied within one or two minutes of onset (50); and after a longer period of time, although the heart could be defibrillated, even central carotid artery infusion with epinephrine and other materials was not successful (50). This approach had limited application clinically and in the field. In the meantime, the investigators at The Johns Hopkins University continued to conduct research on closed chest defibrillation and, unlike Wiggers and Beck, had been unable to restore animals and humans after the development of ventricular fibrillation when closed chest electrical shock alone was provided unless wihin one or two minutes. In 1956, Zoll and associates successfully terminated ventricular fibrillation of several patients in an intensive care monitoring area. They externally applied electrical stimulation without external chest cardiac massage (66).

Kouwenhoven recalled that as a result of Wiggers' demonstration of the importance of restoring coronary flow with cardiac massage *before* countershock, it was no longer necessary to defibrillate within two or three minutes, the limitation of The Johns Hopkins closed chest approach. Beck's first successful defibrillation of a human heart on December 7, 1938 did not result in survival because of brain damage (59).

In 1948 Beck and associates applied Wigger's technique clinically and initiated the era of "Hearts Too Good to Die," (58,67) with successful resuscitation and survival of patients, both without and with intrinsic heart disease (1955) (64). The experience in Cleveland of open chest cardiac massage was so effective that it became "the fashion." The successful transfer of Wiggers' technique by Beck to the clinical arena resulted in widespread acceptance of the open chest approach; open chest cardiac resuscitation took place not only in the operating room, the recovery room, the hallways of hospitals, but also in the community (60). In retrospect Kouwenhoven stated, "I had felt frustrated by our inability to successfully restore patients with ventricular fibrillation unless a countershock was provided within the first two or three minutes," and readily acknowledged his appreciation of the contribution of Wiggers' and Beck's technique.

Kouwenhoven was concerned at the time with methods of providing circulation without resorting to thoracotomy:

> It was clearly recognized that time was the most important factor and that time as measured in seconds, literally. The first method tried was to insert needles through the chest into the myocardium and apply pacemaker shocks to the fibrillating heart. These proved to be ineffective and the method was abandoned (41).
> A series of experiments was conducted in which a brief AC defibrillating shock of one tenth or less seconds was applied to the chest at the rate of a shock per second. In these applications only three dogs were saved in a large group. Many times it was impossible to defibrillate the heart when the stimuli had been applied for several minutes. This scheme was also abandoned. (41).

The potential solution to providing circulation during ventricular fibrillation was initiated by a "misadventure" during open chest cardiac resuscitation at Johns Hopkins, supposedly an indirect result of the influence of Beck's concept of "Hearts Too Good to Die." Kouwenhoven recalled that a young medical officer physician (presumably a graduate of Western Reserve University School of Medicine) when working in The Johns Hopkins Hospital emergency room applied "Claude Beck's approach" to cardiac resuscitation i.e., emergency thoracotomy, manual massage of the fibrillating heart, and successful defibrillation, with survival. This case was presented enthusiastically at grand rounds. Several months later, another case with ventricular fibrillation was presented. Another house officer (not a Western Reserve University graduate) had performed an emergency thoracotomy of a patient with ventricular fibrillation. Unfortunately, in the course of making an incision in the left chest, he had inadvertently cut the heart, almost transecting it, of course, with an unfavorable outcome.

According to Kouwenhoven, at the grand rounds presentation of this case of near-transection of the heart, he stated he was struck by the absurdity of the open chest cardiac massage technique. This misadventure provoked his interest in exploring an earlier *chance* observation that should provide an alternative to open chest cardiac massage. He recalled that when Mine Safety electrodes were pressed on an animal's chest, there was a slight rise in blood pressure before a shock was applied. In 1958, his assistant, Guy Knickerbocker, a 24 year old graduate student of electrical engineering who had joined Kouwenhoven to participate in the program of the Edison project in 1954, also noticed this phenomenon (41). When interviewed in July 1991, Knickerbocker said that with the passage of many years, he presently was not sure who made the observation initially, whether it was he who had made the observation or that he and Kouwenhoven made it together. He did recall looking at the Sanborn record pressure curve which showed a definite rise in the intraarterial femoral pressure. He and Kouwenhoven...

> ...were proceeding with their studies in closed-chest defibrillation when they observed that there was a rise in intra-arterial presssure when the heart defibrillator electrodes were applied to the chest wall of the dog with ventricular fibrillation. A relaxation and push caused additional increase in arterial pressure. They considered that the rhythmic application of pressure to the chest wall might cause the heart to empty and provide circulation. These observations and ideas were discussed with the staff of The John Hopkins Hospital, but they were assured that pressing on the animal's chest was like pressing on a balloon: 'when the pressure was relaxed, the chest expanded and the pressure returned to normal; the rise was not sufficient indication of circulation. (41).

Inadequate consideration was given to the concepts of the production of an artificial circulation by external cardiac compression, because others previously had condemned this technique. Pike and colleagues in 1908 had attempted extrathoracic massage without success.

> They noted that rhythmic manual compression of the thorax of a cat over the heart gave fairly good results in certain stages of heart stoppage, but the time when massage was effective was much too limited to make the method a sure one. They questioned whether, in fact, the loss of the pulse was associated with the heart ceasing to beat ... [Electrocardiograms were not in common use at that time.] Furthermore, they noted that rhythmic compression of the thorax of a large dog at a rate necessary for resuscitation was exceedingly laborious and often could not be kept for a sufficiently long time. (68).

George Crile's report of resuscitation by chest compression was similarly rejected.

> In 1908, Crile, Cleveland, Ohio, had been successful in animals with arterial perfusion and squeezing the unopened chest. He demonstrated the latter before

the Cleveland Academy of Medicine in 1908. As he stated, "This led naturally to the use of adrenalin saline solution intravascularly, combined with rhythmic pressure on the chest as a means of resuscitation." This furnishes an external pseudocardiac reaction. Direct massage is, therefore, not essential. (69).

During the first decade of the twentieth century, three people had been successfully resuscitated. Crile's patient, a 12 year old girl, was one. At one time he referred to this incident as death and resurrection. The medical profession marvelled for a short time, but they were not ready to accept cardiac resuscitation. Acceptance was extended to the Pulmotor, a mechanical device." (69).

Earlier, in 1878, Boehm reported treatment of the arrested heart with a closed chest method of resuscitation. "Working with cats, he grasped the chest in his hand at the area of greatest expansion and applied rhythmic pressure. His results were quite striking in some series of tests. Tournade and his co-workers reported that compression of the thorax of a dog in a cardiac arrest could produce blood pressure of 60 or 100 mm. There were no survival data. In 1933, Killick and Eve reported "that the rocking technique of artificial respiration by which a patient is tilted about 60° in each direction from the horizontal plane will produce a change in the blood pressure at the atrium from 38 to 76 mm Hg. Eve hypothesized that this change will produce sufficient blood flow to nourish the heart and the brain." (70).

At the time (1957) when Knickerbocker and Kouwenhoven were developing their techniques for external cardiac massage, they first became aware of the 1947 publication of N. L. Gurvich and G. S. Yuniev (71), who approximately ten years earlier had found that a capacitor discharge, sent through the chest of a dog, would be followed by resumption of cardiac function if applied not later than one or one and one-half minutes after the onset of induced ventricular fibrillation, and that this time limitation might be extended to as long as eight minutes by rhythmical application of pressure of the thorax by squeezing both sides of the chest in the region of the heart. In tests which lasted 10 to 15 minutes, 19 animals survived and 17 died (71). These authors, however, gave no specific information as to the method of application of the pressure. Their method had not been applied to a patient. According to Knickerbocker in 1958, a Russian delegation of clinicians visited The Johns Hopkins University, and when asked whether any practical use of Gurvich's technique had ever been used in Russia, they indicated that that had not been the case but certainly upon return to Russia they would spread the gospel and, of course, give priority to a fellow Russian! The next day after the Russians left, Kouwenhoven made a hasty visit to Blalock, head of the Department of Surgery and informed him that it was entirely likely that the Russians would claim closed chest cardiac massage as a Russian invention, as they had also made claims of priority in the development of other advances such as the airplane, the automobile, etc. Blalock called the editor of the Journal of the American Medical Association and urged that early publication of the article, which had been already submitted in February 1960, be facilitated. Indeed, the article did appear in July 1960, possibly expedited in order to establish firmly the appropriate priority of this technique to the Johns Hopkins group. Three years later, when Knickerbocker visited Gurvich and Negovsky's Institute in the U.S.S.R., he was pleased to find that an enlarged photograph of the technique of closed chest massage (Figure 9) was prominently displayed.

Kouwenhoven's group began "an extensive series of experiments in which pressure was applied not only to the sternum but also on the sides of the chest (42). In these experiments, it was the practice to give an anesthetized dog a fibrillating shock and wait one minute before starting to press on the sternum and the chest. After applying pressure for a few minutes, a defibrillating shock could be given and attempts made to save the animal. A number of these animal was autopsied and broken costal junctions and ribs, and other injuries were observed. The blood pressure, however, was forty percent of normal.

Henry T. Bahnson joined Kouwenhoven's group, and "when it was found that a dog could be maintained viable for a period of ten minutes by the application of rhythmic pressure on the lower third of the sternum with a force of eighty to one hundred pounds at the rate of one per second, Bahnson was eager to apply the technique to a patient. His opportunity arrived on the night of February 15, 1958 when he resuscitated a two year old child whose heart was in ventricular fibrillation" with the new combined method—external cardiac compression and closed chest defibrillation. "The next day Doctor Blalock directed that external cardiac massage be applied to children where indicated. Doctor James Jude returned from Army service in July 1958, was appointed Resident Surgeon, and was assigned to work with Doctor Kouwenhoven. Systematically, they developed a technique of external cardiac compression. They were able to demonstrate with clever experiments that the compression of the chest was sufficient to augment the arterial blood pressure to a point that adequate coronary artery perfusion took place. Later in 1958, external cardiac massage was applied to an obese woman in her 40s who experienced ventricular fibrillation while undergoing anesthesia. The cardiopulmonary resuscitation was successful (41,70).

A report of the method of closed chest cardiac massage and the results were published on July 9, 1961 in the Journal of the American Medical Assocation. This was a landmark article (72). Longmire reports in his biography of Alfred Blalock that Blalock discussed a paper by Jude, Kouwenhoven

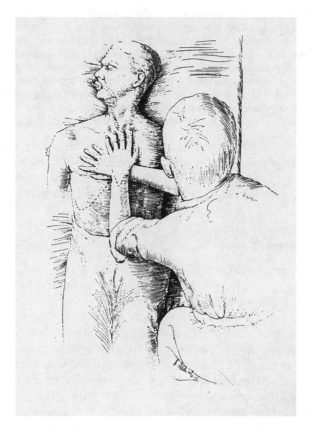

Figure 9. Photograph showing the technique of closed chest cardiac massage in 1960, the landmark article on closed chest cardiac massage. (*Courtesy of the Journal of The American Medical Association, 173:1064–1067, copyright, 1960*)

and Knickerbocker presented before the American Surgical Association in 1961, stated that "There are two things of great interest to me in this project; first, it proves that a man over three score and ten years can still have original ideas, and second, that most really significant contributions are relatively simple in concept" (73).

The new concept of external cardiac compression in association with artificial ventilation as the primary step in the management of a patient with cardiac arrest received wide acceptance, and was successful.

It is almost a quarter of a century since the publication of 'Closed-Chest Cardiac Massage' in JAMA. During this period, thousands and thousands of persons across the whole world have owed their lives to those who were able to show that without special equipment, and using only the two hands, anyone with training can save a life. Only a few years before his death, Kouwenhoven, at the age of 83 years, said that the discovery and development of cardiopulmonary resuscitation made the closed-chest defibrillator a useful and effective device for depolarizing fibrillating human hearts. Many lives have been saved and I thank the Lord for the opportunity that has been granted me. (70).

The development of successful open chest, and subsequently, closed-chest defibrillation provide an excellent example of the value of inter-institutional collaboration of multiple disciplines such as medicine, physiology, surgery, and engineering, working together, sharing goals, knowledge, and experience.

Acknowledgements

It is a pleasure to acknowledge my indebtedness to the archivists, James Stimpert, at The Ferdinand Hamburger, Jr. Archives, The Johns Hopkins University, Nancy C. Erdey. The University Hospitals of Cleveland, and Dennis Harrison, Case Western University; to Robert G. Cheshier, Director, and his Interlibrary Loan Staff, of the Cleveland Health Sciences Library, Doctor Robert M. Hosler, Doctor Mary Elen Beck Wohl, and to the following former members of The John Hopkins Hospital, who kindly provided personal views and impressions of the era of resuscitation and the development of closed chest cardiac massage and defibrillation. The following individuals granted telephone interviews in July, 1991: Doctors Peter Dans, Guy G.Knickerbocker, James R. Jude and McGehee Harvey.

REFERENCES

1. Sue, P. Histoire du galvanisme: et analyse des differens ouvrages publies sur cette decouverte depuis son origine jusqu a ce jour. Paris, Bernard, 1802.
2. Amberson, W.R. The influence of fashion in the development of knowledge concerning electricity and magnetism. Am Sci 46:33–50, 1958.
3. Fleming, J.A. s.v. ("Electricity"). Encyclopedia Britannica. 11th ed.
4. Bidwell, S. s.v. ("Magnetism"). Encyclopedia Britannica 11th ed.
5. Franklin, B. Experiments and observations on electricity made at Phildelphia in America. London, 1769.
5a. Schecter, D.C. Exploring the origins of electrical cardiac stimulation. Medtronics, Minneapolis, MN, 1983.
6. Cohen, L.B. Introduction. In: L. Galvani. Commentary on the effects of electricity on muscular motion Tr. by M.G. Foley; Norwood, Conn., Burndy Library, 1954.

7. Galvani, L. De viribus electritatis in motu musculari commentarius. De Bononiensi Scientarium et Artium. Instituto atque Academia Commentarii, 7:363, 1791.
8. Galvani, L. Dell'uso e dell'attivita dell' arco conduttore nelle contrazioni dei muscoli. Bologna, S. Tommaso d'Aquino, 1794.
9. Du Bois-Reymond, E. Untersuchungen ueber thierische Elektricitaet, Berlin, Reimer, 1848–84.
10. Humboldt, A. von. Versuche ueber die gereizte Muskel und Nervenfaser nebst Vermuthungen ueber den chemischen Process des Lebens in der Thier- und Pflanzenwelt. Posen, Decker, 1797.
11. Oersted, H.C. Galvanic magnetism Phil. Mag. 56: 394, 1820
12. Lippmann, G. Relations entre les phenomenes electriques et capillaires. Ann Chim (Phy), ser. 5, 5: 494, 1875.
13. Waller, A.D. On the electromotive changes connected with the mammalian heart, and of the human heart in particular. Phil. Trans. B, 180: 169, 1889.
14. Ader C. Sur un nouvel appareil enregistreur pour cables sousmarins. C.R. Acad. Sci. (Paris) 124, 1440, 1897.
15. Einthoven W. Die galvanometrische Registrierung des menschlichen Elektrokardiogramms, angleich eine Beurtheilung der Anwendung des Capillar-Elektrometers in der Physiologie. Pfluegers Arch Physiol 99: 472–480, 1903.
16. Einthoven W., G. Fahr and A. de Waart. Ueber die Richtung und die manifeste Groesse der Potentialschwankungen im menschlichen Herzen und ueber den Einfluss der Herzlage auf die Form des Elektrokardiogramms. Pfluegers Arch Physiol, 150:275–315, 1913.
17. Waller, A.D. and E.W. Reid. On the action of the excised mammalian heart. Phil Trans B. 178: 215, 1887.
18. Helmholtz, H. Ueber einige Gesetze der Verteilung elektrischer Stroeme in koerperlichen Leitern, mit Anwendung auf die thierisch elektrischen Versuche. Ann Physik Chem (Ser2) 89:211, 1853.
19. Einthoven, W., G. Fahr and A. de Waart. On the direction and manifest size of the variations of potential in the human heart and on the influence of the position of the heart on the form of the electrocardiogram. Tr. by Hoff HE and P. Sekelj. Am Heart J., 40: 163–211, 1950.
20. Wilson F.N., A.G. Macleod and P.S. Barker. The distribution of the currents of action and of injury displayed by heart muscle and other excitable tissues. Ann Arbor, University of Michigan Press, 1933.
21. Craib, W.H. A study of the electrical field surrounding active heart muscle. Heart, 14:71–109, 1927.
22. Craib, W.H. A study of the electrical field surrounding skeletal muscle. J. Physiol (Lond.), 66:49–73, 1928.
23. Katz, L.N. The genesis of the electrocardiogram. Physiol Rev., 27: 398–435, 1947.
24. Dolgin, M., S. Grau and L.N. Katz. Experimental studies on the validity of the central terminal of Wilson as an indifferent reference point. Am Heart J., 37:868–880, 1949.
25. Wolferth, C.C., M.M. Livezey and F.C. Wood. The relationships of Lead I, chest leads from the C3, C4 and C5 positions, and certain leads made from each shoulder region: the bearing of these observations upon the Einthoven equilat-

eral triangle hypothesis and upon the formation of Lead I. Am Heart J., 21:215–227, 1941.

26. Rosenbaum F.F. Note at end of an article reproduced in Selected Papers of Doctor Frank L. Wilson (eds) Johnston, F.D., Lepeschkin, E., Heart Station, University Hospital, Ann Arbor, Michigan, p. 363, 1954. Wilson, F.N., Johnston, F.D., Cotrim, N., Rosenbaum, F.F.: Relations between the potential variations of the ventricular surfaces and the form ofthe electrocardiogram in leads from the precordium and the extremeties. Trans Assn Am Physicians, 56:258–271, 1941.

27. Brody, D.A. Discussion: Part IV (Distribution of electrical potentials in volume conductors.) Ann NY Acad. Sci., 65: 1051–1072, 1957.

28. Hill, A. The genesis of the normal electrocardiogram. Br. Heart J., 8:147–156, 1946.

29. Bayley, R.H., E.W, Reynolds, Jr., C.L. Kinard and J.F. Head. The zero of potential of the electric field produced by the heart beat. The problem with reference to homogeneous volume conductors. Circ. Res, 2:4–13, 1954.

30. Burger H.C. and J.B. van Milaan. Heart-vector and leads. Br. Heart J., 9: 154, 1947.

31. Burger, H.C. and J.B. van Milaan. Heart-vector and leads. Part II, Br. Heart J., 9:154–160, 1947.

32. Burger, H.C. and J. B. van Milaan and W. Den Boer. Comparison of different systems of vectorcardiography. Br. Heart J., 14:401–405, 1952.

33. Koch-Momm, E. Allgemeine Elektrokardiographie. 2nd ed., Dresden, Steinkopff, T., 1937.

34. Wilson, F.N., F.D. Johnston, F.F., Rosenbaum and P.S. Barker. On Einthoven's triangle, the theory of unipolar electrocardiographic leads, and the interpretation of the precordial electrocardiogram. Am Heart J., 32:277–310, 1946.

35. Wilson, F.N., J.M. Bryant and F.D. Johnston. On the possiblity of constructing an Einthoven triangle for a given subject. Am Heart J., 37:493–522, 1949.

36. Johnston, F.D. The spread of currents and distribution of potentials in homogeneous volule conductors. Ann NY Acad. Sci., 65:963–979, 1957.

37. Lepeschkin, E. Modern electrocardiography. Baltimore, Williams and Wilkins, 1951.

38. Frank, E. Spread of current in volume conductors of finite extent. Ann NY Acad. Sci., 65:980–1002, 1957.

39. McFee, R. Comparison of heart vectors calculated with different systems of leads. Circulation 2:128–133, 1950.

40. Rudy, Y. Critical aspects of the forward and inverse problems in electrocardiography. In: *Simulation and imaging of the cardiac system.* Sideman S. and R. Beyar (Eds), Martinus Nijhoff, Dordrecht, The Netherlands, 1985.

41. Kouwenhoven, W.B. and O.R. Langworthy. Cardiopulmonary resuscitation. An account of forty-five years of research. JAMA 226:877–886, 1973.

42. Kouwenhoven, W.B., W.R. Milnor, G.G. Knickerbocker and W.R. Chesnut. Closed chest defibrillation of the heart. Surgery 42:550–561, 1957.

43. Wiggers, C.J. Reminiscences and adventures in circulation research. New York, Grune E. Stratton, 1958.

44. Wiggers, C.J. The interpretation and treatment of heart failure during anesthesia and operations. Ohio State Med J 46:127, 1950.

45. Wiggers, C.J. Pressure pulses in the cardiovascular system. London, Longmans, Green and Company, 1928.
46. Prevost, J.L. and F. Battelli. Sur quelques effets des echarges électriques sur le coeur des mammiferes. C. R. Acad. Sci. 129: 1267, 1899.
47. Hooker, D.R., W.B. Kouwenhoven, W.B. and O.R. Langworthy. The effect of alternating currents on the heart. Am J Physiol 103:444–454, 1933.
48. Ferris, L.P., B.G. King, P.W. Spence, et al. Effect of electric shock on the heart. Electrical Engineering, May 1936.
49. Wiggers, C.J. Revival of the heart from ventricular fibrillation by successive use of potassium and sodium salts. Am J Physiol 92: 223–239, 1930.
50. Kouwenhoven, W.B., D.R. Hooker and O.R. Langworthy. Recovery of the electrically fibrillated dog heart by electric countershock. Am J Physiol 101:65, 1932.
51. Wiggers, C.J. Cardiac massage followed by countershock in revival of mammalian ventricles from fibrillation due to coronary occlusion. Am J Physiol 116:161–162 1936.
52. Wiggers, C.J. The physiological basis for cardiac resuscitation from ventricular fibrillation-method for serial defibrillation. Am Heart J 20:413–422, 1940.
53. Beck, C.S. Reminiscences of cardiac resuscitation. Rev. Surg. 27:76–86, 1970.
54. Mautz, F.R. Reduction of cardiac instability of the epicardial and systemic administration of drugs as a protection in cardiac surgery. J Thoracic Surg 5:612–628, 1936.
55. Mautz, F.R. Resuscitation of the heart from ventricular fibrillation with drugs combined with electric shock. Proc Soc Exper Biol and Med 36:634–636, 1937.
56. Beck, C.S. Resuscitation for cardiac standstill and ventricular fibrillation occurring during operation. Am J Surg 54:273–279, 1941.
57. Beck, C.S. and F.R. Mautz. The control of the heartbeat by surgeon: with special reference to ventricular fibrillation occurring during operation. Ann Surg 106:525–537, 1937.
58. Beck, C.S., W.H. Pritchard and H.S. Feil. Ventricular fibrillation of long duration abolished by electric shock. J. Am. Med. Assoc. 135:985–986, 1947.
59. Beck, C.S. Historical communication. My life in heart surgery, 1923-1969. Geriatrics 26:84–99, Feb. 1971.
60. Mozen, H., R. Katzman and J. Martin. Successful defibrillation of heart. Resuscitative procedure started on medical ward and completed in operating room. J. Am. Med. Assoc. 161:111, 1955.
61. Beck, C.S. Surgery of the heart. Proceedings of the California Academy of Medicine 1937–1938 (Address delivered February 20, 1937).
62. Beck, C.S. Treatment of cardiac arrest. Veterans Administration Technical Bulletin TB 10—65, July 18, 1950, Washington, D.C.
63. Day, H.A. Letter to Doctor Beck. September 12, 1969.
64. Beck. C.S., E.C. Weckesser and F.M. Barry. Fatal heart attack and successful defibrillation. New concepts of coronary artery disease. J. Am. Med. Assoc. 161:434–436, 1955.
65. Weckesser, E.C. Twenty-eight year survival after myocardial infarction with ventricular fibrillation treated by electrical schock. Letter to the editor. N Eng J Med 312:248, 1985.

66. Zoll, P.M., A.J. Linenthal, W. Gibson, M.H. Paul and L.R. Notman. Termination of ventricular fibrillation in man by externally applied electric countershock. N Eng J Med 254:727–732, 1956.
67. Likoff, W. Hearts too good to die. Editorial Geriatrics 38:35, July 1983.
68. Pike F.H., C.C. Guthrie and G.N. Stewart. Studies of resuscitation: I. The general conditions affecting resuscitation, and the resuscitation of the blood and of the heart. J Exp Med 10: 371–418, 1908.
69. Crile, G. Demonstration of arterial perfusion and compression of unopened chest. Cleveland Academy of Medicine, 1908. Cited by Hosler EM: A concise history of cardiac resuscitation, November 28, 1975 for Archives of the Cleveland Health Museum and Education Center.
70. Sladen, A. Closed-chest massage, Kouwenhoven, Jude, Knickerbocker. JAMA 251:3137–3140, 1984.
71. Gurvich, H.L., G.S. Yuniev. Restoration of heart rhythm during fibrillation by a condenser discharge. Am Rev Soviet Med 4: 252–256, 1947.
72. Kouwenhoven, W.B., J.R. Jude and G.G. Knickerbocker. Cardiac arrest. Report of application of external cardiac massage on 118 patients. JAMA 178:1064–1067, 1960.
73. William P. Longmire, Jr. Alfred Blalock: His Life and Times; 1991. William Longmire Jr., Publisher.

Chapter 13

Cardiac Pacemakers

A. SENNING, I. BABOTAI AND R.J. BING

The most informative and detailed report on the effect of electricity on the heart has been published in a book by Schechter on the origins and developments of electrical cardiac stimulation to the present (1). Schechter relates that Harvey in his book, De Motu Cordis, described experiments on pigeons in which the heart had wholly ceased to pulsate. Harvey wetted his fingers with saliva and placed them for a short time on the heart, obeserving that "under the influence of this procedure the heart recovered new strength and life, so that both ventricles and auricles (atria) pulsated, contracting and relaxing alternately, recalled as it were from death to life."(2). In 1791, Galvani whose work was discussed in the preceeding chapter, applied a live torpedo fish to the nerves, muscle and heart of a dead frog. Convulsive contractions occurred, and ceased after withdrawl of the fish (3). In 1797 von Humboldt experimented on the heart of a carp (4). When the heart was touched with the solution of "protosulphide of potassium" the number of beats declined.

The newly introduced method of execution by guillotine turned out to be a bonanza for the study of the effect of electrical stimulation on the human body. Early experiments were summarized by Schechter (1). Bichat who worked during the French revolution, would avail himself of the bodies of guillotine victims to experiment on the effect of electricity. They were at his disposal thirty or forty minutes after the execution (5). He states that he could not produce motion in the hearts of these executed victims through the spinal marrow or the heart nerves. "However, mechanical excitants directly applied to the flesh fibers produced contractions in them—." In 1802 Nysten, working on a guillotined criminal under dramatic conditions in a Parisian cemetary, found that the contractility of the left ventricle was extinguished soon after death and always before that of other muscle organs, that the right ventricle could be made to contract more than one hour after death, that both atria continued to contract under Galvanic influence long after movement was totally abolished in other muscles, that the contractile faculty of the right atrium was always preserved much more than that of any other part of the heart, that a portion of the superior vena cava adjacent to the right atrium had contractile capacity almost equal to that of the right atrium and finally, that the aorta was unresponsive to electrical stimulation (6). Schechter also describes the activity of a physicians club in Mainz, Germany, engaged in assessing the effects of different kinds of electricity on the body. "A physician's club—received a windfall of study material when on November 21, 1803 there was a mass execution of 20 marauding brigands (7). A hut was erected at 150 feet from the scaffold, so that the corpses could be delivered as quickly as possible to the eager scientists. The bandits were decapitated faster than the experiments could be done, however, so that only a few of the bodies could be examined, at 4 and 22 minutes for the first two, and a couple of hours after death for the other two." Schechter also mentions the observation by Carpne who wrote an article on Galvanic experiments on a hanged man (8). On a corpse which he obtained, he introduced air into the trachea while massaging the chest and passing current from a voltaic pile to the intercostal nerves and the vagi, the phrenic nerves and the rectum during ten minute intervals. Apparently, the cadavers face began to lighten, and when Carpne connected his battery to the pericardium and diaphragm, the pectoral muscles began to move as well as the atria of the heart, but not the ventricles (8).

The first electrical pacing was used in an attempt to resuscitate a patient. Lidwill and Booth (9) succeeded in reviving a stillborn baby with their electric "pacemaker" after "everything else had been tried". The pacing stimulus was supplied to the heart by an insulated needle with a bare tip. Hyman constructed a machine with a magnetic generator in 1932 (10).

Design of an effective method for defibrillation was an important step in the introduction of the pacemaker. Many of these developments have been described in an earlier chapter. The Swiss physiologists Prevost and Batelli (11) in 1900 published a method to defibrillate hearts by means of capacitor discharge. Kouwenhowen and Langworth (12) confirmed this on the closed chest in 1932, and in 1934 Wiggers (13) introduced a technique using serial shocks to the exposed hearts.

Already in 1804, Vasalli (14) had pointed out the necessity to ventilate the lungs during resuscitation; Wiggers stressed the importance of supplying the myocardium with oxygenated blood by cardiac massage before applying a countershock. This technique was crowned with the first successful intraoperative defibrillation by Beck (15) in 1947. Beck subsequently installed defibrillators in the operating and emergency rooms. He was not able to interest his colleagues in this technique. The defibrillator was not accepted as standard equipment in the operating room and intensive care units until 15 to 20 years later.

Senning's group in Stockholm first used electrically induced ventricular fibrillation (16) in order to avoid air embolism during open heart surgery with experimentally unclamped aortas in 1952 (Figure 1). After a period of 3

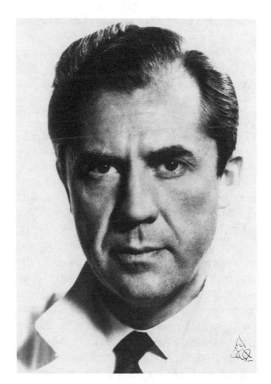

Figure 1. Ake Senning (*with permission*)

to 4 hours of ventricular fibrillation, using 380 Volt/20ms AC countershock, defibrillation was always successful. However, somtimes asystole followed, and pacing for one to two minutes was required.

The background of clinical cardiac electrostimulation is also comprehensively described by Schechter (1). He quotes an article published by Kite on "The Recovery of the Apparently Dead" published in London in 1788, which described electric shock for resuscitation (17). The apparatus consisted of pieces of brass-wire enclosed in glass tubes with knobs at one end, which were to be applied to "those parts between which we intend the electric fluid to pass.... In this manner, shocks may be sent through any part of the body: and their direction constantly varied, without a probablity of the resistance receiving any inconvenience" (17). In 1862, Walshe suggested that irregular movements arising out of "mechanical difficulties and modified innervation of the hearts contractility, impairment and unsteadiness of the nervous force presiding over its tenacity, may be possibly contribute a share of feeble, wavering non-rhthymical motion." He suggested that successive electrical impulses which can succeed at each other at appreciable intervals of time, may be a treatment of "fluttering palpitation" (18).

In 1869 the famous French physician Duchenne treated a patient with . . .

smallness and extreme rapidity of the pulse (136 to 140 pulsations) with such irregularity and intermittences that often 6 or 8 successive pulsations missed; impossible to distinguish the rhythm of valvar sounds on auscultation of the heart;.... however it being urgent to act, I wished to try to modify the morbid condition of the center giving rise to the to nerves of the heart and lungs by electrocutaneous excitation of the region related to that nervous center (19).

It is likely that the patient had diptheria and myocarditis.

The effect of electrocution on the heart was also thoroughly explored by Prevost and Battelli toward the end of the 19th century. They quantitatively demonstrated that fibrillary contraction induced by electricity could be abolished by another powerful discharge of either alternating or direct current, a visionary look into the future (11). Direct stimulation of the beating heart was first carried out by Ziemssen (21). Ziemssen had the advantage of observing a forty-two year old woman who had a huge defect on the anterior left thoracic wall consequent to resection of a chest wall tumor. In this patient the heart covered only by skin was visible and palpable. Ziemssen performed detailed studies most of them electrical on this conveniently exposed normal heart and reported his findings in 1882. The results of these experiments prompted Ziemssen to use electric currents in patients with intact thorax. His main conclusion was that it needed currents of sufficient intensity and frequency to modify the action of the heart (21).

Schechter quoted the work of MacWilliams published from 1887 to 1914 in which the treatment of Adams-Stokes attacks was considered (22).

> But, on the other hand, in certain of forms of cardiac arrest there appears to be a possibility of restoring by artificial means the rhythmic beat and tiding over a sudden and temporary danger—. Now we know that when the mammalian heart has been inhibited through the vagus nerve it is quite possible to excite an immediate renewal of the rhythmic action by direct stimulation of the organ. No doubt it is very possible, as I have already suggested in a former paper, that the fate of the heart may be sealed in cases of fatal inhibitory arrest by the supervention of fibrillar contraction or heart-delirium in the ventricles.

In 1904 Andrew Smith mailed this suggestion to the editor of the *Medical Records*, as quoted by Schechter: "Sir: As a possible successful means of resuscitation in sudden heart-failure I would suggest laying bare the pericardium over the left ventricle and applying electricity at the bottom of the wound" (1). Even more direct was the approach of Robinovitch who in 1907 resuscitated a patient by means of rhythmic electrostimulation (23). The patient as quoted in the book by Schechter was a young woman, a chronic morphine eater. The patient apparently had a cardiac arrest became . . .

> black in the face and none of those present expected any good results from the application of rhythmic electric excitations. We practiced rhythmic excitations during a period of about 30 seconds; the duration of the closure of the circuit was about 1/4 of a second and the period of the opening of the circuit was about 1 second. We shortened the period of the opening of the circuit- as against our own indications and our papers on the subject of resuscitation, because the patient seemed to be thoroughly asphyxiated- as we judged her condition from the color of her face. As the rhythmic excitations were being repeated, it was astonishing to see the accompanying change of color in the patient's face; the dark blue color changed to pale, then to almost natural color; at the end of the 30 seconds of rhythmic excitations, the patient took a long spontaneous breath, opened her eyes and said: "Oh I feel so cold in my back." The cold she felt was the wet cotton of the electrodes. But the interesting point is that the patient felt no other inconvenience during the rhythmic excitations- while she was in profound syncope.(23)

Late in the 16th Century Geronimo of Padua had first described typical Adams-Stokes attacks (24). Subsequently, many others reported the typical symptoms with syncope and slow pulse. Cardiac pacing during Adams-Stokes attacks was first introduced 370 years later by Zoll in 1952 (25), using external thoracic electrodes. Thus the era of cardiac pacing had begun. In 1951, Callaghan and Bigelow (26) described an electrical pacemaker with transvenous electrodes, which they used to pace hypothermic animals in asystole. In patients, however this method was unsuccessful. The tip of the intravenous electrode was introduced into the auricle, "two inches too short" (26).

In 1957, Weirich, Gott, and Lillehei (27) reported the use of myocardial electrodes to pace hearts with iatrogenic A-V block after closure of a ventricular septal defect.

In the late 1950s the treatment of Adams-Stokes syndrome with percutaneous electric stimulation was frequently performed. For this purpose, pacemakers for external use were built by Medtronic in USA and Elema in Sweden. Unfortunately, infection frequently caused abscesses, sepsis, and death. Only implantation of the total pacer assembly solved this problem. Transistors became available in 1956 allowing construction of smaller implantable electrical pacemakers. In 1957, the first experiments on implantation were started in Stockholm. Electrical parameters for clinical cardiac pacing were defined on patients with Adam-Stokes syndrome, who carried external pacemakers. On the basis of these data an artifical pacemaker was constructed together with Elmquist (28). On October 8th, 1958, the unit was implanted in a patient with a total A-V block resulting from a viral myocarditis. During the last weeks the patient had 20 to 30 cardiac arrests a day. In order to avoid publicity, the implantation was carried out in the evening when the operating rooms were empty. The first pacemaker functioned only 8 hours. The second was implanted with better success.

The energy source of the first pacemakers was a rechargeable battery, which was charged once a month by induction from a radio- frequency generator. The energy source was later changed to mercury batteries. In 1960, Chardack (29) implanted pacemakers, which were constructed by Greatbatch (30). Now the doors had opened for the pacemaker industry, with Medtronic in the USA and Elema in Europe leading the way. The early years were full of troubles: rapid threshold rises, electrode displacements, lead and insulation breaks, fast battery depletion and especially a negative attitude on the part of most cardiologists. The first implanted pacemakers were so short lived that our first patient is now equipped with his 24th pacemaker.

Infections fortunately have disappeared. With the use of improved leads and inert platinum electrodes with lithium iodine batteries and metallic housing (30), the pacemaker became a durable and reliable instrument for treating bradycardic arrhythmias.

The first pacemakers had a fixed stimulation rate of 72 beats per minute. The fixed rate occasionally caused ventricular fibrillation, when the stimulus fell into the vulnerable phase of late systole of the patient's own heart beat. These accidents were avoided with the introduction in 1964 of on-demand pacemakers with R-wave inhibition (31) and R-wave triggering in 1966 (32). In 1969, Berkovits (33) reported on the bifocal demand pacing.

In the beginning, pacemaker electrodes were placed by thoracotomy either on or into the myocardium. In 1958, Furman and Schwedel (34) used the transvenous route in two patients; this already had been accomplished by Callaghan and Bigelow in 1951 (26).

Pacemaker implantation without thoracotomy was done in 1962 by Ekestrom, Johansson, and Lagergren (35), who introduced the electrode transvenously with its tip in the right ventricle. In 1963, a trial triggered 100 ms delayed ventricular pacing without thoracotomy was introduced by the same investigators (36). They placed the sensing electrode on the atrium via a mediastinoscope and installed the ventricular electrode transvenously.

The transvenous route of electrode placement is used today in more than 98% of pacemaker implantations. Early reports of a high displacement rate and excessive threshold rise led to the development of electrodes with various types of active and passive fixation mechanism for atrial and ventricular position. Improvement in inert pacemaker electrode designs have reduced the acute and chronic threshold. A lower threshold allows greater patient safety margins and increases the pacemaker's battery life. A new steroid-loaded pacing electrode which was developed by Medtronic, elutes a minimal amount of a steriod compound into cardiac tissue, in order to reduce tissue reaction and thus maintain a low threshold.

With the progress in electronics, the circuits changed from discrete to hybrid to integrated circuits, and finally to microprocessors. Programmability progressed from the simple invasive change of rate and voltage (Medtronic, 1960) to external noninvasive radio-frequency adjustments of all pacing parameters. The ultimate universal pacing system could be achieved in the dual chamber "physiologic" pacing system; it is the ideal treatment of high degree A-V block, reestablishing A-V synchrony. At present, the introduction of rate-responsive sensor-controlled pacemakers allows the patients with chronotropic incompetence or atrial fibrillation to increase their heart rate during exercise.

The automatic implantable defibrillator, which was introduced by Mirowski in 1980 (37), was a device for treatment of patients with ventricular tachycardia and fibrillation using high energy defibrillation shocks via epicardial patch electrodes. The automatic implantable cardioverter defibrillators (AICD) of today detect ventricular tachyarhythmias using a range of detection criteria. The defibrillator delivers support pacing for bradycardia, anti-tachycardia pacing, synchronized low energy cardioversion shocks and snychronized high energy defibrillation shocks. Multiprogrammable telemetry capability allows monitoring and modification of many of the aforementioned parameters.

Development of the modern pacemaker has been the result of teamwork among cardiologists, electrophysiologists, electronic engineers and the industry. Today's technique can respond to most cardiac rhythm disturbances. Hopefully the practice at the bedside can keep up with the rapid technical developments.

REFERENCES

1. David Charles Schechter. Exploring the origins of electrical cardiac stimulation selected works on the history of electrotherapy presented at the Seventh World Symposium in Cardiac Pacing, Vienna, Austria, 1983, Medtronic Inc., Minneapolis, MN 1983.
2. Harvey, W. The circulation of the blood, London, J.M. Dent and Sons Ltd., 1907.
3. Galvani, L. De viribus electricitatis in motu musculari, commentarius, Bologna, Instit. Scient., 1791.
4. Humboldt, F.W.H.A. von. Versuche ueber die gereizte Muskel und Nervenfaser nebst Vermuthungen ueber den chemischen Process des Lebens in der Thier- und Pflanzenwelt, Posen, Decker, 1797, Lettre de Humboldt à Loder sur les applications du Galvanisme, Bibl. germanique 4:301 (1797); Lettre de Humboldt à Blumenbach, Ann. Chim., Paris 64:1(1797).
5. Bichat, X. Recherches Physiologiques sur la Vie et la Mort, Paris, Brosson, Gabon and Cie, 1800.
6. Nysten, P.J. Expériences sur le Coeur et les autres Parties d'un Homme Decapité le 14 Brumaire, An XI, Paris, Levrault, 1802.
7. Vassali-Eandi, Julio, and Rossi. Rapport sue des expériences galvaniques faites sur les têtes et les troncs de trois hommes, peu de temps après leur decapitation, Rep. Acad. of Turin, 1803; Societe de Médicins, Etablis à Mayence: Expériences galvaniques Hommes et des Animaux, Frankfurt, 1804.
8. Carpne., Galvanic experiments on a hanged man, Phil. Magazine, Bible. Brit. 270:373, 1803
9. Lidwill, M.D., H.G. Mond, G.J. Sloman, R.H. Edwards. The first pacemaker. Pace 5:278-281, 1982.
10. Hyman, A.S. Resuscitation of the stopped heart by intracardial therapy. Experimental use of an artificial pacemaker. Arch Intern Med 50:283-305, 1932.
11. Prevost, J.L., F. Battelli. Quelques effects des charges électriques sur le coeur des mammifieres. J. Physiol. Path. Gen. 2:40-41, 1900.
12. Kouwenhoven, W.B., O.R. Langworth. Cardiopulmonary resuscitation. An account of forty-five years of research. JAMA 225:877, 1973.
13. Wiggers, C.J. Physiologic basis for cardiac resuscitation from ventricular fibrillation-method for serial defibrillation. Am. Hrt J. 20:413, 1940.
14. Vasalli. In: Aldini, J. ed. Essai théorique et expérimental sur la galvanisme avec une serie d'expériences. Paris: Fournier, 1804.

15. Beck, C.S. Reminiscences of cardiac resuscitation. Review of Surgery 27:76, 1970.
16. Senning, A. Ventricular fibrillation used as a method to facilitate intracardiac operations. Acta Chir. Scand. 172, 1952.
17. Kite, C. The recovery of the apparently dead, London, C.Dilly, 1788.
18. Walshe, W.H. A practical treatise on the diseases of the heart and great vessels, Philadelphia, Blanchard & Lea, 1862.
19. Duchenne, G. De l'Électrisation localisée et de son application à la pathologie et à le therapeutique, 3rd ed., Paris, J.B. Ballière, 1872.
20. MacWilliam, J.A. Cardiac fibrillation and its relation to chloroform anaesthesia, Brit. Med. J. 2:499, 1914.
21. Ziemssen, H. von. Studien ueber die Bewegungsvorgaenge am menschlichen Herzen, sowie ueber die mechanische und elektrische Erregbarkeit des Herzens und des Nervus phrenicus, angestellt an dem freiliegenden Herzen der Catharina Serafin, Arch. Klin. Med 30:270, 1882.
22. MacWilliam, J.A. Electrical stimulation of the heart in man, Brit. Med. J. 1:348, 1889.
23. Robinovitch, L.G. Resuscitation of a woman in profound syncope caused by chronic morphine poisoning; means used: rhythmic excitations with an induction current; the author's method and model of coil. J. Ment. Path 8:180, 1907.
24. Geronimo Mercuriale (Praelectiones Patavinae). De Cognoscendis et curandis humani corporis affectibus (Venezia 1606), opera postuma, 238-243.
25. Zoll, P.M. Resuscitation of the heart in ventricular standstill by external stimulation. N. Engl J. Med. 247:768, 1952.
26. Callaghan, J.C., W.G. Bigelow. Electrical artificial pacemaker for standstill of the heart. Ann. Surg. 134:8-17, 1951.
27. Weirich, W.L., V.L. Gott, C.W. Lillehei. The treatment of complete heart block by the combined use of a myocardial electrode and an artificial pacemaker. Surg. Forum 8:360-363, 1957.
28. Elmquist, R., A. Senning. Implantable pacemaker for the heart. Medical Electronics. Proc. of the Second International Conference on Medical Electronics, Paris, June 1959.
29. Chardack, W.M., A.E. Gage, W. Greatbatch. A transitorized self-contained implantable pacemaker for long term correction of complete heart block. Surgery 48:643-648, 1960.
30. Greatbatch, W., L.H. Lee, W. Mathias. The solid-state lithium battery: a new improved chemical power source for implantable cardiac pacemakers. Trans. Biomed. Engin 18:317, 1971.
31. Castellanos, A., Jr. L. Lemberg, B.V. Berkovits. The "demand" cardiac pacemaker: a new instrument for the treatment of A-V conduction disturbances. Inter Am Coll. Cardiol. Meeting, Montreal, June 1964.
32. Neville, J.F., K. Millar, W. Keller, J.A. Abildskov. An implantable demand pacemaker. Clin Res 14:256-258, 1966.
33. Berkovits, B.V., A. Castellanos, Jr., L. Lemberg. Bifocal demand pacing. Circulation 39:44-52, 1969.
34. Furman, S., J.B. Schwedel. An intracardiac pacemaker for Stokes-Adam seizures. N. Engl. J. Med 261:943-948, 1959.

35. Ekeström, S., J. Johansson, H. Lagergren. Behandling av Adam Stokes syndrom med intracardiell pacemakerelectrod. Opuscula Medica 7:175-176, 1962.
36. Carlens, E., L. Johansson, I. Karlöf, H. Lagergren. New method for arterial triggered pacemaker treatment without thoracotomy. J. Thorac. Cardiovasc. Surg. 50:229-237, 1965.
37. Mirowski, M., P.R. Reid, M.M. Mower, L. Watkins, V.L., Gott, J.F. Schauble, A. Langer, M.S. Heilman, S.A. Kolenik, R.E. Fischell, M.L. Weisfeldt. Termination of malignant ventricular arrhythmias with an implanted automatic defibrillator in human beings. N. Engl. J. Med. 303:322, 1980.

INDEX